Chronic Stress and Its Effect on Brain Structure and Connectivity

Ana Starcevic
University of Belgrade, Serbia

A volume in the Advances in Psychology, Mental Health, and Behavioral Studies (APMHBS) Book Series

IGI Global
DISSEMINATOR OF KNOWLEDGE

Published in the United States of America by
IGI Global
Medical Information Science Reference (an imprint of IGI Global)
701 E. Chocolate Avenue
Hershey PA, USA 17033
Tel: 717-533-8845
Fax: 717-533-8661
E-mail: cust@igi-global.com
Web site: http://www.igi-global.com

Library of Congress Cataloging-in-Publication Data

Names: Starcevic, Ana, 1979- editor.
Title: Chronic stress and its effect on brain structure and connectivity / Ana Starcevic, editor.
Description: Hershey, PA : Medical Information Science Reference (an imprint of IGI Global), [2019] | Includes bibliographical references.
Identifiers: LCCN 2018029786| ISBN 9781522575139 (hardcover) | ISBN 9781522575146 (ebook)
Subjects: | MESH: Stress, Psychological--complications | Brain--anatomy & histology | Brain Diseases--etiology | Chronic Disease
Classification: LCC RC49 | NLM WM 172.4 | DDC 616.08--dc23 LC record available at https://lccn.loc.gov/2018029786

This book is published in the IGI Global book series Advances in Psychology, Mental Health, and Behavioral Studies (APMHBS) (ISSN: 2475-6660; eISSN: 2475-6679)

British Cataloguing in Publication Data
A Cataloguing in Publication record for this book is available from the British Library.

All work contributed to this book is new, previously-unpublished material.
The views expressed in this book are those of the authors, but not necessarily of the publisher.

For electronic access to this publication, please contact: eresources@igi-global.com.

Advances in Psychology, Mental Health, and Behavioral Studies (APMHBS) Book Series

ISSN:2475-6660
EISSN:2475-6679

MISSION

The complexity of the human mind has puzzled researchers and physicians for centuries. While widely studied, the brain still remains largely misunderstood.

The **Advances in Psychology, Mental Health, and Behavioral Studies (APMHBS)** book series presents comprehensive research publications focusing on topics relating to the human psyche, cognition, psychiatric care, mental and developmental disorders, as well as human behavior and interaction. Featuring diverse and innovative research, publications within APMHBS are ideally designed for use by mental health professionals, academicians, researchers, and upper-level students.

COVERAGE

- Addiction
- Mental Health & Disorders
- Anxiety
- Human Interaction
- Trauma & Stress
- Emotional Health
- Psychiatry
- Socialization
- Human Behavior
- Developmental Disorders

IGI Global is currently accepting manuscripts for publication within this series. To submit a proposal for a volume in this series, please contact our Acquisition Editors at Acquisitions@igi-global.com or visit: http://www.igi-global.com/publish/.

The Advances in Psychology, Mental Health, and Behavioral Studies (APMHBS) Book Series (ISSN 2475-6660) is published by IGI Global, 701 E. Chocolate Avenue, Hershey, PA 17033-1240, USA, www.igi-global.com. This series is composed of titles available for purchase individually; each title is edited to be contextually exclusive from any other title within the series. For pricing and ordering information please visit http://www.igi-global.com/book-series/advances-psychology-mental-health-behavioral/110200. Postmaster: Send all address changes to above address.

Titles in this Series

For a list of additional titles in this series, please visit:
https://www.igi-global.com/book-series/advances-psychology-mental-health-behavioral/110200

Multicultural Counseling Applications for Improved Mental Healthcare Services
Anasuya Jegathevi Jegathesan (HELP University, Malaysia) and Siti Salina Abdullah (University Malaysia Terengganu, alaysia)
Medical Information Science Reference • ©2019 • 302pp • H/C (ISBN: 9781522560739) • US $265.00

Assessing and Averting the Prevalence of Mass Violence
Sarah E. Daly (St. Vincent College, USA)
Information Science Reference • ©2019 • 271pp • H/C (ISBN: 9781522556701) • US $185.00

Scientific Concepts Behind Happiness, Kindness, and Empathy in Contemporary Society
Nava R. Silton (Marymount Manhattan College, USA)
Information Science Reference • ©2019 • 321pp • H/C (ISBN: 9781522559184) • US $185.00

Handbook of Research on Psychosocial Perspectives of Human Communication Disorders
Sanjeev Kumar Gupta (All India Institute of Speech and Hearing, India) and Srinivasan Venkatesan (All India Institute of Speech and Hearing, India)
Medical Information Science Reference • ©2018 • 465pp • H/C (ISBN: 9781522549550) • US $275.00

Deconstructing Stigma in Mental Health
Brittany A. Canfield (Southern New Hampshire University, USA) and Holly A. Cunningham (CPES Inc., USA)
Medical Information Science Reference • ©2018 • 307pp • H/C (ISBN: 9781522538080) • US $225.00

Social, Psychological, and Forensic Perspectives on Sexual Abuse
Rejani Thudalikunnil Gopalan (Gujarat Forensic Sciences University, India)
Information Science Reference • ©2018 • 374pp • H/C (ISBN: 9781522539582) • US $195.00

For an entire list of titles in this series, please visit:
https://www.igi-global.com/book-series/advances-psychology-mental-health-behavioral/110200

IGI Global
DISSEMINATOR OF KNOWLEDGE

701 East Chocolate Avenue, Hershey, PA 17033, USA
Tel: 717-533-8845 x100 • Fax: 717-533-8661
E-Mail: cust@igi-global.com • www.igi-global.com

To Alex, my brother, the brightest scientific mind.

Table of Contents

Detailed Table of Contents

We all know that the baby's world is a 10-20 square foot field, which grows steadily over the years. The small world plays a leading role in shaping the child's mind at a rate inversely proportional to its size. In fact, not only stressful pieces of life but all kinds of experience takes part in the psychosocial development of the child, good or bad. Herewith, the conditions that cause chronic stress such as neglect, abuse, poverty, domestic or societal violence, war, and dislocation leave unfavorable traces that are difficult to change in the human mind. Today, while we, the mental health workers, are more focused on the apparent wounds that such adverse experiences have left in our souls, the unseen wounds continue to shape the child, society, and us all.

As adolescents face new challenges, the prevalence of stress, anxiety, and depression is growing. This chapter presents research on stress, anxiety, and depression as it relates to brain development and treatment options. While prescription medication is a common treatment option, there is concern over use with the development of the adolescent brain and side effects. In addition to, or in place of, medication, other treatment options presented in this chapter include psychotherapy, biofeedback, mindfulness, diet, exercise, and social media use. With advances in technology and increased use among adolescents, the chapter will present new treatment options that are available through apps and social media.

Emotions and mood are complex psychic phenomena that play important roles in everyday behavior. No anatomical structure can be identified as a specific brain center for emotions, and a neurophysiological basis of emotions is unclear and hard to define. Today, it is thought that neurotransmitters such as dopamine, serotonin, and norepinephrine have important roles in mood regulation, and much of the evidence for this assumption is based on the effectiveness of antidepressant medications currently available in psychiatric practice. James-Lange, Cannon-Bard, and Schachter's and other theories historically tried to explain the origin and formation of emotional responses. Despite extensive research efforts on this topic, many aspects regarding the nature of emotional responses remain unclear. Multidisciplinary approach, including the adequate cooperation of psychiatrists, neurophysiologists, and experts from other areas, is needed to provide us with a more comprehensive insight on biological basis of conative psychic functions.

Pain and stress basically overlap in conceptual and physiological perceptions. Chronic stress and chronic pain share a common behavioral model of failure to extinguish negative memories as one of psychological and physiological mechanisms of defense. They also have discrepancies such that the final brain endophenotype of posttraumatic stress disorder (PTSD), depression, and chronic pain appears to be different among the three conditions, and the role of the hypothalamic-pituitary-adrenal axis remains unclear in the physiology of pain. Persistence of either stress or pain is maladaptive and could lead to compromised homeostasis. The effectiveness of interventions that may increase return to work and patient satisfaction in trauma victims should be a future directive of research.

Little is known about the clinical consequences of psychological morbidity associated with orthopedic trauma. Anxiety disorders, depression, bipolar disorder,

Preface

There are many studies conducted that showed how chronic stress and cortisol can damage the brain, so the fact of reducing chronic stress is of great importance in order to maintain healthy brain structure and connectivity.

Neuroscientists found that chronic stress triggers long term changes in brain structure and connectivity, and that explains why early exposure to stress events make those people later in life more vulnerable to anxiety and mood disorders.

Chronic stress triggers long term changes in brain structure and function and has long been established that posttraumatic stress disorder (PTSD) induces changes in the volume of gray matter versus white matter, as well as the size and connectivity of the amygdala.

Stress induces secretion of a stress hormone, cortisol, which create a domino effect activates the connection pathways between hippocampus and amygdala making structures of brain sustainable to constant feeling of fight or flight.

The impact of being under a constant stress damages the natural cell function to malfunction by inhibiting connection pathways to the prefrontal cortex and causing impaired cognitive functions. Sometimes, neuroplasticity makes brain structure and function more resistant generally to clinical manifestation of stress related disorders.

This book presents a brief summary of current tendencies of chronic stress management and its effect on brain structures and their connectivity, also within some clinical stress related manifestations.

In the chapter "Posttraumatic Stress Disorder," the author made a review of literature on chronic stress impact on gene expression alteration during child development.

In the chapter "Adolescent Chronic Stress, Brain Function, and Treatment for Depression and Anxiety," the author explains how important adolescent period is for an individual as it is a time of significant maturation of the brain, marked by structural alterations in many limbic and cortical regions and that stress and adversity could induce depression, which affects most of the population worldwide.

Emotions are probably the most important of all psychological functions as it correlates and induces human behavior and cognitive functions. It presents the base of all personality traits and shades of reasoning, decision making and intervenes in the area of other psychological functions. In the chapter "Neurophysiological and Neurobiological Basis of Emotions and Mood," a complex psychic function for which there is no precise and comprehensive definition is very well described emphasizing the impact of emotions on behavior and differences which appear in different brain structures such as limbic system, brain cortex, thalamus and basal ganglia.

Pain and stress basically overlap in conceptual and physiological perceptions, which was described in the chapter "Chronic Stress and Chronic Pain: Disability After Trauma and Global Trends." Chronic stress and chronic pain share a common behavioral model of failure to extinguish negative memories as one of psychological and physiological mechanisms of defense.

The effectiveness of prevention strategies which could be develop through psychiatrists and orthopaedic surgeons cooperation strategies as well as developing strategies when PTSD occur postoperatively should also be one of the main targets in the near future, as PTSD as an entity presents one of the greatest disability factors in society producibility nowadays, which is also very important from the economy perspective. This was described in the chapter "Orthopaedic Trauma and Posttraumatic Stress Disorder."

The effect of orthodontic therapy of different orthodontic anomalies on life quality referred to one's personality is described in the chapter "Changing the Quality of Life After Orthodontic Inaccuracy Therapy."

The rehabilitation procedures exert significant pressure to cochlear implant recipients resulting to low levels of self-esteem, and therefore, the chapter "Self-Determination Calibration for Cochlear Implant Rehabilitation" explains models that quantify stress as quality of life measurements by using metrics like the Vernier Scale models for self-regulation.

Sex is a basic quality of every living beings, but it is highly controversial to understand and there are lots of speculations, myths, and practices prevailed in the society of particularly developing countries. Sex has a direct and indirect influence of brain, regarding sexual orientations, sexual actions, preferences, and sexualities. This sector of medical science requires more thorough and unbiased studies to simplify this complex matter. This was described in the chapter "Sex and the Brain."

There is a relationship between quantum mind-brain models and psychiatry through cytoskeletal proteins and cell membrane. Brain cell membranes seem to play a key role in psychiatric illness. By combining neurobiological data with facts and ideas from psychology, psychiatry, and quantum mechanics, a new, multidisciplinary view is presented on the relationship between, and the origin of, brain and mind. Very big part of unconscious mental activity may not physically present in the synapse networks of the material brain in medical, anatomical way of explanation but at sub-manifest level, as a new way or perspective and scientific explanation of different brain's structure connectivity and consequence mental behavior. The quantum mind or quantum consciousness group of hypotheses propose that classical mechanics cannot explain consciousness. It posits that quantum mechanical phenomena, such as quantum entanglement and superposition, may play an important part in the brain's function and could form the basis of an explanation of consciousness. This very interesting topic was evaluated in the chapter "Quantum Cognition and Its Influence on Decrease of Global Stress Level Related With Job Improvement Strategies."

"Digital Health Interventions in Mental Health" is the chapter in which the author explains the importance of Health Digitalization globally and its importance and high significance as this scientific area has in medicine and psychiatry.

Due to high media coverage globally, we are all involved in the state of negative influence of constant exposure to negative news to viewers mental state, which was shown in the chapter "The Increase of How Mass Media Coverage Manipulates Our Minds."

I hope you will enjoy reading this book, as it is full of novelties in the multidisciplinary scientific areas connected to neuroscience and psychiatry.

Ana Starcevic
University of Belgrade, Serbia

Chapter 1
Posttraumatic Stress Disorder:
Children and Psychological Trauma

Veysi Çeri
Marmara University, Turkey

ABSTRACT

We all know that the baby's world is a 10-20 square foot field, which grows steadily over the years. The small world plays a leading role in shaping the child's mind at a rate inversely proportional to its size. In fact, not only stressful pieces of life but all kinds of experience takes part in the psychosocial development of the child, good or bad. Herewith, the conditions that cause chronic stress such as neglect, abuse, poverty, domestic or societal violence, war, and dislocation leave unfavorable traces that are difficult to change in the human mind. Today, while we, the mental health workers, are more focused on the apparent wounds that such adverse experiences have left in our souls, the unseen wounds continue to shape the child, society, and us all.

DOI: 10.4018/978-1-5225-7513-9.ch001

INTRODUCTION

"Everything is related to how the world is presented to the child," says Donald Winnicott, to state the importance of the environment on the mental development of the child. We all know that the baby's world is a 10-20 square foot field, which grows steadily over the years. The small world plays a leading role in shaping the child's mind at a rate inversely proportional to its size.

The infant mind, which does not host almost any content, in the beginning, gets a position that affects every area of his later life by being shaped with the effect of its close environment. A position where he can see the world as it passes through its lenses.

In fact, not only stressful piece of life but all kinds of experiences take part in the psychosocial development of the child, good or bad. Herewith, the conditions that cause chronic stress such as neglect, abuse, poverty, domestic or societal violence, war and dislocation leave unfavourable traces that are difficult to change in the hu-man mind. Today, while we, the mental health workers, are more focused on the apparent wounds that such adverse experiences have left in our souls, the unseen wounds continue to shape the child, society and the universe (Terr,1990).

Although the neuroimaging technologies in the years that Winnicott pointed out the importance of the environment were far from showing the effects of such experiences on brain development, today, there is growing evidence that shows the structure of the brain is shaped by one's experiences(Teicher,2016). Today, it is also well known that traumatic experiences such as accidents, sexual or physical abuse, surviving war or maltreatment can lead to structural or functional changes in various brain areas, and may cause suicidal behaviours and PTSD or other psychiatric disorders(Dyregrov,2006).

It is becoming clearer every day that chronic stress which arises from traumatic exposure lead to changes in the brain circuits related to working memory, attention, emotion regulation, cognition and threat detection systems(Teicher,2016) which cause significant deterioration in the detection, integration and representation of internal and external stimulus (Van der Kolk,1996). Although traumatic stress may have negative consequences for everyone, the impact of such incidents in early years which is the most critical time for the brain development is more devastating because of the destructive consequence of the chronic fear response on the development of the central nervous system(Kaufman,2001).

Since the effect of chronic stress on the function and volume of related structures of the brain is addressed in the relevant parts of this book, it will be discussed the impact of traumatic stress on the development of a unique psychiatric disorder, PTSD, in the light of literature findings in the present chapter. The epidemiology and the effect of PTSD on the psychosocial wellbeing and functionality of the child will also be addressed.

DEFINITIONS

Although it was not believed that the diagnosis of PTSD is relevant for children and adolescents, studies by Leonore Terr, David Kinzie, William Sack, William Yule, Van Der Kolk and many others who researched whether mental wellbeing of children is adversely affected by traumatic events proved otherwise. Thanks to the authors, today it is, undisputedly accepted that PTSD could develop in children following life-threatening traumatic incidents(Dyregrov,2006).

The traumatic experience is defined as exposing to an incident that threat person's bodily integrity or his life (Karakaya,2007) Many people are exposed to traumatic incidents such as injuries, violence, natural disasters, fire, traffic accidents or sexual and physical assault during childhood. Besides, witnessing the injuring or killing of someone, and learning death or serious injuring of a close relative or parents after a traumatic event could also be traumatic(Ozgen,1999;DSM 5,2013). Besides, some medical interventions, such as various medical procedures and surgery, are similarly traumatic for children (Ari AB et al,2017).

Psychiatric disorders arise as a result of the complex interaction between social, psychological and biological factors (Cuhadaroglu,2008). An accumulation of ad-verse experiences and risk factors cause greater harm to mental health(Sack,1999). Both the type of event and duration of exposure may increase risk by intensifying personal threat (Hodes,2008). It has been showed that the number of exposures to traumatic incidents is associated with increased PTSD probability (Laufer,2009; Thabet,2000).

It must be known that PTSD mean neither ''as a normal response to stressful situations or events'' nor the person with PTSD is ''emotionally weak'' or "mentally ill''. But it could be conceptualized as an "information-processing disorder that interferes with the processing and integration of current life experience"(Vander Kolk,1996).

CHILDHOOD TRAUMATIC EXPERIENCES

Epidemiologic studies have revealed that two-thirds of US population survive at least one traumatic severe incident at one point of their life. However, when it is taken in to account that the most of the community in many countries live in areas under conflict and expose to violence, it is estimated that the global prevalence of experiencing traumatic incidents worldwide might be higher than in the US(Galea,2005)

Many people are exposed to traumatic incidents in their childhood. In a national study conducted in the UK, the prevalence of exposure to a traumatic event was found to be around 8.7% in children 5-10 years of age, and about 12.6% in children aged 10-15 years. (Ford,2003). It is estimated that children in underdeveloped countries are exposed to more traumatic experiences. Given that a considerable part of the world's children's population is gathered in developing or underdeveloped countries, it is estimated that traumatic experiences are more than an exception for children.

Unintentional injuries which increase gradually after the age of five are the leading cause of traumatic experiences and one of the main causes of mortality and morbidity during childhood and adolescence(Minino,Peden 2008). Just traffic accidents, each year, lead death of over a million, and injuring of nearly 50 million people worldwide (WHO,2015), while, every day, 2000 children lose their lives as a result of unintentional injuries (Branche,2008).

The data show that millions of children are treated in emergency services every year due to various accidents. For example in 1997, in England, more than 72 thousand children were treated in emergency services because of a traffic accident, and 16 per cent of these children had fatal injuries. Beyond causing death, injuries are also the leading reason for permanent disabilities in children and adolescents (Peden,2008). Literature shows that the number of children who die from accidents and injuries is higher than the total number of children who die from various infectious diseases (Molnar,2001).

Sexual and physical abuse are also common during childhood. Epidemiological studies indicate that child sexual abuse (CSA) is far from being an exception (Molnar,2001). A review of community–based studies that investigate CSA from various countries reported a range of 7% to 36% for females and 3% to 29% for males (Finkelhor,1994). Another review revealed that 12% to 35% of girls and 4% to 9% of boys were forced to have sexual involvement before age 18 years(Putnam,2003). Nevertheless, the fact that child sexual abuse is largely hidden and never disclosed suggests that childhood sexual abuse might be at the epidemic level. Over 2 million cases of child physical abuse reported in the US in 2008, which estimated to represent only a small part of the actual incident rates(Nooner,2012).

Violence is also one of the significant traumatic experiences of childhood. War by its nature is one of the prominent reason for chronic stress for people who survive it. It has been estimated that more than 160 wars which caused the death of 24 million people have taken place since 1945 (Pedersen,2002). Although fatalities are the worst toll of the wars, the adverse impacts of conflicts are not limited to deaths and physical destruction. It also leads to the displacement of many people and devastated and everlasting psychological wounds. As a consequence of war, conflicts and violence, every minute, 24 people were forced to flee their homes in 2015. Accordingly, the number of displaced people has risen from 37 million to 65 million in the past two decades (UNHCR,2015).

Today, 352 million children are trying to grow up in areas under conflict which are mostly underdeveloped countries. Living in the conflict zone does not just mean exposing violence. It brings with it many negative experiences such as the violation of human rights, maltreatment, the attainment of basic physiological needs, uncertainty, inability to reach educational opportunities. However, children in underdeveloped countries expose to many other traumatic incidents. For example, it is also reported that accidents and unintentional injuries are more common among children living in these countries

Refugee and asylum-seeking children also constitute another group of children ex-posed to intense traumatic experiences. Today, children account for more than half of the refugee population, which has reached the highest number of all time, rising to 65 million. Findings of investigations with refugee children indicate that these children have been exposed to a large number of traumatic experiences which are not limited to the pre-migration period and continue after the resettlement. It has been showed that various traumatic and adverse life experiences such as violence, loss, physical, emotional or sexual assaults, uncertainty, poverty, overcrowded and unsafe housing, domestic violence, impaired parenting, limited access to education and health services, discrimination, stigma or social exclusion by new culture are all very common among refugee children (Fazel,2005; Heptinstal,2004; Ibrahim,2017; Ahmad,2008; Kinzie,1986)

As mentioned above, children worldwide expose to various traumatic events which is at the epidemic level. Although the adverse effects of traumatic events on children's mental and psychosocial well-being are better understood day by day, we must accept that we have failed to protect children from such traumatic experiences.

Post-Traumatic Stress Reactions in Children

Following traumatic events, various stress symptoms such as excessive fear, shock, crying, intrusive thoughts, hyperarousal, unable to calm, sleeping problems, impatience, nervousness, abdominal or muscle pain, stomach cramps, irritability, fatigue, dizziness, unwillingness to go out, school refusal, loneliness, social isolation, enuresis, sudden change in preferred games and activities may develop in children and adolescents. Additionally, memory and concentration difficulties and attention problems are also observed frequently. Suicidal thoughts and sense of worthlessness are other significant symptoms that can develop in children and adolescents after traumatic events.

Symptom cluster may vary with age and by gender. And it may manifest with classic attention deficit hyperactivity disorder (ADHD) symptoms such as hyperactivity, restlessness, impulsivity, irritability or distractibility in younger children (De Bellis,2013;De Bellis,1999), and "unless a careful history of traumatic exposure is taken in relation to the timing of the onset or worsening of symptoms, these conditions may be difficult to distinguish"(Cohen,2010).

Although externalizing problems, repetitive plays (and drawing) or behavioral re-enactments could be seen in all ages; younger children more commonly exhibit such behaviors(Dyregrov,2006). Irritability and feeding problems might be seen during infancy. Problems in emotional regulation, irritability, intense fear, regression, sleep and eating problems and are common in the early childhood period. Pre-school children may manifest the overwhelming stress by repeated games, aggression, difficulties in impulse control, separation anxiety, enuresis or encopresis and night fears. Attention and concentration problems, peer problems, separation anxiety, somatic symptom, drop in school achievement, isolation and various fears could be observed in school-age children. Despite the fact that, most of these symptoms disappear within 2-4 weeks, these symptoms may increase rather than diminish, and they can reach dimensions that threaten the child's functioning over time. Although such symptoms could be alarming for children, it could be tough for parents to be aware of these symptoms because of children's unwillingness to talk about these symptoms to not upset their parents.

Physiological and Biochemical Measures

It is suggested that "fight and flight" response to traumatic incidents are less compatible with younger children(Perry,1995). When exposed to a traumatic event, children tend to respond with irritability at the beginning, which is to attract the attention of adults. But if traumatic exposure or threats persist without help, the response might switch immobilizing or freezing and then dissociation or surrendering(Tebbit,1997).

Traumatic exposure triggers physiological and biological changes in traumatized children. These changes can forward to mobilize the child to escape from the traumatic exposure. However, these changes may normalize if the traumatic exposure persists for a period or the child start to dissociate. (McFarlane et al., 1987; Shaw et al., 1995),

Post-Traumatic Stress Disorder

Although the negative outcome of traumatic experiences on mental well-being has been recognized for a long time, systematic research has carried out for the last 50 years. In 1952, post-traumatic reactions conceptualized as the "Great Stress Reaction" in the Diagnostic and Statistical Manual of Mental Disorders (DSM) –I.. It took place in DSM-III, with the name of "Post-traumatic Stress Disorder", especially after the monitoring of soldiers injured in the Vietnam war. The PTSD diagnosis has come up with some minor changes but has remained in all subsequent DSM updates including DSM-V.

In DSM V, post-traumatic stress disorder is defined as a psychological disorder characterized with intrusive (repetitive, involuntary images, memory and emotions associated with the event etc), avoidance (situations associated with the trauma or emotional numbness etc.) and hyperarousal (irritability, anger, sleep and concentration problems etc) and negative alteration in mood and cognitions that occur after encountering one or more traumatic events and persist for at least one month. The diagnostic criteria were separated for children under the age of 6 and people older than six years in DSM-V as shown below:

DSM-V posttraumatic stress disorder diagnostic criteria for people older than 6 years:

1. Exposure to actual or threatened death, serious injury, or sexual violence in one (or more) of the following ways:
    a. Directly experiencing the traumatic event(s).
    b. Witnessing, in person, the event(s) as it occurred to others.
    c. Learning that the traumatic event(s) occurred to a close family member or close friend. In cases of actual or threatened death of a family member or friend, the event(s) must have been violent or accidental.
    d. Experiencing repeated or extreme exposure to aversive details of the traumatic event(s) (e.g., first responders collecting human remains: police officers repeatedly exposed to details of child abuse).

Note: Criterion A4 does not apply to exposure through electronic media, television, movies, or pictures, unless this exposure is work related.

2. Presence of one (or more) of the following intrusion symptoms associated with the traumatic event(s), beginning after the traumatic event(s) occurred:
    a. Recurrent, involuntary, and intrusive distressing memories of the traumatic event(s).
    b. Note: In children older than 6 years, repetitive play may occur in which themes or aspects of the traumatic event(s) are expressed.
    c. Recurrent distressing dreams in which the content and/or affect of the dream are related to the traumatic event(s).

Note: In children, there may be frightening dreams without recognizable content. Dissociative reactions (e.g., flashbacks) in which the individual feels or acts as if the traumatic event(s) were recurring. (Such reactions may occur on a continuum, with the most extreme expression being a complete loss of awareness of present surroundings.)

Note: In children, trauma-specific reenactment may occur in play. Intense or prolonged psychological distress at exposure to internal or external cues that symbolize or resemble an aspect of the traumatic event(s). Marked physiological reactions to internal or external cues that symbolize or resemble an aspect of the traumatic event(s).

3. Persistent avoidance of stimuli associated with the traumatic event(s), beginning after the traumatic event(s) occurred, as evidenced by one or both of the following:

   a. Avoidance of or efforts to avoid distressing memories, thoughts, or feelings about or closely associated with the traumatic event(s).
   b. Avoidance of or efforts to avoid external reminders (people, places, conversations, activities, objects, situations) that arouse distressing memories, thoughts, or feelings about or closely associated with the traumatic event(s).
4. Negative alterations in cognitions and mood associated with the traumatic event(s), beginning or worsening after the traumatic event(s) occurred, as evidenced by two (or more) of the following:
   a. Inability to remember an important aspect of the traumatic event(s) (typically due to dissociative amnesia and not to other factors such as head injury, alcohol, or drugs).
   b. Persistent and exaggerated negative beliefs or expectations about oneself, others, or the world (e.g., "I am bad," "No one can be trusted," 'The world is completely dangerous," "My whole nervous system is permanently ruined").
   c. Persistent, distorted cognitions about the cause or consequences of the traumatic event(s) that lead the individual to blame himself/herself or others.
   d. Persistent negative emotional state (e.g., fear, horror, anger, guilt, or shame).
   e. Markedly diminished interest or participation in significant activities.
   f. Feelings of detachment or estrangement from others.
   g. Persistent inability to experience positive emotions (e.g., inability to experience happiness, satisfaction, or loving feelings).
5. Marked alterations in arousal and reactivity associated with the traumatic event(s), beginning or worsening after the traumatic event(s) occurred, as evidenced by two (or more) of the following:
   a. Irritable behavior and angry outbursts (with little or no provocation) typically expressed as verbal or physical aggression toward people or objects.
   b. Reckless or self-destructive behavior.
   c. Hypervigilance.
   d. Exaggerated startle response.
   e. Problems with concentration.
   f. Sleep disturbance (e.g., difficulty falling or staying asleep or restless sleep).
6. Duration of the disturbance (Criteria B, C, D, and E) is more than 1 month.

7. The disturbance causes clinically significant distress or impairment in social, occupational, or other important areas of functioning.
8. The disturbance is not attributable to the physiological effects of a substance (e.g., medication, alcohol) or another medical condition.

DSM-V posttraumatic stress disorder diagnostic criteria for children younger than 6 years:

1. Exposure to actual or threatened death, serious injury, or sexual violence in one (or more) of the following ways:

    a. Directly experiencing the traumatic event(s).
    b. Witnessing, in person, the event(s) as it occurred to others, especially primary care givers.
    c. Learning that the traumatic event(s) occurred to a parent or caregiving figure.

Note: Witnessing does not include events that are witnessed only in electronic media, television, movies, or pictures.

2. Presence of one (or more) of the following intrusion symptoms associated with the traumatic event(s), beginning after the traumatic event(s) occurred:
    a. Recurrent, involuntary, and intrusive distressing memories of the traumatic event(s).
    b. Recurrent distressing dreams in which the content and/or affect of the dream are related to the traumatic event(s).
    c. Dissociative reactions (e.g., flashbacks) in which the child feels or acts as if the traumatic event(s) were recurring. (Such reactions may occur on a continuum, with the most extreme expression being a complete loss of awareness of present surroundings.) Such trauma-specific reenactment may occur in play.
    d. Intense or prolonged psychological distress at exposure to internal or external cues that symbolize or resemble an aspect of the traumatic event(s).
    e. Marked physiological reactions to reminders of the traumatic event(s).

Note: Spontaneous and intrusive memories may not necessarily appear distressing and may be expressed as play reenactment.

Note: It may not be possible to ascertain that the frightening content is related to the traumatic event.

3. One (or more) of the following symptoms, representing either persistent avoidance of stimuli associated with the traumatic event(s) or negative alterations in cognitions and mood associated with the traumatic event(s), must be present, beginning after the event(s) or worsening after the event(s):
   a. Persistent Avoidance of Stimuli
   b. Avoidance of or efforts to avoid activities, places, or physical reminders that arouse recollections of the traumatic event(s).
   c. Avoidance of or efforts to avoid people, conversations, or interpersonal situations that arouse recollections of the traumatic event(s).
   d. Negative Alterations in Cognitions
   e. Substantially increased frequency of negative emotional states (e.g., fear, guilt, sadness, shame, confusion).
   f. Markedly diminished interest or participation in significant activities, including constriction of play.
   g. Socially withdrawn behavior.
   h. Persistent reduction in expression of positive emotions.
4. Alterations in arousal and reactivity associated with the traumatic event(s), beginning or worsening after the traumatic event(s) occurred, as evidenced by two (or more) of the following:
   a. Irritable behavior and angry outbursts (with little or no provocation) typically ex pressed as verbal or physical aggression toward people or objects (including extreme temper tantrums).
   b. Hypervigilance.
   c. Exaggerated startle response.
   d. Problems with concentration.
   e. Sleep disturbance (e.g., difficulty falling or staying asleep or restless sleep).
5. The duration of the disturbance is more than 1 month.
6. The disturbance causes clinically significant distress or impairment in relationships with parents, siblings, peers, or other caregivers or with school behavior.

7. The disturbance is not attributable to the physiological effects of a substance (e.g., medication or alcohol) or another medical condition.

The lifetime prevalence of PTSD was estimated in The National Comorbidity Survey (NCS) as 7.8% (Kesssler,1995). However, prevalence rates vary from study to study widely related to, sample selection, the type of trauma and methodology of the survey. For example, it has been reported that higher rates of PTSD are observed following man-made traumatic incidents and sexual abuse, than exposure to natural disasters (Donnelly 2002).

Clinical presentation of post-traumatic stress varies widely. For example, hyper-arousal can be manifest as, concentration problems, irritability, anger outbursts or problems in emotion regulation. Difficulties in sustaining attention may also observe as a consequence of reexperiencing the traumatic event. Thus, children may look like having hyperactivity(Donelly,2002)

Although many children who experienced a traumatic event will develop PTSD, this rate varies considerably from study to study. It has been suggested that the differences between the results may be related to the traumatized person and the nature of the traumatic event (De Bellis,1999). Thus, the nature of the traumatic event, individual's physical or emotional proximity to the incident, person's age, psychological development and previous experiences family characteristics and cultural factors can influence the development of PTSD (Langeland,2008;Kilptrik,2003; Olofsson,2009;Pfefferbaum,1997). The physical proximity is described as physical distance from the traumatic event, while emotional proximity is characterized as emotional involvement with the survivors of the incident(Pynoos,1987).

PTSD has been criticized for being a culturally constructed disorder which does not have validity in other nations (Summerfield,2000). However, high rates of PTSD has been shown in many non-western countries (Fazel,2005;Heptinstal,2004;Ibrahim,2017;Ahmad,2008;Kinzie,1986) which showed that PTSD is not limited to any culture, and it is universal among all cultures which were exposed to traumatic events (Mollica,2001;Yule,2015).

Although PTSD has been reported to have severe negative impacts on self-control, concentration, attention, cognition, emotion regulation, memory and learning that may threat children's school attendance and academic achievement, the impact of PTSD on academic functionality has not been adequately studied (Heringa,2017). However, studies which investigated the impact of traumatic experiences on school drop out or academic problems among children have shown the negative outcome of such experiences on the academic life of survivors (Broberg,2005;De Prince,2009).

Complex PTSD

The psychiatry field had ignored the effects of psychological trauma on mental health for long years. However, it was eventually wiped out with the involvement of PTSD in DSM-III. Discussions are not finished after accepting the PTSD diagnosis in the DSM-III. Some authors argue that PTSD symptoms are normal reactions against an abnormal situation, while others say that DSM criteria are from covering the effect of psychological trauma in depth. In addition, studies have shown that there is a significant difference between stress reactions that develop following a single traumatic event and reactions which develop after exposing repetitive and prolonged traumas. However, the trauma literature suffices to focus on PTSD that develops after a single trauma for many years. However, studies in recent years have revealed that the traumatic events are not causing just classical PTSD. In light of these new findings, a new diagnosis, Complex PTSD, has been suggested. Although there have been many studies on the validity of Complex PTSD and serious studies have been undertaken to include it in DSM 5 as a different diagnosis from PTSD, this diagnosis has not been included in DSM 5. However, the diagnosis of Complex PTSD has taken part as a different disorder than TSSB in ICD-11.

Complex post-traumatic stress disorder (Complex PTSD) is conceptualized as a "disorder that may develop following exposure to an event or series of events of an extremely threatening or horrific nature, most commonly prolonged or repetitive events from which escape is difficult or impossible (e.g., torture, slavery, genocide campaigns, prolonged domestic violence, repeated childhood sexual or physical abuse)." And it is characterized by "1) severe and pervasive problems in affect regulation; 2) persistent beliefs about oneself as diminished, defeated or worthless, ac-companied by deep and pervasive feelings of shame, guilt or failure related to the traumatic event; and 3) persistent difficulties in sustaining relationships and in feeling close to others" in addition to all diagnostic requirements for PTSD.

EPIDEMIOLOGY

Almost all children exposed to traumatic events develop some of the post-traumatic reactions mentioned above, most of these symptoms disappear in a couple of weeks. However, a considerable proportion of these children develop

PTSD which characterized by re-experiencing, avoidance, hyperarousal and negative alterations in cognition and mood (DSM-5,2013).

PTSD is not a rare or occasional disorder. However, the prevalence of PTSD in the community sample varies considerably from country to country ranging from 7 to 12%(Breslau,2012). The differences in study findings are acknowledged with methodological or sample differences, the nature of the traumatic incident, assessment tool, cultural differences, time of assessment, and demographical characteristics of the investigated population (age, economical or educational situation etc.) (Dyregrov,2006).

Prevalence of PTSD in Community

In a study of 490 adolescents aged 16-22 years evaluated with a semi-structured interview tool, 3% of girls and 1% of boys were found to have PTSD (Olofsson,2009). The results of a study of 287 children in Afghanistan showed that more than one in four men (26%) had PTSD. In the same study, it was found that 14% of the girls had PTSD(Catani,2009). The lifetime prevalence of PTSD which is reported to be as high as 8.7%, is estimated to be higher in the USA than in Europe (dsm-5,2013). It is concluded that 61% of children will experience a potentially traumatic event and PTSD will develop in 4.7% of them by the age of 18(Mc Laughlin,2013).

Although it is reported that PTSD is less prevalent in children and adolescents than adults. This might be because of previous criteria did not fully account for develop-mental differences (DSM-5,2013). In a child and adolescent psychiatric epidemiology study in the UK that assessed 10,438 children aged 5 to 15 years, PTSD was found to be around 0.14% of this age interval (Ford,2003).

It has been reported that adolescents might be at higher risk of experiencing trauma than either adults or children (Nooner,2012). In a study of adolescents aged 12-17 in the United States, the 12-month prevalence of PTSD was determined to be 6.3% in girls and 3.7% in males, and the co-morbidity of depression and substance use with PTSD was also high, Thus, it is noted that PTSD may also be a risk factor for substance use in children and adolescents (Kilpatrick,2003). Nooner et al., by evaluating studies from 2000 to 2011, reported that the prevalence of PTSD among adolescents is 3–57% (Nooner,2012).

The results of a study with 8th Grade students in Denmark show that the lifetime prevalence of PTSD of these kids is around 9%. And, another community study in the United States reported that one out of every ten children had PTSD (Kessler,1995). The results of a comprehensive meta-analytic study examining the development of PTSD in children and assessing a total of more than 2500 children revealed that more than a third of children (36%) developed PTSD after exposure to a traumatic event (Fletcher,1996).

"Traumatization within attachment relationships has profoundly different impacts on affect regulation, self-concept, and management of interpersonal relationships than do disasters and motor vehicle accidents"(Van der Kolk,1996). The incidence of PTSD after different traumatic events vary enormously which explained with differing methodologies, different types of traumatic events or cultures (Dyregrov,2006).

Traffic Accidents

It is known that traffic accidents are the main factors causing PTSD development in adults (Blanchard,1997). In a follow-up study in which adults were evaluated, the incidence of PTSD was 32% one year after the traffic accidents, and the stress symptoms of the person following the accident were more correlated with the development of later PTSD than the severity of the injury by accident (Koren,1999). However, it is not known exactly how much such traumatic experiences lead to the development of PTSD in children (Keppel-Berison,2002). The results of studies conducted with children who were evaluated following traffic accidents indicate that a quarter to one-third of these children suffers from PTSD (Langeland,2008).

The results of a study with children showed that 24% of children who were assessed after 9 months of traffic accident had stress symptoms and 14% had PTSD (Keppel-Benson,2002). An-other important finding in the same study is that the supportive approach of the police or health team after the incident has been effective in preventing the development of PTSD symptomatology in children. This result shows the importance of the supportive attitude of the team that interferes with accidents or injuries when it comes to children.

In another study, 35% of the children reported having PTSD (Stallard,1998), while another study findings revealed that PTSD developed in 50% of the children (Milgram,1988). In a follow-up study in which the children were evaluated immediately after the accident and at 1, 6 and 18 months, symptoms of PTSD in children were observed in 69%, 57%, 59% and 38%, respectively

(Schreirer,2005). In a review included twelve studies, it was reported that PTSD was observed around 30% of children over the period of 1-2 months after the event (Qouta,2003).

War and Violence

Another group of children with a very high prevalence of PTSD is the children who live in areas under conflict. The studies which carried out with children exposed to violence, war or terrorism have revealed a high prevalence rate of PTSD among child survivors (Thabet,2008).

In one of the first study which carried out with children from areas under conflict Kinzie et al. revealed that one out of two Cambodian refugee children residing in the US has PTSD (32). The findings of a study of 121 children living near a bombardment area in Palestine revealed severe PTSD symptoms in 51% of the child (Qouta,2003). PTSD was found in 87% of children in a study conducted 5 years later with children in the Halabja region of Kurdistan where the Iraqi Ba'as regime carried out genocide with chemical weapons (Ahmat,2000). Seventy per cent of Kuwaiti children evaluated after the Gulf War was also observed to have significant PTSD symptoms (Nader,1993). The results of a comprehensive community sampling study which carried out in Algeria, Cambodia, Ethiopia and Gaza with people older than16 years revealed that the proportions of PTSD in these places were 37.4%, 28.4%, 15.8% and 17.8%, respectively(De Jong,2001). The results of a study with child survivors of the Bosnian war suggest that 28% of children have PTSD (Papageorgieu,2000). In a research that evaluates children aged 1.5-5 years, there was PTSD in more than one third (37.8%) of children living near a conflict area (Feldman,2011). The results of a study which carried out with 99 Cambodian children aged 18-25 showed that 86% of these children had PTSD or PTSD-NOS (Savin,1996). Another study with Cambodian children also reported high rates of PTSD (%37) among child survivors (Realmuto,1992). Results of Kızılhan et al.'s fascinating investigation with child warriors showed that 48.3% of these children had PTSD. They also revealed that PTSD rates in child soldiers were higher than other child survivors of the war (Kizilian,2018). Ceri et al. also reported high rates of PTSD and Acute Stress Disorders among Yazidi child survivors (Ceri,2016). The finding of a systematic review reported PTSD ranging from 4.5 to 89.3%, with an overall pooled estimate of 47% among children exposed to war (Attanayake,2009).

Displaced Children

Study results with refugee children indicate increased PTSD rates in these children (Bronstein,2011). This increase is reported to be ten times higher than non-refugee children. Studies from various countries such as Uganda (Betancourt,2009), Somalia (Betancourt,2009), Darfur (Morgos,2008), Cambodia(Kinzie,1986), Bosnia(Goldin,2008), Syria (Kandemir,2018) and Iraq (Ahmad,2008) have shown high rates of PTSD among displaced children.

In a review that evaluate 260 refugee children, Fazel and his friends reported the TSSB rate as 11%. Dyregrov and Yule (2006) report that 25% to 70% of refugee children have PTSD in conclusion of their review on PTSD in children (Dyregrov,2006). Another comprehensive review which included 22 studies concerning refugee children from over 40 different countries reported that 19 to 54% of refugee children residing in Western countries had PTSD (Bronstein,2011).

The results of a series of studies with refugee children in Turkey have shown that, even after years of resettlement, PTSD was observed in 9% to 43% of these children (Ceri,2016;Yalin,2017; Nasiroglu,2016). Çeri et al. in their study which carried out with Yazidi children immediately after their arrival to Turkey revealed that 18% of these children had acute stress symptoms, and, PTSD was diagnosed in 10% the children (Ceri,2016). In another study, Nasıroğlu and Çeri reported that 36% of refugee children have PTSD (Nasiroglu,2018). Another study found that more than half (55%) of refugee children had PTSD (Hodes,2008). The results of a study with Bosnian children showed that 65% of these children had PTSD even after one year of their journey to the US (Weine,1995). The result of a follow-up study in Netherland indicated that the psychological distress of refugee children are severe and It has a chronic nature (Bean,2007).

Child Abuse

High rates of PTSD have been reported among victim of CSA (Rowan,1993). A national cohort study revealed increased lifetime PTSD diagnosis for females (39%) and males (29%) who sexually abused during childhood. The lifetime PTSD diagnosis was 5.7% and 3.8% among for females and males who have not childhood sexual abuse (Molnar,2001). Finding of a meta analysis which included thirty-seven studies involving 25,367 people indicated that "there is a 143% increase in the risk of developing PTSD symptoms following CSA among the general population"(Paolucci,2001). Another study which carried out with child survivors of sexual abuse reported one out of two (48%) children suffer from PTSD (McLEER,1988).

Natural Disasters

Post-traumatic stress reactions which develop following disasters is a serious public health problem as millions of children are affected each year (Nooner,2012). In a review which investigates the epidemiology of PTSD after disasters Galea et al. (2005) revealed that PTSD rates are ranging from five to sixty per cent among child survivors(Galea,2005).

A study which carried out with children who survived a hurricane reported that 56% of children have PTSD 3 months after the incident. The PTSD prevalence was found as high as 34% 10 months after the hurricane (LAGRECA,1996). Another study revealed that 20 per cent of children who survive an earthquake have PTSD (Hsu,2002). A meta-analysis which consists of forty-six articles involving 76,101 earthquake survivors indicated a 23.6% prevalence rates for PTSD (Dai,2016). Another study which investigates psychological problems among children after hurricane Katrina reported a 32% of PTS symptoms (Lai,2015). Seventy per cent of the children who live in an area impacted by a tsunami in India also reported suffering posttraumatic stress symptoms two months after the disaster (John,2007).

Various Traumatic Incidents

A study which carried with children who affected by the 11/09 terrorist attacks revealed that 84% of children had experienced moderate or severe posttraumatic stress reactions (Fairbrother,2003). 37% of children aged 2 to 15 years who survived the demolition of a dam, were found to have PTSD symptoms two years after the incident (Green,1991). Another study which carried out with children who survive a sniper attack in school revealed that 38% of the children had a significant level of PTSD symptoms (Hinton,2009). Reports have shown that one out of two children exposed to physical abuse also has PTSD (Dubner,1999). Domestic violence is another common kind of traumatic experience for exposed children that associated with high PTSD rates of about 36% (De Bellis,2009).

PTSD AND FUNCTIONALITY

Childhood PTSD does not only lead to psychological difficulties in the child but affects the child's academic life and is associated with increased depression, sub-stance use and suicidal behaviors. (Warshaw,1993) PTSD, which develops after a traumatic experience, can seriously disrupt the developmental process of the child and can negatively affect the social and academic life of the child by causing considerable loss in functionality (Karakaya,2007). It has been reported that survivors were more easily annoyed, had more difficulty controlling their emotions, and were more aggressive towards family members after a traumatic experience (Hinton,2009; Abe,1994). It was found that when people with PTSD are nervous, their heart rate increases more (Beckham,2002). Several studies have also shown that PTSD has a detrimental effect on cognitive functions (Gil,1990;Kocak,2017). It is therefore understood that PTSD has a serious negative impact on children's social and academic functioning (Ainmani,2017). It is stated that early treatment may prevent the later negative out-comes by preventing further functionality loss (Olofsson,2009). However, it is stated that PTSD in children is not well recognized in the society and treatment can be delayed (Ceri,2018; Ceri,2017).

Children's immediate attention may switch on physical safety or survival after ex-posing a life-threatening event and may not turn to the normal function for a while (Pfefferbaum,2016). Even though a traumatic event will not lead the development of PTSD among all of the exposed children, partial symptomatology could be debilitating and should be the target for treatment even in the absence of full syndrome criteria(Pfefferbaum,2016). Several studies have investigated whether traumatic events have an adverse effect on concentration or attention of child survivors. A study which Sprung carried out with children exposed to a hurricane reported lower concentration levels among child survivors (Sprung,2010). Another study also reported attention problems among children who indirectly exposed to 11/09 attacks (Hock,2004). Problems in attention, memory, learning and concentration were reported in several other studies that carried out with children exposed to traumatic incidents (Scrimmin,2009; Vasterling,2009; Chemtob,2008). Another study findings revealed significant deterioration in verbal intelligence scores of children who survive an earthquake (Chetomb,2008). Other studies also reported a decline in school achievement in children exposed to various disasters (Pérez-Pereira,2012; Ward,2008). It is also reported that adolescents with PTSD are under risk to failed a grade or suspended from school (Nooner,2012). Another study revealed a drop in attention and executive functions of children with PTSD (Beers,2002).

A study which conducted with children witnessed domestic violence revealed that those children had diminished executive functioning. Their attention and IQ also tended to be lower (Samuelson,2010). Another study which carried out with the child survivor of sexual abuse showed reduced ability to inhibit automatic responses in the Stroop test (Barrera, 2013). Findings of another study reported diminished cognitive skills or neuropsychological deficits among children with PTSD (De Bellis,2013). A study which assessed executive functions such as automatic response inhibition, self-regulation, monitoring, and cognitive flexibility, indicated significant difficulties in women who had a history of CSA (Navalta,2006). Worsened performance in the visuospatial domain task also revealed among children with PTSD (De Bellis,1999)

PTSD, Brain Development and Neural Circuitry

The development of the brain and central nervous system which is associated with the progression of cortical myelinization continue during childhood and adolescence (Sowell,2001). Pediatric PTSD causes structural and functional abnormalities in neural circuits that regulate distress and emotion. It is also stated that abnormalities are observed in the development of frontolimbic circuits in these children and that abnormalities in these pathways make emotional control difficult and lead to increased perception. It is also reported that children and adolescents with PTSD have a decreased hippocampal volume and an increase in amygdala reactivity (Herringa,2017).

Neuroimaging studies have revealed an association between PTSD and emotion regulation, dopamine, and norepinephrine activation (Nooner,2012). Reduced grey matter volume in the anterior cingulate cortex, ventromedial prefrontal cortex, and hippocampus have also been showed (O'Doherty,2015). Functional brain imaging studies have revealed hyper-activation in the amygdala, insula and mid Anterior cingulate cortex, whereas hypo-activation is indicated in the medial prefrontal areas and Dorsal Anterior Cingulate Cortex (Hayes,2012). The effect of traumatic exposure on brain might vary according to the age of survivor. In a study conducted with victims of sexual abuse, it was reported that abuse before age 14 effect hippocampus volume, while abuse that exposed between 10-11 years of age is associated with amygdala volume and aged 14-16 years with prefrontal cortex volume (Teicher,2016).

Risk Factors

An accumulation of adverse experiences and risk factors cause elevated harm to mental health (Sack,1999). Both the duration of exposure and proximity to the event may increase risk by intensifying the threat on the survivor (Hodes,2008). The number of exposures to traumatic incidents is reported to be associated with PTSD (Laufer,2009; Thabet,2000),

In a meta-analysis, Cox and colleagues reported that eight factors are associated with higher PTSD rates among traumatised children after traffic accidents such as threat to life, previous psychopathology, younger age, female gender, previous traumatic exposure, severity of injury, involvement of a family member or a close friend in the accident (Cox,2008). Another meta-analysis which involved 32,238 children aged 6-18 years and investigated twenty five possible risk factors for PTSD revealed race, younger age, female gender, low intelligence scores, low SES, pre and post-traumatic adverse events, low social support, peritrauma fear, perceived life threat, social withdrawal, comorbid psychological problem, poor family functioning, distraction, previous psychological problems in the individual or parent, low self-esteem before trauma, post-traumatic parental psychological problems, bereavement, time, trauma severity and exposure to the event by media as risk factors for PTSD (Trickey,2012).

Another research that aims to investigate risk factors for the development of PTSD pointed out the nature and impact of the traumatic event, physical proximity, expo-sure time, children's and parents previous experiences as important factors in the development of PTSD in children and adolescents (Pfefferbaum,1997). Nooner et al. in their review revealed that 4 out of 5 adolescents had been exposed to a serious traumatic event, while PTSD developed in 3 to 57% of them. Gender, type and number of traumatic exposure and age were associated with increased rates of PTSD (Nonner,2012). Gekker et al. suggested that child abuse is leading to more severe PTSD which is associated with more comorbid disorders and resistant to treatment (Gekker,2018). Level of exposure (Pine,2002), age, ethnicity(Meiser,2002), lack of social support, problems in family cohesion, female gen-der, prior exposure to trauma, prior psychiatric problems, and strong peritraumatic reactions (Pine,2002) have also reported to have an association with development of PTSD after various traumatic events in children. Although risk factors vary across studies, previous psychopathology and personal threat to life were found to be significant in all studies (Trickey,2012). The miscognitions or misinterpretation of the event, extreme worry about the safety of family, disruption in parental relationship, relocation, neglect, and avoidance-focused coping methods are also stated as risk factors for the development of PTSD in children following a traumatic event.

Course

It is stated that negative childhood experiences are the main cause of preventable mental disorders and substance use (Teicher,201).

Exposure to traumatic events in early childhood is particularly toxic due to its devastating effects on healthy development. The traumatic experiences in early childhood may prepare the ground for the development of other debilitating conditions. Toxic stress might lead to severe biological changes that cause problems in cognition, emotion and behavioral regulation which are associated with impaired social skills, aggression, violence and impulsivity (Donelly,2002).

It has been showed that childhood onset PTSD could persist for as long as 33 years (Morgan,2003). A follow-up study which carried out with adolescent survivors of a ship sinking revealed that 34% of survivors have PTSD years after the event (Yule,2000). Another study which assessed child survivors of a landslide disaster, 33 years after the incident, found that 29% of children still have PTSD (Morgan,2003). Sack et al. in their follow up study which carried out with refugee children of Cambodia reported that the onset of PTSD was quite variable, with 18% of subjects developing PTSD at least five years after cessation of the traumatic exposure (Sack,1999). They also reported that PTSD persists in one out of every three children even a decade later (Sack,1999). A study which carried out 20 years after an earthquake showed that 30% of children have full PTSD, the prevalence of partial PTSD symptoms were as high as 56% among the survivors (Najarian,2017).

New findings point out that the effects of toxic stress may extend its influence be-yond the survivor into next generations by leading behavioural changes in the ex-posed person or epigenetic changes that transmit directly to the offspring of the survivor (Neigh,2009). Furthermore, when left untreated PTSD may lead the development of affective or anxiety disorders, and substance use and impair their psychosocial and academical functioning in the later time course (Bolton,2000). Psychiatric comorbidity is as common as a norm rather than an exception in people with PTSD (Creamer et al., 2001). Even adult-onset PTSD patients who have a history of child abuse may represent a subgroup with a more severe form of the disorder that is associated with a higher comorbid depression, psychotic symptoms and phobic disorder, severe clinical course, treatment resistance and poorer outcome (Gekker,2018). Findings of National Comorbidity Survey showed that lifelong PTSD is associated with increased mood, anxiety disorders and substance abuse (Kessler et al., 1995, (Jeon et al., 2007). Comorbid psychiatric conditions lead to more functional impairment and treatment resistance and worse quality of life in PTSD patients (Post et al., 2011; Araujo et al., 2014; Pagotto et al., 2015; Gekket 2018).

It has been shown that lifetime traumatic event exposure increases suicidal thoughts, substance abuse and binge drinking in adults (Forman-Hoffman,2012). It was reported that the history of having traumatic exposure or PTSD might lead a three times increase in suicide attempts in adolescents (Nonner,2012).

Individuals with a history of child abuse, as compared to their counterparts without such history, showed a more severe comorbidity profile in general, characterized by a higher mean number of lifetime and current comorbid disorders and a greater life-time and current prevalence of panic disorder (Gekker,2018).

TREATMENT

Early Interventions

Although prevention is better than treatment, it is a hard task to achieve in most of the disorders which arise as a result of complex interaction of social, psychological and biological factors (Cuhadaroglu,2008). However, the preventing of PTSD may be achieved very easily by ending the happening of traumatic incidents or the exposure of children to such events. Thus making policies and arrangements to decrease accidents, child abuse or maltreatment and exposing violence may have a significant effect on reducing rates of children who suffer from PTSD

In case of exposure to traumatic events, early interventions will also be very useful if its effect on preventing the development of PTSD could be shown. Like the ABC of first aid in medical support, the psychological first aid starts with ensuring that the child feels secure and safe and to make certain that the child knows what is happening around him and provides information and explanation about the status of family members and his/her friends(3).

Despite strong evidence have shown that traumatic events increase psychiatric morbidity and the initial distress might be far greater than PTSD, there is no effective way to protect children from developing PTSD after traumatic exposure (Rose,2002).

Various preventing or supportive interventions have been developed to support children to cope with post-traumatic stress (Rose,2002). A program which teaches cognitive behavioral coping strategies to prevent the development of psychopathology following stressful events results indicated a significant decline in depressive and externalising symptoms (Jaycox,1994). Crisis Intervention Program for Children and Adolescents (CIPCA) has been recently developed by Abdulbaghi Ahmad to prevent post-traumatic psychopathology among displaced children and adolescents (Ahmad,2014). The findings of a recent study pointed out that a single session of CIPCA might be effective in preventing and/ or relieving the symptoms of PTSD in displaced kids (Ceri,2108). Debriefing is also a psychological intervention that aims to reduce the psychological morbidity after traumatic exposure (Hodgkinson,1991). It consists of encouraging of the survivor to express his emotion, support to process the traumatic event and increase social connectedness (Rose,2002). However, meta-analysis fails to show the effectiveness of such preventive interventions, and it is recommended to carry out further investigation to evaluate whether preventive intervention programs are efficient (Rose,2002; March,1998). Although the efficacy of these interventions has not been showed systemically, it is important to be aware of that reduction of even one symptom of PTSD might have notable favourable effect on the functionality of children (Donelly,2002).

Partial symptomatology is widespread in kids exposed to traumatic events and may impair the functioning of the individual even if the exact criteria are not met (Giaconia et al., 1995). Thus, it is crucial to recognise all symptoms and to think about treatment even when the full PTSD symptoms have not developed. This is especially critical for children whom PTSD might undermine their development (Tebutt,1997).

Study findings have revealed that psychological interventions might be useful in relieving posttraumatic stress symptoms. Results of a recent meta-analysis have indicated a significant weighted mean effect size in PTSD improvement as a result of psychosocial treatment, which pointed out a 74% reduction in PTSD. Furthermore, kids getting any psychological intervention improved considerably better than those children not get an intervention (Newman,2014).

Treatment of PTSD

Because even partial PTSD symptoms may lead significant impairment in the child's social, emotional or academic functionality, "treatment decisions should take into account functional impairment and symptom severity regardless of whether or not they have an actual PTSD diagnosis" (Cohen,2010).

Treatment of PTSD start with education of parents and the child about PTSD. School teachers also should be involved. PTSD treatment requires trauma-focused approaches such as trauma-focused cognitive-behavioral (CBT), psychodynamic, or family therapy (Cohen,2010).

Trauma-focused CBT which has a sizeable supporting data about its effectiveness in school-age and older children is recommended as the first choice in PTSD (March,1998). Pharmacological interventions are not suggested as an initial treatment option. How-ever, using pharmacological agents as an adjunct (Cohen,2010). Deblinger, Stauffer and Steer (2001) revealed better outcomes among children enrolled in group CBT than children enrolled in a support group (Deblinger,2001). Another study also showed the effectiveness of CBT in PTSD among sexually abused children (King,2000). A study which carried out with 229 children with PTSD reported better outcomes for PTSD and depression symptoms in children assigned to Trauma-Focused CBT, compared to those as-signed to child centered therapy (March,1998). Findings of a (Cohen,2004) meta-analysis revealed that CBT, EMDR, Exposure, and Eclectic with CBT interventions are all effective for children and adolescents (Newman,2104). Another meta-analysis also give some evidence for the effectiveness of psychological therapies in both prevention PTSD and treatment of PTSD in children and adolescents (Deblinger,2010)

Cohen et al stated that a trauma-focused psychotherapy should directly address children's traumatic experiences, include parents in treatment, not focus only relieving PTSD symptoms but also enhancing the child's functionality and resilience capacity, and supporting his/her developmental trajectory(Cohen,2010).

Neither therapies nor medications expected to be useful in settings where traumatic exposure is ongoing in the life of a child (Gillies,2016). The pharmacological interventions should be considered in the early phases of the treatment when severe and debilitating symptoms such as hyperarousal or avoidance are limiting the child's functionality or interfering with therapy (Donelly,2002).In a review that aimed to assess the effectiveness of pharmacotherapy in the treatment of PTSD in 1999, Donelly et al. concluded that there were not enough studies in the Pediatric PTSD literature to confirm treatment recommendations(Donelly,1999). Although there have been two decades passed, we still don't have adequate evidence for pharmacological interventions in PTSD treatment in children and adolescents.

In conclusion of a meta analysis concerning treatment of PTSD in adults Trauma Focused Psychotherapies (TFP) were recommended as first-line interventions. Stress inoculation training and potentially sertraline or venlafaxine, rather than entire classes of selective serotonin reuptake inhibitors (SSRIs) or serotonin-norepinephrine reuptake inhibitors (SNRIs) were suggested as a second-line treatment option (Lee,2016). A meta-analysis on pharmacotherapy of PTSD in adults also reported favourable results with selective serotonin reuptake inhibitors compared to placebo in reduction of PTSD symptoms (Hoskins,2015). Another review which aims to assess medication options for treatment of PTSD in adults concluded that medical treatments could be useful for the treatment of PTSD and to reduce its core symptoms and functionality loss (Stein,2000).

Adrenergic agents such as clonidine and guanfacine and the β-adrenoceptor antagonist propranolol could be useful in the treatment of hyperarousal and impulsivity in PTSD by reducing sympathetic arousal (De Bellis,1994). However, there are not adequate data to recommend such agents in children with PTSD. Similarly there is no evidence about dopamine blocking agents in the treatment of pediatric PTSD. However, these agents could be used for patients with PTSD who exhibit paranoid behaviors, para-hallucinatory phenomena or intense flashbacks, anger, self-destructive behavior, or psychotic symptoms (Donelly,1999).

Psychotherapy and pharmacotherapy is represented as the twin cornerstones of intervention for PTSD (Stein,2009). And, it is stated that "regardless of what type of treatment intervention is preferred for treatment of PTSD, the ultimate goal of the intervention should be symptom reduction, and ideally, resolution, as well as a full return of optimal psychosocial functioning (Stein,2009)

Donelly et al. recommended a stepwise work in selecting pharmacological agents for treatment of PTSD in children and adolescents which start with accurate diagnosis and recognizing even partial PTSD symptoms that lead significant functionality loss in the child's social, emotional or academic life.

The second step is focusing comorbid conditions which are very common with PTSD such as depression, anxiety disorders and ADHD etc. Thirdly, target symptoms and reasonable treatment goals must be identified (e.g. reduction in sleep latency, frequency of nightmares, or avoidance behavior). The fourth and final step is selection of therapeutics. However, it must not be forget that psychosocial support, psychoeducation and CBT is the first choice and such interventions must always be in mind before consideration is given to pharmacotherapy (Donelly,2002).

A gradual approach should be followed in pharmacological treatment of PTSD in children which begins with the treatment of the most disabling symptoms first. It also must be taken into account that reduction of even a single symptom, might lead considerable relief and improvement in overall functioning of the child (Donelly,2002).

Summary

Growing amount of evidence showing that traumatic experiences have a devastating impact on the child, by deteriorating their physical, cognitive, emotional, and social development. Beside causing psychiatric disorders such adverse experiences shaping the whole community by leading disruption in traumatized children's way of life, sense of self, other and community. However, the findings of research on effect of traumatic stress on the child could be summarized in five measurable areas stated below

- Leading severe mental, interpersonal and behavioral problems such as PTSD, depression, suicidal ideation, affect regulation, poor judgement, peer and relationship problems and substance use
- Academic and occupational problems, deterioration in language use, literacy and math skills
- Changes in brain structure and neuronal circuits, volume and functional changes in distinct brain structures such as hippocampus, amygdala, dorsal prefrontal cortex and anterior cingulate cortex
- Increased risk for physical health and lowered life expectancy due to various medical conditions

REFERENCES

Abe, J., Zane, N., & Chun, K. (1994). Differential responses to trauma: Migration-related discriminants of post-traumatic stress disorder among Southeast Asian refugees. *Journal of Community Psychology*, *22*(2), 121–135. doi:10.1002/1520-6629(199404)22:2<121::AID-JCOP2290220208>3.0.CO;2-D

Ahmad, A. (2008). Posttraumatic stress among children in Kurdistan. *Acta Paediatrica (Oslo, Norway)*, *97*(7), 884–888. doi:10.1111/j.1651-2227.2008.00873.x PMID:18532935

Ahmad, A. (2014). Crisis intervention program for children and adolescents (CIPCA) to prevent posttraumatic psychopathology, preliminary report. *Duhok Medical Journal*, *8*(2), 1–11.

Ahmad, A., Sofi, M., Sundelin-Wahlsten, V., & Von Knorring, A.-L. (2000). Posttraumatic stress disorder in children after the military operation "Anfal" in Iraqi Kurdistan. *European Child & Adolescent Psychiatry*, *9*(4), 235–243. doi:10.1007007870070026 PMID:11202098

Ainamani, H. E., Elbert, T., Olema, D. K., & Hecker, T. (2017). PTSD symptom severity relates to cognitive and psycho-social dysfunctioning–a study with Congolese refugees in Uganda. *European Journal of Psychotraumatology*, *8*(1), 1283086. doi:10.1080/20008198.2017.1283086 PMID:28326164

Ari, A. B., Peri, T., Margalit, D., Galili-Weisstub, E., Udassin, R., & Benarroch, F. (2017). Surgical procedures and pediatric medical traumatic stress (PMTS) syndrome: Assessment and future directions. *Journal of Pediatric Surgery*. PMID:29129330

Attanayake, V., McKay, R., Joffres, M., Singh, S., Burkle, F. Jr, & Mills, E. (2009). Prevalence of mental disorders among children exposed to war: A systematic review of 7,920 children. *Medicine, Conflict, and Survival*, *25*(1), 4–19. doi:10.1080/13623690802568913 PMID:19413154

Barrera, M., Calderón, L., & Bell, V. (2013). The cognitive impact of sexual abuse and PTSD in children: A neuropsychological study. *Journal of Child Sexual Abuse*, *22*(6), 625–638. doi:10.1080/10538712.2013.811141 PMID:23924174

Bean, T. M., Eurelings-Bontekoe, E., & Spinhoven, P. (2007). Course and predictors of mental health of unaccompanied refugee minors in the Netherlands: One year follow-up. *Social Science & Medicine*, *64*(6), 1204–1215. doi:10.1016/j.socscimed.2006.11.010 PMID:17188787

Beckham, J. C., Vrana, S. R., Barefoot, J. C., Feldman, M. E., Fairbank, J., & Moore, S. D. (2002). Magnitude and duration of cardiovascular responses to anger in Vietnam veterans with and without posttraumatic stress disorder. *Journal of Consulting and Clinical Psychology*, *70*(1), 228–234. doi:10.1037/0022-006X.70.1.228 PMID:11860049

Beers, S. R., & De Bellis, M. D. (2002). Neuropsychological function in children with maltreatment-related posttraumatic stress disorder. *The American Journal of Psychiatry*, *159*(3), 483–486. doi:10.1176/appi.ajp.159.3.483 PMID:11870018

Betancourt, T. S., Abdi, S., Ito, B. S., Lilienthal, G. M., Agalab, N., & Ellis, H. (2015). We left one war and came to another: Resource loss, acculturative stress, and caregiver–child relationships in Somali refugee families. *Cultural Diversity & Ethnic Minority Psychology*, *21*(1), 114–125. doi:10.1037/a0037538 PMID:25090142

Betancourt, T. S., Speelman, L., Onyango, G., & Bolton, P. (2009). A qualitative study of mental health problems among children displaced by war in northern Uganda. *Transcultural Psychiatry*, *46*(2), 238–256. doi:10.1177/1363461509105815 PMID:19541749

Blanchard, E., & Hickling, E. (1997). *After the crash: assessment and treatment of motor vehicle accident survivors*. Washington, DC: APA.

Bolton, D., O'Ryan, D., Udwin, O., Boyle, S., & Yule, W. (2000). The long-term psychological effects of a disaster experienced in adolescence: II: General psychopathology. *Journal of Child Psychology and Psychiatry, and Allied Disciplines*, *41*(4), 513–523. doi:10.1111/1469-7610.00636 PMID:10836681

Branche, C., Oyebite, K., Hyder, A., Ozanne-Smith, J., Bartolomeos, K., & Rivara, F. (2008). *World report on child injury prevention*. World Health Organization.

Breslau, N. (2012). *Epidemiology of posttraumatic stress disorder in adults*. In *The Oxford Handbook of Traumatic Stress Disorders* (pp. 84–97). New York: Oxford University Press. doi:10.1093/oxfordhb/9780195399066.013.0007

Broberg, A. G., Dyregrov, A., & Lilled, L. (2005). The Göteborg discotheque fire: Posttraumatic stress, and school adjustment as reported by the primary victims 18 months later. *Journal of Child Psychology and Psychiatry, and Allied Disciplines*, *46*(12), 1279–1286. doi:10.1111/j.1469-7610.2005.01439.x PMID:16313428

Bronstein, I., & Montgomery, P. (2011). Psychological distress in refugee children: A systematic review. *Clinical Child and Family Psychology Review*, *14*(1), 44–56. doi:10.100710567-010-0081-0 PMID:21181268

Catani, C., Schauer, E., Elbert, T., Missmahl, I., Bette, J. P., & Neuner, F. (2009). War trauma, child labor, and family violence: Life adversities and PTSD in a sample of school children in Kabul. *Journal of Traumatic Stress: Official Publication of The International Society for Traumatic Stress Studies*, *22*(3), 163–171. doi:10.1002/jts.20415 PMID:19462436

Ceri, V., & Ahmad, A. (2018). Exploring Psychological Vaccination for Potentially Traumatized Children. *Journal of Psychology and Clinical Psychiatry*, *9*(1), 143–147. doi:10.15406/jpcpy.2018.09.00512

Çeri, V., Beşer, C., Fiş, N. P., & Arman, A. (2018). Findings From A Specialized Child Psychiatry Unit For Care of Refugee Children in Istanbul. *J Clin Psy*, *21*(2), 113–121. doi:10.5505/kpd.2018.57070

Ceri, V., Özlü-Erkilic, Z., Özer, Ü., Kadak, T., Winkler, D., Dogangün, B., & … . (2017). Mental health problems of second generation children and adolescents with migration background. *International Journal of Psychiatry in Clinical Practice*, 1–6. PMID:28498088

Ceri, V., Özlü-Erkilic, Z., Özer, Ü., Yalcin, M., Popow, C., & Akkaya-Kalayci, T. (2016). Psychiatric symptoms and disorders among Yazidi children and adolescents immediately after forced migration following ISIS attacks. *Neuropsychiatrie, 30*(3), 145-50.

Chemtob, C. M., Nomura, Y., & Abramovitz, R. A. (2008). Impact of conjoined exposure to the World Trade Center attacks and to other traumatic events on the behavioral problems of preschool children. *Archives of Pediatrics & Adolescent Medicine*, *162*(2), 126–133. doi:10.1001/archpediatrics.2007.36 PMID:18250236

Cohen, J. A. (2010). Practice parameter for the assessment and treatment of children and adolescents with posttraumatic stress disorder. *Journal of the American Academy of Child and Adolescent Psychiatry, 49*(4), 414–430. PMID:20410735

Cohen, J. A., Deblinger, E., Mannarino, A. P., & Steer, R. A. (2004). A multisite, randomized controlled trial for children with sexual abuse–related PTSD symptoms. *Journal of the American Academy of Child and Adolescent Psychiatry, 43*(4), 393–402. doi:10.1097/00004583-200404000-00005 PMID:15187799

Cox, C. M., Kenardy, J. A., & Hendrikz, J. K. (2008). A meta-analysis of risk factors that predict psychopathology following accidental trauma. *Journal for Specialists in Pediatric Nursing, 13*(2), 98–110. doi:10.1111/j.1744-6155.2008.00141.x PMID:18366377

Çuhadaroğlu Çetin, F., Coşkun, A., & İşeri, E. (2008). *Çocuk ve ergen psikiyatrisi temel kitabı. 1.* Ankara: Baskı Hekimler Yayın Birliği.

Dai, W., Chen, L., Lai, Z., Li, Y., Wang, J., & Liu, A. (2016). The incidence of post-traumatic stress disorder among survivors after earthquakes: A systematic review and meta-analysis. *BMC Psychiatry, 16*(1), 188. doi:10.118612888-016-0891-9 PMID:27267874

De Beilis, M. D., & Putnam, F. W. (1994). The psychobiology of childhood maltreatment. *Child and Adolescent Psychiatric Clinics of North America, 3*(4), 663–678. doi:10.1016/S1056-4993(18)30463-2

De Bellis, M. D., Hooper, S. R., Spratt, E. G., & Woolley, D. P. (2009). Neuropsychological findings in childhood neglect and their relationships to pediatric PTSD. *Journal of the International Neuropsychological Society, 15*(6), 868–878. doi:10.1017/S1355617709990464 PMID:19703321

De Bellis, M. D., Keshavan, M. S., Clark, D. B., Casey, B., Giedd, J. N., Boring, A. M., ... Ryan, N. D. (1999). Developmental traumatology part II: Brain development. *Biological Psychiatry, 45*(10), 1271–1284. doi:10.1016/S0006-3223(99)00045-1 PMID:10349033

De Bellis, M. D., Woolley, D. P., & Hooper, S. R. (2013). Neuropsychological findings in pediatric maltreatment: Relationship of PTSD, dissociative symptoms, and abuse/neglect indices to neurocognitive outcomes. *Child Maltreatment*, *18*(3), 171–183. doi:10.1177/1077559513497420 PMID:23886642

De Jong, J. T., Komproe, I. H., Van Ommeren, M., El Masri, M., Araya, M., & Khaled, N. (2001). Lifetime events and posttraumatic stress disorder in 4 postconflict settings. *Journal of the American Medical Association*, *286*(5), 555–562. doi:10.1001/jama.286.5.555 PMID:11476657

Deblinger, E., Stauffer, L. B., & Steer, R. A. (2001). Comparative efficacies of supportive and cognitive behavioral group therapies for young children who have been sexually abused and their nonoffending mothers. *Child Maltreatment*, *6*(4), 332–343. doi:10.1177/1077559501006004006 PMID:11675816

DePrince, A. P., Weinzierl, K. M., & Combs, M. D. (2009). Executive function performance and trauma exposure in a community sample of children. *Child Abuse & Neglect*, *33*(6), 353–361. doi:10.1016/j.chiabu.2008.08.002 PMID:19477515

Donnelly, C., Amaya-Jackson, L., & March, J. (1999). Psychopharmacology of pediatric posttraumatic stress disorder. *Journal of Child and Adolescent Psychopharmacology*, *9*(3), 203–220. doi:10.1089/cap.1999.9.203 PMID:10521013

Donnelly, C. L., & Amaya-Jackson, L. (2002). Post-traumatic stress disorder in children and adolescents. *Paediatric Drugs*, *4*(3), 159–170. doi:10.2165/00128072-200204030-00003 PMID:11909008

DSM-5®. (2013). *Diagnostic and Statistical Manual of Mental Disorders (DSM-5®)*. American Psychiatric Publication.

Dubner, A., & Motta, R. (1999). Sexually and physically abused foster care children and posttraumatic stress disorder. *Journal of Consulting and Clinical Psychology*, *67*(3), 367–373. doi:10.1037/0022-006X.67.3.367 PMID:10369057

Dyregrov, A., & Yule, W. (2006). A review of PTSD in children. *Child and Adolescent Mental Health*, *11*(4), 176–184. doi:10.1111/j.1475-3588.2005.00384.x

Fairbrother, G., Stuber, J., Galea, S., Fleischman, A. R., & Pfefferbaum, B. (2003). Posttraumatic stress reactions in New York City children after the September 11, 2001, terrorist attacks. *Ambulatory Pediatrics*, *3*(6), 304–311. doi:10.1367/1539-4409(2003)003<0304:PSRINY>2.0.CO;2 PMID:14616045

Fazel, M., & Betancourt, T. S. (2017). *Preventive mental health interventions for refugee children and adolescents in high-income settings*. The Lancet Child & Adolescent Health.

Fazel, M., Wheeler, J., & Danesh, J. (2005). Prevalence of serious mental disorder in 7000 refugees resettled in western countries: A systematic review. *Lancet*, *365*(9467), 1309–1314. doi:10.1016/S0140-6736(05)61027-6 PMID:15823380

Feldman, R., & Vengrober, A. (2011). Posttraumatic stress disorder in infants and young children exposed to war-related trauma. *Journal of the American Academy of Child and Adolescent Psychiatry*, *50*(7), 645–658. doi:10.1016/j.jaac.2011.03.001 PMID:21703492

Finkelhor, D. (1994). The international epidemiology of child sexual abuse. *Child Abuse & Neglect*, *18*(5), 409–417. doi:10.1016/0145-2134(94)90026-4 PMID:8032971

Finkelhor, D., Hotaling, G., Lewis, I. A., & Smith, C. (1990). Sexual abuse in a national survey of adult men and women: Prevalence, characteristics, and risk factors. *Child Abuse & Neglect*, *14*(1), 19–28. doi:10.1016/0145-2134(90)90077-7 PMID:2310970

Fletcher, K. E. (1996). Childhood posttraumatic stress disorder. *Child Psychopathology*, 242-76.

Ford, T., Goodman, R., & Meltzer, H. (2003). The British child and adolescent mental health survey 1999: The prevalence of DSM-IV disorders. *Journal of the American Academy of Child and Adolescent Psychiatry*, *42*(10), 1203–1211. doi:10.1097/00004583-200310000-00011 PMID:14560170

Forman-Hoffman, V., Bose, J., Batts, K., Glasheen, C., Hirsch, E., & Karg, R. (2012). *Correlates of lifetime exposure to one or more potentially traumatic events and subsequent posttraumatic stress among adults in the United States: results from the Mental Health Surveillance Study, 2008-2012*. Academic Press.

Galea, S., Nandi, A., & Vlahov, D. (2005). The epidemiology of post-traumatic stress disorder after disasters. *Epidemiologic Reviews*, *27*(1), 78–91. doi:10.1093/epirev/mxi003 PMID:15958429

Gekker, M., Coutinho, E., Berger, W., Luz, M., Araújo, A., Pagotto, L., ... Mendlowicz, M. V. (2018). Early scars are forever: Childhood abuse in patients with adult-onset PTSD is associated with increased prevalence and severity of psychiatric comorbidity. *Psychiatry Research*, *267*, 1–6. doi:10.1016/j.psychres.2018.05.042 PMID:29879599

Gil, T., Calev, A., Greenberg, D., Kugelmass, S., & Lerer, B. (1990). Cognitive functioning in post-traumatic stress disorder. *Journal of Traumatic Stress*, *3*(1), 29–45. doi:10.1002/jts.2490030104

Gillham, J. E., Reivich, K. J., Jaycox, L. H., & Seligman, M. E. (1995). Prevention of depressive symptoms in schoolchildren: Two-year follow-up. *Psychological Science*, *6*(6), 343–351. doi:10.1111/j.1467-9280.1995.tb00524.x

Gillies, D., Maiocchi, L., Bhandari, A. P., Taylor, F., Gray, C., & O'Brien, L. (2016). Psychological therapies for children and adolescents exposed to trauma. *The Cochrane Library*. PMID:27726123

Goldin, S., Hägglöf, B., Levin, L., & Persson, L. Å. (2008). Mental health of Bosnian refugee children: A comparison of clinician appraisal with parent, child and teacher reports. *Nordic Journal of Psychiatry*, *62*(3), 204–216. doi:10.1080/08039480801983604 PMID:18622884

Green, B. L., Korol, M., Grace, M. C., Vary, M. G., Leonard, A. C., Gleser, G. C., & Smitson-Cohen, S. (1991). Children and disaster: Age, gender, and parental effects on PTSD symptoms. *Journal of the American Academy of Child and Adolescent Psychiatry*, *30*(6), 945–951. doi:10.1097/00004583-199111000-00012 PMID:1757444

Hayes, J. P., Hayes, S. M., & Mikedis, A. M. (2012). Quantitative meta-analysis of neural activity in posttraumatic stress disorder. *Biology of Mood & Anxiety Disorders*, *2*(1), 9. doi:10.1186/2045-5380-2-9 PMID:22738125

Heptinstall, E., Sethna, V., & Taylor, E. (2004). PTSD and depression in refugee children. *European Child & Adolescent Psychiatry*, *13*(6), 373–380. doi:10.100700787-004-0422-y PMID:15619050

Herringa, R. J. (2017). Trauma, PTSD, and the developing brain. *Current Psychiatry Reports, 19*(10), 69. doi:10.100711920-017-0825-3 PMID:28823091

Hinton, D. E., Rasmussen, A., Nou, L., Pollack, M. H., & Good, M.-J. (2009). Anger, PTSD, and the nuclear family: A study of Cambodian refugees. *Social Science & Medicine, 69*(9), 1387–1394. doi:10.1016/j.socscimed.2009.08.018 PMID:19748169

Hock, E., Hart, M., Kang, M. J., & Lutz, W. J. (2004). Predicting children's reactions to terrorist attacks: The importance of self-reports and preexisting characteristics. *The American Journal of Orthopsychiatry, 74*(3), 253–262. doi:10.1037/0002-9432.74.3.253 PMID:15291702

Hodes, M. (2008). Psychopathology in refugee and asylum seeking children. In Rutter's Child and Adolescent Psychiatry (5th ed.). Wiley.

Hodes, M., Jagdev, D., Chandra, N., & Cunniff, A. (2008). Risk and resilience for psychological distress amongst unaccompanied asylum seeking adolescents. *Journal of Child Psychology and Psychiatry, and Allied Disciplines, 49*(7), 723–732. doi:10.1111/j.1469-7610.2008.01912.x PMID:18492037

Hodgkinson, P. E., & Stewart, M. (1991). Coping with catastrophe: A handbook of disaster management. Taylor & Frances/Routledge.

Hoskins, M., Pearce, J., Bethell, A., Dankova, L., Barbui, C., Tol, W. A., ... Bisson, J. I. (2015). Pharmacotherapy for post-traumatic stress disorder: Systematic review and meta-analysis. *The British Journal of Psychiatry, 206*(2), 93–100. doi:10.1192/bjp.bp.114.148551 PMID:25644881

Hsu, C.-C., Chong, M.-Y., Yang, P., & Yen, C.-F. (2002). Posttraumatic stress disorder among adolescent earthquake victims in Taiwan. *Journal of the American Academy of Child and Adolescent Psychiatry, 41*(7), 875–881. doi:10.1097/00004583-200207000-00022 PMID:12108814

Ibrahim, H., & Hassan, C. Q. (2017). Post-traumatic stress disorder symptoms resulting from torture and other traumatic events among Syrian Kurdish refugees in Kurdistan Region, Iraq. *Frontiers in Psychology, 8*, 241.

Jaycox, L. H., Reivich, K. J., Gillham, J., & Seligman, M. E. (1994). Prevention of depressive symptoms in school children. *Behaviour Research and Therapy, 32*(8), 801–816. doi:10.1016/0005-7967(94)90160-0 PMID:7993324

John, P. B., Russell, S., & Russell, P. S. S. (2007). The prevalence of posttraumatic stress disorder among children and adolescents affected by tsunami disaster in Tamil Nadu. *Disaster Management & Response*, *5*(1), 3–7. doi:10.1016/j.dmr.2006.11.001 PMID:17306747

Kandemir, H., Karataş, H., Çeri, V., Solmaz, F., Kandemir, S. B., & Solmaz, A. (2018). Prevalence of war-related adverse events, depression and anxiety among Syrian refugee children settled in Turkey. *European Child & Adolescent Psychiatry*, 1–5. PMID:29948231

Karakaya, I., & Çolak, B. (2007). Çocuk ve Ergenlerde Travma Sonrası Stres Bozukluğu ve Adli Tıbbi Değerlendirme. *The Bulletin of Legal Medicine*, *12*(2), 82–87. doi:10.17986/blm.2007122642

Kaufman, J., & Charney, D. (2001). Effects of early stress on brain structure and function: Implications for understanding the relationship between child maltreatment and depression. *Development and Psychopathology*, *13*(3), 451–471. doi:10.1017/S0954579401003030 PMID:11523843

Keppel-Benson, J. M., Ollendick, T. H., & Benson, M. J. (2002). Post-traumatic stress in children following motor vehicle accidents. *Journal of Child Psychology and Psychiatry, and Allied Disciplines*, *43*(2), 203–212. doi:10.1111/1469-7610.00013 PMID:11902599

Kessler, R. C., Sonnega, A., Bromet, E., Hughes, M., & Nelson, C. B. (1995). Posttraumatic stress disorder in the National Comorbidity Survey. *Archives of General Psychiatry*, *52*(12), 1048–1060. doi:10.1001/archpsyc.1995.03950240066012 PMID:7492257

Kilpatrick, D. G., Ruggiero, K. J., Acierno, R., Saunders, B. E., Resnick, H. S., & Best, C. L. (2003). Violence and Risk of PTSD, Major Depression, Substance Abuse/Dependence, and Comorbidity: Results From the National Survey of Adolescents. *Journal of Consulting and Clinical Psychology*, *71*(4), 692–700. doi:10.1037/0022-006X.71.4.692 PMID:12924674

King, N. J., Tonge, B. J., Mullen, P., Myerson, N., Heyne, D., Rollings, S., ... Ollendick, T. H. (2000). Treating sexually abused children with posttraumatic stress symptoms: A randomized clinical trial. *Journal of the American Academy of Child and Adolescent Psychiatry*, *39*(11), 1347–1355. doi:10.1097/00004583-200011000-00008 PMID:11068889

Kinzie, J. D., Sack, W. H., Angell, R. H., Manson, S., & Rath, B. (1986). The psychiatric effects of massive trauma on Cambodian children: I. The children. *Journal of the American Academy of Child Psychiatry*, *25*(3), 370–376. doi:10.1016/S0002-7138(09)60259-4

Kizilhan, J. I., & Noll-Hussong, M. (2018). Post-traumatic stress disorder among former Islamic State child soldiers in northern Iraq. *The British Journal of Psychiatry*, 1–5. PMID:29852882

Koçak, E. E., & Kılıç, C. (2017). Travma Sonrası Stres Bozukluğunda Bilişsel Bozukluklar. *Türk Psikiyatri Dergisi*, *28*(2), 124–131. PMID:29192945

Koren, D., Arnon, I., & Klein, E. (1999). Acute stress response and posttraumatic stress disorder in traffic accident victims: A one-year prospective, follow-up study. *The American Journal of Psychiatry*, *156*(3), 367–373. PMID:10080550

La Greca, A. M., Silverman, W. K., Vernberg, E. M., & Prinstein, M. J. (1996). Symptoms of posttraumatic stress in children after Hurricane Andrew: A prospective study. *Journal of Consulting and Clinical Psychology*, *64*(4), 712–723. doi:10.1037/0022-006X.64.4.712 PMID:8803361

Lai, B. S., Kelley, M. L., Harrison, K. M., Thompson, J. E., & Self-Brown, S. (2015). Posttraumatic stress, anxiety, and depression symptoms among children after Hurricane Katrina: A latent profile analysis. *Journal of Child and Family Studies*, *24*(5), 1262–1270. doi:10.100710826-014-9934-3 PMID:25892902

Langeland, W., & Olff, M. (2008). Psychobiology of posttraumatic stress disorder in pediatric injury patients: A review of the literature. *Neuroscience and Biobehavioral Reviews*, *32*(1), 161–174. doi:10.1016/j.neubiorev.2007.07.002 PMID:17825911

Laufer, A., & Solomon, Z. (2009). Gender differences in PTSD in Israeli youth exposed to terror attacks. *Journal of Interpersonal Violence*, *24*(6), 959–976. doi:10.1177/0886260508319367 PMID:18663245

Lee, D. J., Schnitzlein, C. W., Wolf, J. P., Vythilingam, M., Rasmusson, A. M., & Hoge, C. W. (2016). Psychotherapy versus pharmacotherapy for posttraumatic stress disorder: Systemic review and meta-analyses to determine first-line treatments. *Depression and Anxiety*, *33*(9), 792–806. doi:10.1002/da.22511 PMID:27126398

March, J. S., Amaya-Jackson, L., Murray, M. C., & Schulte, A. (1998). Cognitive-behavioral psychotherapy for children and adolescents with posttraumatic stress disorder after a single-incident stressor. *Journal of the American Academy of Child and Adolescent Psychiatry*, *37*(6), 585–593. doi:10.1097/00004583-199806000-00008 PMID:9628078

Mc, L. E. E. R. S. V., Deblinger, E., Atkins, M. S., Foa, E. B., & Ralphe, D. L. (1988). Post-traumatic stress disorder in sexually abused children. *Journal of the American Academy of Child and Adolescent Psychiatry*, *27*(5), 650–654. doi:10.1097/00004583-198809000-00024 PMID:3182633

McLaughlin, K. A., Koenen, K. C., Hill, E. D., Petukhova, M., Sampson, N. A., & Zaslavsky, A. M. (2013). Trauma exposure and posttraumatic stress disorder in a national sample of adolescents. *Journal of the American Academy of Child & Adolescent Psychiatry, 52*(8), 815-30.

Meiser-Stedman, R. (2002). Towards a cognitive–behavioral model of PTSD in children and adolescents. *Clinical Child and Family Psychology Review*, *5*(4), 217–232. doi:10.1023/A:1020982122107 PMID:12495267

Milgram, N. A., Toubiana, Y. H., Klingman, A., Raviv, A., & Goldstein, I. (1988). Situational exposure and personal loss in children's acute and chronic stress reactions to a school bus disaster. *Journal of Traumatic Stress*, *1*(3), 339–352. doi:10.1002/jts.2490010306

Mills, R., Kisely, S., Alati, R., Strathearn, L., & Najman, J. (2016). Self-reported and agency-notified child sexual abuse in a population-based birth cohort. *Journal of Psychiatric Research*, *74*, 87–93. doi:10.1016/j.jpsychires.2015.12.021 PMID:26774419

Mollica, R., Culhane, A., & Hovelson, D. (2001). The special psychiatric problems of refugees. In M. Gelder, N. Andreasen, J. Lopez-Ibor, & J. Geddes (Eds.), New Oxford Textbook of Psychiatry (2nd ed.; pp. 1493–1500).Oxford University Press.

Molnar, B., Buka, S., & Kessler, R. (2001). Child sexual abuse and subsequent psychopathology: Results from the national comorbidity survey. *American Journal of Public Health*, *91*(5), 753–760. doi:10.2105/AJPH.91.5.753 PMID:11344883

Morgan, L., Scourfield, J., Williams, D., Jasper, A., & Lewis, G. (2003). The Aberfan disaster: 33-year follow-up of survivors. *The British Journal of Psychiatry*, *182*(6), 532–536. doi:10.1192/bjp.182.6.532 PMID:12777345

Morgos, D., Worden, J. W., & Gupta, L. (2008). Psychosocial effects of war experiences among displaced children in southern Darfur. *Omega*, *56*(3), 229–253. doi:10.2190/OM.56.3.b PMID:18300649

Nader, K. O., Pynoos, R. S., Fairbanks, L. A., Al-Ajeel, M., & Al-Asfour, A. (1993). A preliminary study of PTSD and grief among the children of Kuwait following the Gulf crisis. *British Journal of Clinical Psychology*, *32*(4), 407–416. doi:10.1111/j.2044-8260.1993.tb01075.x PMID:8298537

Najarian, L. M., Majeed, M. H., & Gasparyan, K. (2017). Effect of relocation after a natural disaster in Armenia: 20-year follow-up. *Asian Journal of Psychiatry*, *29*, 8–12. doi:10.1016/j.ajp.2017.03.030 PMID:29061434

Nasıroğlu, S., & Ceri, V. (2016). Posttraumatic stress and depression in Yazidi refugees. *Neuropsychiatric Disease and Treatment*, *12*, 2941–2948. doi:10.2147/NDT.S119506 PMID:27881919

Nasıroğlu, S., Çeri, V., Erkorkmaz, Ü., & Semerci, B. (2018). Determinants of psychiatric disorders in children refugees in Turkey's Yazidi refugee camp. *Psychiatry and Clinical Psychopharmacology*, 1-9.

Navalta, C. P., Polcari, A., Webster, D. M., Boghossian, A., & Teicher, M. H. (2006). Effects of childhood sexual abuse on neuropsychological and cognitive function in college women. *The Journal of Neuropsychiatry and Clinical Neurosciences*, *18*(1), 45–53. doi:10.1176/jnp.18.1.45 PMID:16525070

Neigh, G. N., Gillespie, C. F., & Nemeroff, C. B. (2009). The neurobiological toll of child abuse and neglect. *Trauma, Violence & Abuse*, *10*(4), 389–410. doi:10.1177/1524838009339758 PMID:19661133

Newman, E., Pfefferbaum, B., Kirlic, N., Tett, R., Nelson, S., & Liles, B. (2014). Meta-analytic review of psychological interventions for children survivors of natural and man-made disasters. *Current Psychiatry Reports*, *16*(9), 462. doi:10.100711920-014-0462-z PMID:25085234

Nooner, K. B., Linares, L. O., Batinjane, J., Kramer, R. A., Silva, R., & Cloitre, M. (2012). Factors related to posttraumatic stress disorder in adolescence. *Trauma, Violence & Abuse*, *13*(3), 153–166. doi:10.1177/1524838012447698 PMID:22665437

O'Doherty, D. C., Chitty, K. M., Saddiqui, S., Bennett, M. R., & Lagopoulos, J. (2015). A systematic review and meta-analysis of magnetic resonance imaging measurement of structural volumes in posttraumatic stress disorder. *Psychiatry Research: Neuroimaging*, *232*(1), 1–33. doi:10.1016/j.pscychresns.2015.01.002 PMID:25735885

Olofsson, E., Bunketorp, O., & Andersson, A. L. (2009). Children and adolescents injured in traffic–associated psychological consequences: A literature review. *Acta Paediatrica (Oslo, Norway)*, *98*(1), 17–22. doi:10.1111/j.1651-2227.2008.00998.x PMID:18795910

Özgen, F., & Aydın, H. (1999). Travma sonrası stres bozukluğu. *Klinik Psikiyatri.*, *1*, 34–41.

Paolucci, E. O., Genuis, M. L., & Violato, C. (2001). A meta-analysis of the published research on the effects of child sexual abuse. *The Journal of Psychology*, *135*(1), 17–36. doi:10.1080/00223980109603677 PMID:11235837

Papageorgiou, V., Frangou-Garunovic, A., Iordanidou, R., Yule, W., Smith, P., & Vostanis, P. (2000). War trauma and psychopathology in Bosnian refugee children. *European Child & Adolescent Psychiatry*, *9*(2), 84–90. doi:10.1007007870050002 PMID:10926057

Peden, M. (2008). *World report on child injury prevention.* World Health Organization.

Peden, M. (2008). World report on child injury prevention appeals to "Keep Kids Safe". *Injury Prevention*, *14*(6), 413–414. doi:10.1136/ip.2008.020693 PMID:19074252

Pedersen, D. (2002). Political violence, ethnic conflict, and contemporary wars: Broad implications for health and social well-being. *Social Science & Medicine*, *55*(2), 175–190. doi:10.1016/S0277-9536(01)00261-1 PMID:12144134

Pérez-Pereira, M., Tinajero, C., Rodríguez, M. S., Peralbo, M., & Sabucedo, J. M. (2012). Academic effects of the Prestige oil spill disaster. *The Spanish Journal of Psychology, 15*(3), 1055–1068. doi:10.5209/rev_SJOP.2012.v15.n3.39396 PMID:23156914

Perry, B. D., Pollard, R. A., Blakley, T. L., Baker, W. L., & Vigilante, D. (1995). Childhood trauma, the neurobiology of adaptation, and "use-dependent" development of the brain: How "states" become "traits". *Infant Mental Health Journal, 16*(4), 271–291. doi:10.1002/1097-0355(199524)16:4<271::AID-IMHJ2280160404>3.0.CO;2-B

Pfefferbaum, B. (1997). Posttraumatic stress disorder in children: A review of the past 10 years. *Journal of the American Academy of Child and Adolescent Psychiatry, 36*(11), 1503–1511. PMID:9394934

Pfefferbaum, B., Noffsinger, M. A., Jacobs, A. K., & Varma, V. (2016). Children's cognitive functioning in disasters and terrorism. *Current Psychiatry Reports, 18*(5), 48. doi:10.100711920-016-0685-2 PMID:26997166

Pine, D. S., & Cohen, J. A. (2002). Trauma in children and adolescents: Risk and treatment of psychiatric sequelae. *Biological Psychiatry, 51*(7), 519–531. doi:10.1016/S0006-3223(01)01352-X PMID:11950454

Putnam, F. W. (2003). Ten-Year Research Update Review: Child Sexual Abuse. *Journal of the American Academy of Child and Adolescent Psychiatry, 42*(3), 269–278. doi:10.1097/00004583-200303000-00006 PMID:12595779

Pynoos, R. S., Frederick, C., Nader, K., Arroyo, W., Steinberg, A., Eth, S., & … . (1987). Life threat and posttraumatic stress in school-age children. *Archives of General Psychiatry, 44*(12), 1057–1063. doi:10.1001/archpsyc.1987.01800240031005 PMID:3689093

Qouta, S., Punamäki, R.-L., & El Sarraj, E. (2003). Prevalence and determinants of PTSD among Palestinian children exposed to military violence. *European Child & Adolescent Psychiatry, 12*(6), 265–272. doi:10.100700787-003-0328-0 PMID:14689258

Realmuto, G. M., Masten, A., Carole, L. F., Hubbard, J., Groteluschen, A., & Chhun, B. (1992). Adolescent survivors of massive childhood trauma in Cambodia: Life events and current symptoms. *Journal of Traumatic Stress, 5*(4), 589–599. doi:10.1002/jts.2490050408

Rose, S. C., Bisson, J., Churchill, R., & Wessely, S. (2002). Psychological debriefing for preventing post traumatic stress disorder (PTSD). *The Cochrane Library*. PMID:12076399

Rowan, A. B., & Foy, D. W. (1993). Post-traumatic stress disorder in child sexual abuse survivors: A literature review. *Journal of Traumatic Stress*, *6*(1), 3–20. doi:10.1002/jts.2490060103

Sack, W. H., Him, C., & Dickason, D. (1999). Twelve-year follow-up study of Khmer youths who suffered massive war trauma as children. *Journal of the American Academy of Child and Adolescent Psychiatry*, *38*(9), 1173–1179. doi:10.1097/00004583-199909000-00023 PMID:10504817

Samuelson, K. W., Krueger, C. E., Burnett, C., & Wilson, C. K. (2010). Neuropsychological functioning in children with posttraumatic stress disorder. *Child Neuropsychology*, *16*(2), 119–133. doi:10.1080/09297040903190782 PMID:19787496

Savin, D., Sack, W. H., Clarke, G. N., Meas, N., & Richart, I. (1996). The Khmer Adolescent Project: III. A study of trauma from Thailand's Site II refugee camp. *Journal of the American Academy of Child and Adolescent Psychiatry*, *35*(3), 384–391. doi:10.1097/00004583-199603000-00021 PMID:8714328

Schreier, H., Ladakakos, C., Morabito, D., Chapman, L., & Knudson, M. M. (2005). Posttraumatic stress symptoms in children after mild to moderate pediatric trauma: A longitudinal examination of symptom prevalence, correlates, and parent-child symptom reporting. *The Journal of Trauma and Acute Care Surgery*, *58*(2), 353–363. doi:10.1097/01.TA.0000152537.15672.B7 PMID:15706200

Scrimin, S., Moscardino, U., Capello, F., & Axia, G. (2009). Attention and memory in school-age children surviving the terrorist attack in Beslan, Russia. *Journal of Clinical Child and Adolescent Psychology*, *38*(3), 402–414. doi:10.1080/15374410902851689 PMID:19437300

Sowell, E. R., Thompson, P. M., Tessner, K. D., & Toga, A. W. (2001). Mapping continued brain growth and gray matter density reduction in dorsal frontal cortex: Inverse relationships during postadolescent brain maturation. *The Journal of Neuroscience*, *21*(22), 8819–8829. doi:10.1523/JNEUROSCI.21-22-08819.2001 PMID:11698594

Sprung, M., & Harris, P. L. (2010). Intrusive thoughts and young children's knowledge about thinking following a natural disaster. *Journal of Child Psychology and Psychiatry, and Allied Disciplines*, *51*(10), 1115–1124. doi:10.1111/j.1469-7610.2010.02273.x PMID:20840501

Stallard, P., Velleman, R., & Baldwin, S. (1998). Prospective study of post-traumatic stress disorder in children involved in road traffic accidents. *BMJ (Clinical Research Ed.)*, *317*(7173), 1619–1623. doi:10.1136/bmj.317.7173.1619 PMID:9848900

Stein, D., Zungu-Dirwayi, N., & Seedat, S. (2000). Pharmacotherapy for posttraumatic stress disorder. *Cochrane Database of Systematic Reviews*, (4), CD002795. PMID:11034765

Stein, M. B., & Ravindran, L. N. (2009). Pharmacotherapy of posttraumatic stress disorder. In Post Traumatic Stress Disorder (pp. 125–135). CRC Press.

Summerfield, D. (2000). Childhood, war, refugeedom and 'trauma': Three core questions for mental health professionals. *Transcultural Psychiatry*, *37*(3), 417–433. doi:10.1177/136346150003700308

Tebbutt, J., Swanston, H., Oates, R. K., & O'toole, B. I. (1997). Five years after child sexual abuse: Persisting dysfunction and problems of prediction. *Journal of the American Academy of Child and Adolescent Psychiatry*, *36*(3), 330–339. doi:10.1097/00004583-199703000-00011 PMID:9055513

Teicher, M. H., Samson, J. A., Anderson, C. M., & Ohashi, K. (2016). The effects of childhood maltreatment on brain structure, function and connectivity. *Nature Reviews. Neuroscience*, *17*(10), 652–666. doi:10.1038/nrn.2016.111 PMID:27640984

Terr, L. (1990). *Too scared to cry: How trauma affects children and ultimately us all*. New York: Basic.

Thabet, A. A., Tawahina, A. A., El Sarraj, E., & Vostanis, P. (2008). Exposure to war trauma and PTSD among parents and children in the Gaza strip. *European Child & Adolescent Psychiatry*, *17*(4), 191–199. doi:10.100700787-007-0653-9 PMID:18365135

Thabet, A. A., & Vostanis, P. (2000). Post traumatic stress disorder reactions in children of war: A longitudinal study. *Child Abuse & Neglect*, *24*(2), 291–298. doi:10.1016/S0145-2134(99)00127-1 PMID:10695524

Trickey, D., Siddaway, A. P., Meiser-Stedman, R., Serpell, L., & Field, A. P. (2012). A meta-analysis of risk factors for post-traumatic stress disorder in children and adolescents. *Clinical Psychology Review*, *32*(2), 122–138. doi:10.1016/j.cpr.2011.12.001 PMID:22245560

UNHCR. (2015). *UNHCR Global Trends*. Retrieved from http://www.unhcr.org/576408cd7

Van der Kolk, B. A., & McFarlane, A. C. (1996). *Traumatic stress: The effects of overwhelming experience on mind, body, and society*. Guilford Press.

Vasterling, J. J., Brailey K. (2005). *Neuropsychological Findings in Adults With PTSD*. Academic Press.

Ward, M. E., Shelley, K., Kaase, K., & Pane, J. F. (2008). Hurricane Katrina: A longitudinal study of the achievement and behavior of displaced students. *Journal of Education for Students Placed at Risk*, *13*(2-3), 297–317. doi:10.1080/10824660802350391

Warshaw, M. G., Fierman, E., Pratt, L., Hunt, M., Yonkers, K. A., Massion, A. O., & … . (1993). Quality of life and dissociation in anxiety disorder patients with histories of trauma or PTSD. *The American Journal of Psychiatry*, *150*(10), 1512–1516. doi:10.1176/ajp.150.10.1512 PMID:8379556

Weine, S., Becker, D., McGlashan, T., Laub, D., Lazrove, S., & Vojvoda, D. (1995). Psychiatric consequences of" ethnic cleansing": Clinical assessments and trauma testimonies of newly resettled Bosnian refugees. *The American Journal of Psychiatry*, *152*(4), 536–542. doi:10.1176/ajp.152.4.536 PMID:7694901

WHO. (2015). *Global status report on road safety*. Geneva: World Health Organization.

Yalın, Ş. S., Uzel, B. T., Öztürk, M., Gözaçanlar, Ö., Yörük, G. Ü., & Özkan, Y. (2017). Immigration-related mental health disorders in refugees 5–18 years old living in Turkey. *Neuropsychiatric Disease and Treatment*, *13*, 2813–2821. doi:10.2147/NDT.S150592 PMID:29180867

Yule, W., Bolton, D., Udwin, O., Boyle, S., O'Ryan, D., & Nurrish, J. (2000). The long-term psychological effects of a disaster experienced in adolescence: I: The incidence and course of PTSD. *Journal of Child Psychology and Psychiatry, and Allied Disciplines, 41*(4), 503–511. doi:10.1111/1469-7610.00635 PMID:10836680

Yule, W., & Smith, P. (2015). Post traumatic stress disorder. In A. Thapar, D. S. Pine, J. F. Leckman, S. Scott, M. J. Snowling, & E. Taylor (Eds.), *Rutter's Child and Adolescent Psychiatry* (6th ed.; pp. 806–821). John Wiley & Sons, Ltd. doi:10.1002/9781118381953.ch59

Chapter 2
Adolescent Chronic Stress: Brain Function and Treatment for Depression and Anxiety

Danielle McKain
Beaver Area School District, USA

ABSTRACT

As adolescents face new challenges, the prevalence of stress, anxiety, and depression is growing. This chapter presents research on stress, anxiety, and depression as it relates to brain development and treatment options. While prescription medication is a common treatment option, there is concern over use with the development of the adolescent brain and side effects. In addition to, or in place of, medication, other treatment options presented in this chapter include psychotherapy, biofeedback, mindfulness, diet, exercise, and social media use. With advances in technology and increased use among adolescents, the chapter will present new treatment options that are available through apps and social media.

DOI: 10.4018/978-1-5225-7513-9.ch002

INTRODUCTION

Adolescent development is associated with major changes in emotional and cognitive functions, as well as, a rise in stress-related psychological disorders, such as anxiety and depression. It is also a time of significant maturation of the brain, marked by structural alterations in many limbic and cortical regions (Romeo, 2017). Stress and adversity can cause depression, which, worldwide affects approximately 350 million people (Wu et al., 2017).

Stress significantly contributes to mood, well-being, behavior, and health (Schneiderman, Ironson, & Siegel, 2005). Depression can have a negative impact on growth and development, performance in school, relationships, and may lead to suicide (Bhatia & Bhatia, 2007).

Ross, Foster, and Ionescu (2017) studied how chronic stress can lead to anxious depression through behaviors, physiology, circuits, and molecules. Anxiety and depression among U.S. teenagers increased 33% from 2010-2015, while suicide attempts increased 23%, and suicide increased 31% (Twenge, Joiner, Rogers, & Martin, 2017). Furthermore, the Royal Society for Public Health (2017) states that rates of anxiety and depression in young people have risen 70% since 1992.

Romeo (2017) presents the potential impact of stress on the structure of the adolescent brain and implications for adolescent mental health, emphasizing that adolescence is often a time of stress related anxiety and depression and the adolescent brain could be sensitive to stressors leading to changes in structure. Research is lacking on how chronic stress could disrupt the maturation of the brain in limbic and cortical regions (Romeo, 2017).

As undertreated depression and anxiety present a growing health crisis, Steffen, Austin, and DeBarros (2016) suggest that an effective approach for reducing anxiety and depression is to reduce chronic stress; furthermore, they argue that typical treatment methods like antidepressants and psychotherapy are not working and suggest biofeedback and mindfulness as simple, effective preventative measures for treating chronic stress to address the growing problem. Additional studies suggest treating depression and anxiety with diet and social media (Wu et al., 2017; Royal Society for Public Health, 2017). The mission of this chapter is to discuss existing research on the brain development of adolescents with chronic stress. Additionally, the chapter will present the increase in antidepressant use and some of the advantages and disadvantages of treating depression and anxiety with antidepressants. Lastly, the chapter will present research on six other treatments for depression and anxiety including (1) Psychotherapy (2) Biofeedback (3) Mindfulness (4) Diet (5) Exercise and (6) Social Media.

The objectives of this chapter include:

1. Adolescent Chronic Stress and Depression: Providing an overview of adolescent chronic stress and research on adolescent depression.
2. Adolescent Stress as it Relates to Brain Development: Providing research on the effects of chronic stress on brain development.
3. Prescription Treatment for Chronic Stress: Providing current research on prescription treatment.
4. Other treatment options and apps: Providing other treatment options and apps for stress, depression, and anxiety including (1) Psychotherapy (2) Biofeedback (3) Mindfulness (4) Diet (5) Exercise and (6) Social Media.
5. Limitations of Current Research: Providing limitations of current research.

BACKGROUND: ADOLESCENT CHRONIC STRESS AND DEPRESSION

The Centers for Disease Control and Prevention (CDC) defines depression as more than just feeling down or having a bad day. Depression is described as a sad mood that lasts for an extended time and interferes with normal, everyday functioning (What is depression, n.d.). Symptoms of depression include feeling sad or anxious most or all of the time, not wanting to participate in things that used to bring joy, irritability, frustration, restlessness, insomnia, changes in appetite, aches, pains, headaches, stomach problems, trouble concentrating, fatigue, feelings of guilt, worthlessness, or helplessness, and suicidal thoughts (What is depression, n.d.). Although the exact cause of depression is unknown, causes can be a combination of genetic, biological, environmental, and psychological factors that include a relative with depression, experiencing a traumatic or stressful event, going through a major life change, having a medical problem, and certain medications (What is depression, n.d.). Based on a national sample of over 4,000 adolescents, exposure to interpersonal violence was found to increase the risk of posttraumatic stress disorder, major depressive episode, and substance abuse (Kilpatrick et al., 2003). Symptoms of depression in adolescents often include aggressive behavior, irritability, and poor school performance (Cipriani et al., 2018).

The CDC recommends psychotherapy and setting goals to cope with stress. Suggestions for goals include things such as getting healthier, quitting smoking, stopping drug and alcohol use, overcoming fears and insecurities, coping with stress, making sense of past events, identify triggers, improving relationships with family and friends, understanding and creating a plan to cope with causes. The CDC also recommends medication to improve mood and coping skills, but warns of side effects.

National Center for Health Statistics (NCHS) revealed that mental health problems are common in children and medication is often prescribed; however, there are few studies that have examined the use of prescription medication in adolescents (Howie, Pastor, & Lukacs, 2014). The data from a 2011-2012 National Health Interview Survey found that 1 out of 7 U.S. children ages 2 to 8 were diagnosed with a mental, behavioral, or developmental disorder (MBDD). Furthermore, 7.5% of children ages 6 to 17 were prescribed medication for emotional or behavioral problems. The study also found children insured by Medicaid or the Children's Health Insurance Program were more likely to be prescribed medication for behavioral or emotional problems (Howie, Pastor, & Lukacs, 2014).

Dubicka and Brent (2017) explain that the rate of depression and suicide in adolescents have been increasing over the past decade. Meanwhile, the rate of diagnosis and referral for depression in adolescents has decreased. There is controversy over the best ways to treat adolescent stress and depression and a need for research to identify best treatment practices. Individualized treatments are recommended for adolescents to find a balance between possible risks and benefits from antidepressants, as well as suicide risks; antidepressants and psychological treatment should be carefully considered (Dubicka & Brent, 2017).

Vertical health outlines the pros and cons of medication for teen depression. The pros include improved mood, improved appetite, increased focus, improved sleep, less anxiety, and fewer depressive symptoms. Cons include gastrointestinal symptoms, insomnia, dry mouth, dizziness, changes in weight, headaches, and sexual side effects (Teen Depression: The Pros and Cons of Medication, n.d.). Many sources also emphasize that antidepressants take time to relieve symptoms and that it is important to remain in contact with the physician, if considering stopping treatment (What is depression, n.d.; Teen Depression: The Pros and Cons of Medication, n.d.).

ADOLESCENT STRESS AS IT RELATES TO BRAIN DEVELOPMENT

Teenagers and young adults are particularly vulnerable to chronic stress and depression which can potentially lead to changes in endocrine and brain function (Wu et al., 2017). The development of depression involves neuroendocrine and central nervous system dysfunction. In addition, neurobiological and morphological changes in brain regions that are vulnerable to stress, particularly, the hippocampus, the part of the brain responsible for learning, memory, and emotion (Wu et al., 2017). Stress early in life can affect the development of the amygdala and striatum, the parts of the brain that support valuation and learning and impact cognitive, behavioral, and socioemotional development, but research is lacking (Fareri & Tottenham, 2016). Literature review on the association between stress and development of the amygdala, prefrontal cortex, and ventral striatal dopaminergic systems in adolescents found consistent vulnerability to stress during development (Tottenham & Galván, 2016).

Teens are often prescribed antidepressants for stress, anxiety, and depression. Cipriani et al. (2018) found that most antidepressants given to adolescents are ineffective. Antidepressants are believed to trigger new brain cell growth and connections in older people; however, this may not be effective with adolescents whose brains are still developing (Cipriani et al., 2018).

Prescription Treatment for Chronic Stress

In the 2013 report, Health at a Glance, the Organization for Economic Cooperation and Development (OECD) presented data on Pharmaceutical consumption and specifically, antidepressant consumption. Data presented for developed countries revealed a significant increase in the consumption of antidepressants since 2000. Iceland reported the highest antidepressant use in 2011. Australia, Canada, Denmark, Sweden, Portugal, United Kingdom, Finland, Belgium, Spain, and Norway were all above the OECD average of 5.6% of adults taking a dose of antidepressant medication daily (Health at a Glance, 2013). The United States was not part of the 2013 OECD report, but the National Health and Nutrition Examination Survey revealed that 12.7% of people age 12 and over took antidepressant medication between 2011 and 2014 (Pratt, Brody, & Qiuping, 2017).

Antidepressants are being prescribed more than ever across the world (Health at a Glance, 2013). There is a great deal of controversy concerning antidepressant medication for children and adolescents. While antidepressant consumption increases worldwide, many patients discontinue use due to side effects (Rheker, Winkler, Doering, & Rief, 2016). Antidepressant prescription medication treatment is often successful in adults with severe depression, yet, research on adolescents reveals conflicting results. In 2004, the US Food and Drug Administration started requiring manufacturers of antidepressants to provide a warning label on antidepressants regarding an increased risk for suicidal behavior in children and adolescents taking antidepressants (Dubicka & Brent, 2017).

Other Treatment Options

Other treatment options for adolescent chronic stress, depression, and anxiety that will be discussed in this chapter include psychotherapy, biofeedback, mindfulness, diet, exercise, and social media. These treatment options are intended to be used in addition to professional treatment and are often used in conjunction with or in place of prescription medication.

Psychotherapy

Psychotherapy is a common option that can be used as an alternative or in conjunction with prescription treatment for anxiety, depression, and stress. Dopheide (2006) suggests that psychotherapeutic interventions are effective for prepubertal children and emphasizes the importance of including cognitive behavioral therapy in addition to antidepressants for older adolescents. Bhatia and Bhatia (2007) suggest cognitive behavior therapy and counseling for mild to moderate childhood depression and emphasize the need for a safety plan for adolescents taking antidepressants.

The National Institute of Mental Health explains how depression can cause significant problems in mood, thinking, and behavior at home and school (Antidepressant Medications for Children and Adolescent, n.d.). Psychotherapy is explained as an initial treatment for mild depression that can help determine the severity and persistence of the depression. Psychotherapies can include cognitive behavioral therapy to help people learn new ways of thinking and behaving and interpersonal therapy to help people understand and work through troubled relationships. In a major clinical trial, the National Institute of Mental Health found that a combination of psychotherapy and medication was the most effective treatment for adolescents with depression; the results suggest suggest psychosocial treatments can improve mental disorders and support scientific findings in the area of cognitive-emotional psychology as a way to learn more about the relationships between stress and health (Schneiderman et al., 2005). "Psychosocial interventions have proven useful for treating stress-related disorders and may influence the course of chronic diseases" (Schneiderman et al., 2005, p. 607).

Using Apps for Treatment

Biofeedback, mindfulness, diet, exercise, and social media are all treatment options that have apps available. Huguet et al. (2016) identified 117 self-help apps that are available in Canada for depression and offer cognitive behavioral therapy or behavioral activation and emphasized the need for scientific, technological, and legal knowledge to improve the accessibility, development, and testing. Since both depression and mobile phone use are highly reported in adolescents, these apps have potential. Mobile apps for treating depression that are based on best practices, meet usability standards, have a privacy policy, and safety measures have the potential to help at a low cost (Huguet et al., 2016).

Bakker, Kazantzis, Rickwood, and Rickard (2016) formulated the following 16 recommendations for mental health smartphone apps: cognitive behavioral therapy based, designed for use by nonclinical populations, reporting of thoughts, feelings, or behaviors, recommend activities, activities directly enhance mood improvement, coping skills training, mental health information, real-time engagement, activities explicitly linked to specific reported mood problems, gamification and intrinsic motivation to engage, log of past app use, reminders to engage, links to crisis support services, experimental trails to establish efficacy, ecological momentary assessment, and app usage data.

Arean et al. (2016) used a clinical trial to study the impact of three different mobile apps for depression and found the apps had the greatest impact on those with moderate levels of depression. A survey of Australian general public revealed that people are willing to use apps for mental health and in a systematic review, they found app use can reduce depression, stress, and substance use (Donker et al., 2013). Potential benefits included accessibility, real-time monitoring and tracking, personalized feedback, support, flexibility, and cost. Possible disadvantages included technical problems, privacy, and security.

Biofeedback

Biofeedback is changing one's physiology often through monitoring breathing and heart rate. Biofeedback is said to reduce stress, depression, and anxiety (Steffen et al., 2016). Biofeedback can build stress resilience and is a low-cost treatment.

There are a variety of apps for Biofeedback:

Breathe Deep

Breathe Deep is an app for breath visualization, relaxation, sleep improvement practices, stress reduction, breathing meditations, breath in yoga, breathing training exercises, and health improvement. Sessions range from one to fifteen minutes with different breathing techniques. There are flexible settings of inhalation, inhalation hold, exhalation, and exhalation hold, optimal breathing visualization with nose or mouth, breathing lessons, reset breathing, sounds and vibration cues, statistics and graphs for usage information, and helpful reminders.

Elite HRV

Elite HRV is an app for true heart rate variability. The emphasis of the app is on accuracy, professional quality, and ease of use. Recovery and true stress levels can be tracked, and resilience and nervous system can be boosted with guided breathing and live feedback. The app also gives autonomic nervous system balance gauge, guided breathing and provides exportable data, secure backup, and privacy settings. It provides a deeper understanding of the body's ability to handle stress and state of recovery.

Delta Waves

Delta Waves are the high amplitude brain waves associated with REM sleep. The Delta waves app recreates that sound. Delta waves are the slowest waves with a frequency between 1 and 4 Hz. The app allows users to set the range and offers seven different songs and five ambient sounds of nature with a built-in timer.

BioBreathing

Biobreathing is a breath pacer app that allows the user to count inhale and exhale breathing cycles. The user can select different tones for the inhale and exhale phases and the length of each phase can be set to a maximum of 10 seconds.

Resility Personal Biofeedback

Resility provides relaxation exercises with Xen health's bluetooth Muscle activity monitor to provide real-time biofeedback. Using electromyography, the muscle monitor measures the activity in a muscle to teach the user how to control muscle activity. The app also includes a guided relaxation training, real-time monitoring, alarm alert for when muscle activity exceeds a selected threshold, and record keeping to track history and progress.

Breath~onome

Breath~onome is a customizable timer for yoga and biofeedback breathing exercises that allows the user to learn common breathing patterns or create their own. It provides scientific-based breathing exercises and allows personalized breathing patterns to be saved while tracking sessions and progress.

Brighthearts

Brighthearts uses biofeedback data with sounds and interactive designs to help users relax, reflect, and relate to their body's patterns. It can be used to regulate breathing and increase Heart Rate Variability (HRV). The wave-shaped pattern that is created from heart rhythm is known as respiratory sinus arrhythmia. Increasing HRV through biofeedback training is stated to be an effective treatment for stress and anxiety. The app is available in English, Catalan, Croatian, Czech, Danish, Dutch, Finnish, French, German, Greek, Hungarian, Indonesian, Italian, Japanese, Korean, Malay, Norwegian Bokmal, Polish, Portuguese, Romanian, Russian, Simplified Chinese, Slovak, Spanish, Swedish, Thai, Traditional Chinese, Turkish, Ukrainian, and Vietnamese.

Mindfulness

Steffen et al. (2016) recommend practicing Mindfulness when dealing with stressful situations. The focus of Mindfulness is to be aware of one's body and mind in the present, rather than worrying about the past or future, which the authors suggest exacerbate depression and anxiety. Practicing Mindfulness regularly is said to calm the mind and body as well as reduce stress, depression, and anxiety.

There are a variety of apps for Mindfulness:

Calm

Calm was Apple's 2017 app of the year. It is the number one app for meditation and mindfulness. It is designed to bring more clarity, joy, and peace to daily life. Calm provides guided meditations, sleep stories, breathing programs, and relaxing music to reduce anxiety and promote better sleep. It is recommended as a way to de-stress by psychologists and mental health experts. Guided meditation sessions are offered in a variety of lengths (3, 5, 10, 15, 20, or 25 minutes). The topics of the meditation sessions are calming anxiety, managing stress, deep sleep, focus and concentration, relationships, breaking habits, happiness, gratitude, self-esteem, body scan, loving-kindness, forgiveness, non-judgement, commuting to work or school, mindfulness at college, walking meditation, calm kids, and more. Other features of Calm include daily calm, a ten-minute program to help ease into the day or unwind at the end of the day, sleep stories, 7 and 21-day programs, masterclass, breathing exercises, music, timed meditation, and nature sounds.

With the mission of making the world a happier and healthier place, Calm started with tools and resources for adults, but now has a goal to empower kids to thrive, not just survive. The Calm School Initiative is giving free Mindfulness training tools to every teacher in the world. Acknowledging that as children face unique social and emotional challenges, greater pressures earlier in life, and face more stress and anxiety than ever before, Calm promotes mindfulness education as a way to develop a lifelong capacity for greater self-awareness, concentration, patience, and resilience. Calm research shows the benefits of teaching mindfulness to children, but teachers often face time and budget constraints. Calm Kids offers the app free to teachers in an attempt to empower teachers with mindfulness tools and resources to help kids learn the skill of mindfulness. Calm suggests that school days begin with a few moments of quiet and stillness. The app uses the Dalai Lama's quote "if every 8-year-old is taught meditation, we will eliminate violence from the world within one generation."

Headspace: Meditation

Headspace offers guided meditations on sleep, focus, and exercise. Everyday headspace provides daily meditations on new topics. The app offers 2-3-minute mini meditations and SOS sessions for moments of stress, anxiety, or panic. Sleep sounds are helpful for falling asleep and headspace animations teach new skills pertaining to mindfulness. Progress can be tracked and synced with apple health. Specific sessions are offered for kids on kindness, calmness, and focus.

Mindfulness Daily

Mindfulness daily gives gentle reminders to pause for mindful breaths in meaningful moments. It has effective guided practices for reducing stress and anxiety, improving performances, and enhancing sleep.

Relax Meditation: Mindfulness, Sleep Sounds, Noise

Relax Meditation promotes learning and practicing meditation to increase overall quality of life, stating benefits include boosting overall health, finding happiness, improving relationships, increased focus and awareness, improved productivity, better knowledge of self, and better sleep. Programs are offered in five-day increments on topics including self-esteem, relationships, success, creativity, and new content each month. In addition, there are over 50 free sounds that can be used to create custom melodies or community melodies can be searched and shared. The app also includes brainwave frequencies and a meditation reminder.

Breeth: Meditation and Music

Breeth provides 10-minute sessions of soothing music and guided meditations to de-stress and sleep better. The app promotes more happiness, calmness, and peace of mind, in addition to relaxation, weight loss, sharpened mind, and improved relationships. It includes hundreds of daily meditations and other guided meditations on specific topics including weight loss, insomnia, anxiety, work performance, sleep, and offers a program specifically for kids.

3 Minute Mindfulness

3 Minute Mindfulness is an app for quick meditations and breathing exercises to help deal with stress, anxiety, sleep, and more. It is advertised as a way to be happier, calmer, and more at peace in just 3 minutes and describes mindfulness as paying attention in the present moment, without judgment and noticing what is happening around you. In addition, mindfulness will improve sleep, reduce stress, relieve anxiety, increase positive feelings, calm the mind, and increase focus. Breathing exercises include square breathing and 4-7-8 breathing, as well as the option to create your own.

Zen Mindfulness

Zen Mindfulness offers quotes for inspiration, and over 400 teachings for reflection and inspiration. Start bells, interval bells, and end bells are offered for silent meditation, as well as 27 guided meditations of various lengths. The app also includes instructions for beginners and mindfulness techniques for living a more mindful life.

Mindful Meditation Hypnosis

Mindful Meditation Hypnosis features soothing, therapeutic hypnotherapy tracks that can be customized. Meditation power, deep peace and relaxation, connection to higher self, positive thinking, mental clarity, and better sleep are advertised as benefits. Options include positive thinking, financial success, attract good luck, law of attraction, relaxation, focus, face your fears, mindful eating, deep sleep, seduction, intimacy, inner peace and calm, confidence and inner strength, and lucid dreaming.

Mindfulness Lifestyle

Mindfulness Lifestyle is an app for mindfulness exercises. Mindfulness meditation is described as a way to develop focusing skills, resilience, and well-being. Furthermore, mindfulness can improve abilities to pay attention, calm down, and make better decisions. Mindfulness Lifestyle is designed to increase well-being through teaching mindfulness-based meditation on the go. The sessions include the raisin exercise, dealing with anger, mindful seeing, anxiety reduction meditation, mindful listening, meditation on love, peace, and happiness, the self-compassion pause, self-inquiry meditation, five senses exercise, the mini-mindfulness exercise, stare at the center, meditation on depression, controlling negative thoughts, meditation on joy, mindful walking down the street technique, the three-minute breathing space, dialectical behavioral therapy, observe a leaf for five minutes, mindful eating for four minutes, observe your thoughts for fifteen minutes, mindfulness bell exercise for five minutes, stare at the center, mindfulness techniques for depression, mindfulness techniques for anger, mindfulness techniques for anxiety, mindfulness-based eating awareness training, mindfulness techniques for addiction, mindful breathing, mindful awareness, mindful listening, mindful immersion, mindful appreciation, the body scan, and mindful observation.

Guided Mindfulness Meditation

Guided Mindfulness Meditation is a way to learn to meditate in five minutes per day. The app provides guided meditations that can be used for different needs of everyday life. It promotes an increase in concentration, reduced stress, improved cognitive abilities, help with attention deficit and anxiety, memory, decrease in anger and stress, and increase in happiness. This app is available in English, French, German, Italian, Japanese, Korean, Russian, Simplified Chinese, Spanish, and Traditional Chinese.

Mindfulness: The Art of Being Human

Mindfulness: The Art of Being Human is based on Western psychology and Eastern mindfulness practices and promotes improved mood, better concentration, increased creativity, reduced stress, and managing emotions. The app was researched and written by Reuben Lowe, a mindfulness therapist and clinical practitioner specializing in contextual psychology.

MindPilot: Mindfulness Course and Meditation

MindPilot: Mindfulness and Meditation course helps de-stress, promotes better sleep, and a greater sense of well-being. There are over 20 how to meditate audio tools with a special section on performing better each day and successfully meeting daily challenges. The mindful moments section includes mindful eating, mindful walking, and other exercises.

Mindfulness: Mindfullness and Meditation for dummies

Mindfulness: Mindfullness and Meditation for dummies provides quick and simple one minute mindfulness exercises for every day.

Pacifica for Stress and Anxiety

The Pacifica app was designed from psychologist tools based on Cognitive Behavioral Therapy, mindfulness meditation, relaxation, and mood and health tracking. Stating that stress, anxiety, and depression can be caused by cycles of negative thoughts, that can lead to actions from physical feelings and emotions, the app helps break the cycle through managing stress, anxiety, and depression. The app includes over 30 audio exercises for relaxation and mindfulness including soundscapes, deep breathing, muscle relaxation, and mindfulness meditations. Self-help paths are guided audio lessons designed to help with stress, anxiety, and depression with an introductory path, two paths focused on Cognitive Behavioral Therapy, and one mindfulness path. There is also a mood tracker that can be used to rate mood and feelings throughout the day and make a note of any triggers. The psychologist designed analysis tools are for recording thoughts and using journaling for analyzing distorted thinking patterns. Cognitive Behavioral Therapy then helps break negative thought cycles through promoting balanced thinking. The daily challenges and goal tracking uses a one day at a time approach to facing anxiety and working towards long-term goals. There is also a built-in health tracker to record exercise, sleep, and food that could affect anxiety and mood. The community component allows individuals to offer support, share stories, and advice.

Diet

Stress can cause cortisol levels to increase. When cortisol levels increase, food cravings also increase. These cravings are often for carbohydrates, creating a vicious cycle. Prevention magazine suggests eating foods that are rich in nutrients and energy to help stress instead of comfort foods that are often high fat and sugar (Glassman, 2017). Eating the right foods can help bring focus and balance to stressful situations. Wu et al. (2017) explain that the development of depression is associated with dysfunction in the central nervous system and found that taurine can provide an antidepressant effect and protect brain development while improving learning and memory. Furthermore, they propose that functional food could prevent depression.

Prevention magazine suggests eating the following foods to fight stress: asparagus due to the high folate content, avocados due to glutathione content, berries for anthocyanins (antioxidants that help the brain produce dopamine) cashews and oysters for zinc, chamomile tea for its calming effect, chocolate for polyphenols and flavanols, garlic and grass-fed beef for antioxidants, green tea for theanine, oatmeal for complex carbohydrates, oranges for vitamin C, and walnuts for alpha-linolenic acid (Glassman, 2017).

Mercola (2015) suggests ten superfoods to relieve stress. He emphasizes that healthy foods can affect mood, relieve stress and tension, and stabilize blood sugar. Dark green leafy vegetables are high in folate that help produce neurotransmitters like serotonin and dopamine. Organic turkey breast is a source of tryptophan that is converted to serotonin. Fermented foods promote a healthy gut and healthy brain from good bacteria. Wild Alaskan salmon contains omega-3 fatty acids that have been known to contribute to emotional well-being. Blueberries, as recommended by Prevention are good for anthocyanins. Pistachios can lower vascular constriction and can also be therapeutic to shell. Dark chocolate, also recommended by Prevention, is recommended by Mercola for the neurotransmitter, anandamide, that is produced in the brain. Foods high in vitamin D like egg yolks and mushrooms are also recommended. Seeds are good for magnesium to help regulate emotions and promote a healthy well-being. Lastly, avocados are again recommended for a variety of nutrients including potassium, vitamin E, B, and folate. Mercola recommends staying away from sugar and starch when dealing with stress. Sugar can cause fluctuation in blood sugar which can lead to mood swings. Gluten is also said to be a poor choice when dealing with stress as it inhibits the production of serotonin. The synthetic ingredients in processed foods should also be avoided as they are also known to lower moods.

The use of mobile phone apps for diet and weight loss is relatively new. Zaidan and Roehrer (2016) studied the usability of Australian mobile phone apps for socially focused weight loss and diet wellness apps. A justification evaluation framework resulted from their study and found that ease of use, bar code scanning, reminder, synchronization, and motivation were significant attributes and recommended for weight loss and diet apps.

There are a variety of apps to help track food and keep dieting on track:

Lose It!: Calorie Counter

Lose It calorie counter is a tool for tracking meals, exercise, and nutrition. It provides a barcode scanner, searchable list of common items, and database of popular restaurant meals. The app also has a social feature to find inspiration from others.

My Diet Coach: Weight Loss

My diet coach is described as easy, fun, and motivating. Goals can be set through the app and progress can be tracked. It also offers reminders, inspiring tips, and daily quotes. This app is available in English, French, German, Italian, Polish, Portuguese, Russian, and Spanish.

MyFitnessPal

MyFitnessPal makes tracking food fast and easy with a large food database and barcode scanner. There is also a recipe importer, restaurant logger, water tracker, step tracker, exercise log, community feature, chart progress, and goal setter. This app is available in English, Danish, Dutch, Filipino, French, German, Indonesian, Italian, Japanese, Korean, Malay, Norwegian Bokmal, Polish, Portuguese, Russian, Simplified Chinese, Spanish, Swedish, Traditional Chinese, and Turkish.

8fit Workouts and Meal Planner

8fit has a community of over 20 million users. The app offers customized workout and meal plans to help reach wellness goals. Features include wellness goals, fitness level measurement, and custom workouts and meal plans. Proper exercise form and progression is explained, and ingredient alternatives are provided for all recipes. This app is available in English, Spanish, German, French, Portuguese, and Italian.

MyPlate Calorie Counter

MyPlate allows users to set a personalized calorie goal, keep track of weight and progress, track calories, and set meal reminders. This app also features in-app workouts, a macronutrient snapshot of daily protein, carbs, and fat, an eight-week meal plan, and community support.

Exercise

In addition to eating foods that promote good mood and emotional health, exercise is known to have a positive effect on stress, anxiety, and depression. Young (2007) explains how exercise can increase serotonin in the brain and treat depression without drugs. Craft and Perna (2004) suggest exercise as behavioral therapy for depression. Mangerud, Bjerkese, Lydersen, and Indredavik (2014) found lower levels of physical activity in adolescent psychiatric patients compared to the general population and emphasize the importance of promoting mental and physical health early in life. Although studies on using apps to promote exercise are limited, Middelweerd, Mollee, Wal, Brug, and Velde (2014) studied the behavior techniques commonly used in exercise apps and found self-monitoring, feedback on performance, and goal setting to be the most frequently used.

There are a variety of apps for tracking exercise and exercise programs:

BodBot Personal Trainer

BodBot is a digital personal trainer app that is customizable for individual fitness goals, resources, physical abilities, and more. The workouts are designed to meet the user's level and adapts over time. This app is available in English, Arabic, Catalan, Croatian, Czech, Danish, Dutch, Finnish, French, German, Greek, Hebrew, Hungarian, Indonesian, Italian, Japanese, Korean, Malay, Northern Sami, Norwegian Bokmal, Polish, Portuguese, Romanian, Russian, Simplified Chinese, Slovak, Spanish, Swedish, Thai, Traditional Chinese, Turkish, Ukrainian, and Vietnamese.

Fit30: Home Workouts Exercise

Fit30 is an app for in-home workouts that do not require any equipment. The workouts are designed to maximize fat loss, tone abdominals, buttocks, and leg muscles. The program is designed to be completed in 30 days with intensity increasing and recovery days built in. The high-intensity training is supposed to boost metabolism. This app is available in English, Danish, Dutch, Finnish, French, German, Greek, Indonesian, Italian, Japanese, Korean, Malay, Norwegian Bokmal, Portuguese, Russian, Simplified Chinese, Spanish, Swedish, Thai, Traditional Chinese, Turkish, and Vietnamese.

Sworkit: Workouts and Plans

Sworkit offers a variety of types and lengths of body weight exercises. Features include guided workout plans, custom exercise intervals, unlimited workouts, and trainer advice. The app is available in English, French, German, Hindi, Italian, Japanese, Korean, Portuguese, Russian, Simplified Chinese, Spanish, and Turkish.

Daily Workouts Fitness Trainer

Daily Workouts Fitness Trainer offers fast and effective workouts including targeted workouts that are 5 or 10 minutes in length, full body workouts that are 10 to 30 minutes each, video demonstrations, on-screen instructions with timer, and an integrated health app. This app does not require internet access for most of the workouts and is available in English, Arabic, Catalan, Croatian, Czech, Danish, Dutch, Finnish, French, German, Greek, Hebrew, Hindi, Hungarian, Indonesian, Italian, Japanese, Korean, Malay, Norwegian Bokmal, Polish, Portuguese, Romanian, Russian, Simplified Chinese, Slovak, Spanish, Swedish, Thai, Traditional Chinese, Turkish, Ukrainian, Vietnamese, and Welsh.

Weight Loss Fitness

Weight loss fitness is a six-week program that provides easy workouts for home in as little as six minutes per day. The app provides music and reminders, as well as progress and tips. It can also be synchronized with Apple Health and is available in French, Japanese, Portuguese, Korean, Simplified Chinese, Italian, Spanish, Russian, and German.

30 Day Fitness Challenge Log

The 30-day fitness challenge log is a trainer and tracker that increases counts per set. The program is personalized based on fitness level and offers 80 professional workouts. This app is only available in English.

Social Media

The Royal Society for Public Health report, Status of Mind (2017), found social media can improve access to health information and emotional support for young people. Over 90% of 16 to 24-year olds reported using the internet for social networking. Those who use social media reported feeling emotionally supported by their contacts; however, social media use was also linked to poor sleep and increased rates of anxiety and depression. The report calls social media platforms to identify and offer support for users who may be suffering from mental illness. The report also recommended posting warnings for heavy social media use and alerts for digitally manipulated photos. Appropriate social media use could be taught to youth and those working with youth could also be trained on social media use. The report calls for more research on the effects of social media on young people's health.

LIMITATIONS OF CURRENT RESEARCH

In the fast-paced world adolescents are growing up in, they face more stressors than ever before. At the same time, technology provides more treatment options than ever before. Studies on prescription antidepressant use by adolescents are limited and raise concerns for privacy and safety. Brain development research is complex and limited. Many of the treatment app options discussed in this chapter are new and have limited research. Furthermore, many research studies are limited to adults, and many apps are designed for adults. These apps are difficult to study due to the variety of options available and the fact that they change quickly.

SOLUTIONS AND RECOMMENDATIONS

The impact adolescent chronic stress has on the brain, depression, and anxiety is concerning. The relationship between psychosocial stressors and disease is affected by the number, nature, and persistence of stressors, in addition to an individual's vulnerability, psychosocial resources, and patterns of coping (Schneiderman et al., 2005). Research is needed for the impact chronic stress has on brain development in adolescents, and while there are many associations between chronic stress, depression, and anxiety, the solutions and treatment options are complicated. Much of the existing research recommends professional treatment. It is recommended that the treatment options presented in this chapter are used in addition to professional treatment. While some may benefit from one app, others may find another more helpful or benefit from something completely different. As every individual's situation and circumstances are unique, so are the best treatments.

FUTURE RESEARCH DIRECTIONS

Future research is needed on using biofeedback, mindfulness, diet, exercise, and social media to treat chronic stress and depression. These treatments could be researched alone or in combination with psychotherapy and or medication. These treatments could be further studied more specifically by incorporating app use. Apps like Calm, Headspace, and Breeth have specific options for kids. There is research potential for determining how the problems adolescents face are created and treated with technology. Tottenham and Galván (2016) suggest future research on adolescent stress and affective, motivational, and cognitive systems to study how alterations in one region of the brain affect others through the use of fMRI data. Research is limited on mobile apps for mental health. Donker et al. (2013) suggest research to develop and test evidence-based programs for mental health apps. The variables for future research studies are complex, and as technology offers more options for self-help, research becomes more challenging.

CONCLUSION

Children and adolescents who deal with chronic stress deserve the best treatment possible. The impact stress could have on adolescent brain development is alarming, and the growing number of adolescents prescribed antidepressants raises concern over effectiveness, suicide and other side effects. Psychotherapy, biofeedback, mindfulness, diet, exercise, and social media use are worth investigating. Based on the limited studies available, apps for biofeedback, mindfulness, diet, and exercise are promising, but require more research. Many of these apps include a community feature which supports social media use as a treatment option, but also requires more research.

REFERENCES

Antidepressant Medications for Children and Adolescents: Information for Parents and Caregivers. (n.d.). Retrieved 1 April 2018 from https://www.nimh.nih.gov/health/topics/child-and-adolescent-mental-health/antidepressant-medic ations-for-children-and-adolescents-information-for-parents-and-caregivers.shtml

Arean, P. A., Hallgren, K. A., Jordan, J. T., Gazzaley, A., Atkins, D. C., Heagerty, P. J., & Anguera, J. A. (2016). The use and effectiveness of mobile apps for depression: Results from a fully remote clinical trial. *Journal of Medical Internet Research, 18*(12), e330. doi:10.2196/jmir.6482 PMID:27998876

Bakker, D., Kazantzis, N., Rickwood, D., & Rickard, N. (2016). Mental health smartphone apps: Review and evidence-based recommendations for future developments. *JMIR Mental Health, 3*(1). Retrieved 30 March 2018 from https://www.ncbi.nlm.nih.gov/pmc/articles/PMC4795320/

Bhatia, S. K., & Bhatia, S. C. (2007). Childhood and adolescent depression. *American Family Physician, 75*(1), 73–80. Retrieved from http://citeseerx.ist.psu.edu/viewdoc/download?doi=10.1.1.629.8098&rep=rep1&type=pdf PMID:17225707

Cipriani, A., Furukawa, T. A., Salanti, G., Chaimani, A., Atkinson, L. Z., Ogawa, Y., . . . Geddes, J. R. (2018). Comparative efficacy and acceptability of 21 antidepressant drugs for the acute treatment of adults with major depressive disorder: A systematic review and network meta-analysis. *The Lancet*. Retrieved 1 April 2018 from http://www.thelancet.com/pdfs/journals/lancet/PIIS0140-6736(17)32802-7.pdf

Craft, L. L., & Perna, F. M. (2004). The benefits of exercise for the clinically depressed. *Primary Care Companion to the Journal of Clinical Psychiatry, 6*(3), 104–111. doi:10.4088/PCC.v06n0301 PMID:15361924

Depression, T. (n.d.). *The Pros and Cons of Medication*. Retrieved 1 April 2018 from https://www.psycom.net/depression.central.teens.medication.html

Donker, T., Petrie, K., Proudfoot, J., Clarke, J., Birch, M., & Christensen, H. (2013). Smartphones for smarter delivery of mental health programs: A systematic review. *Journal of Medical Internet Research, 15*(11), e247. doi:10.2196/jmir.2791 PMID:24240579

Dopheide, J. A. (2006). Recognizing and treating depression in children and adolescents. *American Journal of Health-System Pharmacy*, *63*(3), 233–243. doi:10.2146/ajhp050264 PMID:16434782

Dubicka, B., & Brent, D. (2017). Editorial: Pharmacotherapy and adolescent depression - an important treatment option. *Child and Adolescent Mental Health*, *22*(2), 59–60. doi:10.1111/camh.12223

Fareri, D. S., & Tottenham, N. (2016). Effects of early life stress on amygdala and striatal development. *Developmental Cognitive Neuroscience*, *19*, 233–247. doi:10.1016/j.dcn.2016.04.005 PMID:27174149

Glassman, K. (2017). *13 Foods That Fight Stress*. Retrieved 2 April 2018 from https://www.prevention.com/mind-body/emotional-health/13-healthy-foods-that-reduce-stress-an d-depression/slide/4

Health at a Glance. (2013). *OECD indicators*. Retrieved 30 March 2018 from https://www.oecd.org/els/health-systems/Health-at-a-Glance-2013.pdf

Howie, L., Pastor, P., & Lukacs, S. (2014). *Use of Medication Prescribed for Emotional or Behavioral Difficulties Among Children Aged 6–17 Years in the United States, 2011–2012*. Retrieved 8 March 2018 from https://www.cdc.gov/nchs/data/databriefs/db148.htm

Huguet, A., Rao, S., Mcgrath, P. J., Wozney, L., Wheaton, M., Conrod, J., & Rozario, S. (2016). A systematic review of cognitive behavioral therapy and behavioral activation apps for depression. *PLoS One*, *11*(5), e0154248. doi:10.1371/journal.pone.0154248 PMID:27135410

Kilpatrick, D. G., Ruggiero, K. J., Acierno, R., Saunders, B. E., Resnick, H. S., & Best, C. L. (2003). Violence and risk of PTSD, major depression, substance abuse/dependence, and comorbidity: Results from the National Survey of Adolescents. *Journal of Consulting and Clinical Psychology*, *71*(4), 692–700. doi:10.1037/0022-006X.71.4.692 PMID:12924674

Mangerud, W., Bjerkeset, O., Lydersen, S., & Indredavik, M. (2014). Physical activity in adolescents with psychiatric disorders and in the general population. *Child and Adolescent Psychiatry and Mental Health*, *8*(1), 2. doi:10.1186/1753-2000-8-2 PMID:24450542

Mercola, J. (2015). *10 Superfoods That Reduce Stress*. Retrieved 2 April 2018 from https://articles.mercola.com/sites/articles/archive/2015/04/27/10-stress-relieving-superfoods.aspx

Middelweerd, A., Mollee, J. S., Wal, C. N., Brug, J., & Velde, S. J. (2014). Apps to promote physical activity among adults: A review and content analysis. *The International Journal of Behavioral Nutrition and Physical Activity*, *11*(1), 97. doi:10.118612966-014-0097-9 PMID:25059981

Pratt, L., Brody, D., & Qiuping, G. (2017). *NCHS Data Brief. U.S. Department of Health and Human Services. No. 283. Centers for Disease Control and Prevention National Center for Health Statistics Antidepressant Use Among Persons Aged 12 and Over: United States 2011–2014*. Retrieved 30 March 2018 from https://www.cdc.gov/nchs/data/databriefs/db283.pdf

Rheker, J., Winkler, A., Doering, B. K., & Rief, W. (2016). Learning to experience side effects after antidepressant intake – Results from a randomized, controlled, double-blind study. *Psychopharmacology*, *234*(3), 329–338. doi:10.100700213-016-4466-8 PMID:27807605

Romeo, R. D. (2017). The impact of stress on the structure of the adolescent brain: Implications for adolescent mental health. *Brain Research*, *1654*, 185–191. doi:10.1016/j.brainres.2016.03.021 PMID:27021951

Ross, R. A., Foster, S. L., & Ionescu, D. F. (2017). The role of chronic stress in anxious depression. *Chronic Stress*. Retrieved 30 March 2018 from http://journals.sagepub.com/doi/pdf/10.1177/2470547016689472

Royal Society for Public Health. (2017). Retrieved 30 March 2018 from https://www.rsph.org.uk/our-work/campaigns/status-of-mind.html

Schneiderman, N., Ironson, G., & Siegel, S. D. (2005). Stress and health: Psychological, behavioral, and biological determinants. *Annual Review of Clinical Psychology*, *1*(1), 607–628. doi:10.1146/annurev.clinpsy.1.102803.144141 PMID:17716101

Steffen, P. R., Austin, T., & Debarros, A. (2016). Treating chronic stress to address the growing problem of depression and anxiety. *Policy Insights from the Behavioral and Brain Sciences*, *4*(1), 64–70. doi:10.1177/2372732216685333

Tottenham, N., & Galván, A. (2016). Stress and the adolescent brain. *Neuroscience and Biobehavioral Reviews*, *70*, 217–227. doi:10.1016/j.neubiorev.2016.07.030 PMID:27473936

Twenge, J. M., Joiner, T. E., Rogers, M. L., & Martin, G. N. (2017). Increases in depressive symptoms, suicide-related outcomes, and suicide rates among U.S. adolescents after 2010 and links to increased new media screen time. *Clinical Psychological Science*, *6*(1), 3–17. doi:10.1177/2167702617723376

What is depression? (n.d.). Retrieved 20 March 2018 from https://www.cdc.gov/tobacco/campaign/tips/diseases/depression-anxiety.html

Wu, G., Ren, S., Tang, R., Xu, C., Zhou, J., Lin, S., ... Yang, J. (2017). Antidepressant effect of taurine in chronic unpredictable mild stress-induced depressive rats. *Scientific Reports*, *7*(1). PMID:28694433

Young, S. (2007). How to increase serotonin in the human brain without drugs. *Journal of Psychiatry & Neuroscience*, *32*(6), 394–399. PMID:18043762

Zaidan, S., & Roehrer, E. (2016). Popular mobile phone apps for diet and weight loss: A content analysis. *JMIR mHealth and uHealth*, *4*(3), e80. doi:10.2196/mhealth.5406 PMID:27400806

ADDITIONAL READING

Andersen, S. L. (2016). Commentary on the special issue on the adolescent brain: Adolescence, trajectories, and the importance of prevention. *Neuroscience and Biobehavioral Reviews, 70*, 329–333. doi:10.1016/j.neubiorev.2016.07.012 PMID:27423540

Andersen, S. L., & Teicher, M. H. (2008). Stress, sensitive periods and maturational events in adolescent depression. *Trends in Neurosciences, 31*(4), 183–191. doi:10.1016/j.tins.2008.01.004 PMID:18329735

Auerbach, R. P., Admon, R., & Pizzagalli, D. A. (2014). Adolescent depression. *Harvard Review of Psychiatry, 22*(3), 139–148. doi:10.1097/HRP.0000000000000034 PMID:24704785

Bitsko, R. H., Holbrook, J. R., Robinson, L. R., Kaminski, J. W., Ghandour, R., Smith, C., & Peacock, G. (2016). Health care, family, and community factors associated with mental, behavioral, and developmental disorders in early childhood — United States, 2011–2012. *MMWR. Morbidity and Mortality Weekly Report, 65*(9), 221–226. doi:10.15585/mmwr.mm6509a1 PMID:26963052

Dinas, P. C., Koutedakis, Y., & Flouris, A. D. (2010). Effects of exercise and physical activity on depression. *Irish Journal of Medical Science, 180*(2), 319–325. doi:10.100711845-010-0633-9 PMID:21076975

Galván, A., & Mcglennen, K. M. (2011). Daily stress increases risky decision-making in adolescents: A preliminary study. *Developmental Psychobiology, 54*(4), 433–440. doi:10.1002/dev.20602 PMID:22012864

Goff, B., & Tottenham, N. (2014). Early-life adversity and adolescent depression: Mechanisms involving the ventral striatum. *CNS Spectrums, 20*(04), 337–345. doi:10.1017/S1092852914000674 PMID:25511634

KEY TERMS AND DEFINITIONS

Antidepressants: Pharmaceutical treatment for depression.

Biofeedback: The use of breathing and heart rate to change physiology.

Centers for Disease Control and Prevention (CDC): United States government health protection agency.

Cognitive Behavioral Therapy: A talk form of psychotherapy.

Major Depressive Disorder (MDD): A mood disorder that interferes with day to day life.

Mindfulness: Awareness of body and mind in the present.

National Center for Health Statistics (NCHS): An agency in the United States that is responsible for statistical information that is used to set policies and guidelines to improve health.

Organization for Economic Cooperation and Development (OECD): An intergovernmental economic organization consisting of 35 countries promoting economic progress and trade.

Psychotherapy: Psychological mental health treatment, sometimes referred to as talk therapy.

Social Media: Platforms that allow users to share information through social networking.

Chapter 3
Neurophysiological and Neurobiological Basis of Emotions and Mood

Igor V. Pantic
University of Belgrade, Serbia

ABSTRACT

Emotions and mood are complex psychic phenomena that play important roles in everyday behavior. No anatomical structure can be identified as a specific brain center for emotions, and a neurophysiological basis of emotions is unclear and hard to define. Today, it is thought that neurotransmitters such as dopamine, serotonin, and norepinephrine have important roles in mood regulation, and much of the evidence for this assumption is based on the effectiveness of antidepressant medications currently available in psychiatric practice. James-Lange, Cannon-Bard, and Schachter's and other theories historically tried to explain the origin and formation of emotional responses. Despite extensive research efforts on this topic, many aspects regarding the nature of emotional responses remain unclear. Multidisciplinary approach, including the adequate cooperation of psychiatrists, neurophysiologists, and experts from other areas, is needed to provide us with a more comprehensive insight on biological basis of conative psychic functions.

DOI: 10.4018/978-1-5225-7513-9.ch003

INTRODUCTION

Emotions are a complex psychic function for which there is no precise and comprehensive definition. Emotions reflect the individual's mental attitude towards an object (i.e. another individual) or a phenomenon, as well as a consequent mental reaction that influences an opinion about that object or phenomenon (or interaction with it). Mood differs from emotions in terms that it lasts longer, is less intense and less focused on a particular object. In mammals, it is considered that the limbic system is the main structure in the central nervous system responsible for the emergence of emotions. However, with regard to the maintenance and modulation of emotions, many regions in the cortex, thalamus and basal ganglia are also of great significance.

There are numerous classifications of emotions according to the level of intensity, or satisfaction associated with them. Paul Ekman, a famous American psychologist, defined six basic emotions in the middle of the twentieth century: anger, disgust, fear, happiness, sorrow and surprise. These emotions are present in every person, regardless of their affiliation to a particular culture / subculture, religion, customs and attitudes.

Positron emission tomography (PET) technique, as well as various other methods for in vivo monitoring the activity of the brain regions, have opened new possibilities in researching the neurophysiological basis of emotions. A number of experimental animal models have also been developed to examine oxygen consumption, glucose metabolism and other substances in the central nervous system, and based on their conclusions, the specific regions of the brain were proposed to be involved in the modulation of emotions and mood (Young et al., 2018).

There are three major brain neurotransmitters that have been suggested to have an important impact on mood regulation in physiological and pathological conditions: dopamine, serotonin and norepinephrine. Dopamine is the most important neurotransmitter in brain reward circuits, and regions that act as the "pleasure centers" of the central nervous system are abundant with dopaminergic neurons. Norepinephrine has a major role in arousal and sleep/wake cycles, but is also a potentially important mood regulator in both mentally healthy and depressed individual. Today, one of the most frequently prescribed classes of antidepressant medications are selective serotonin reuptake inhibitors which may increase serotonergic brain transmission. However, despite significant advances in the field of neuropharmacology, it is still impossible to fully understand the relation between brain neurotransmitter activity and emotion/mood (Bressan & Crippa, 2005; Drevets et al., 2007; Stahl, 2013).

BRAIN REGIONS RELATED TO EMOTIONS AND MOOD

Over the past few years, in many publications, the importance of the prefrontal cortex in the modulation of both positive and negative emotions has been highlighted. Left prefrontal cortex, as well as the nerve pathways in the nearby white mass of the brain seem to be of particular importance. Harmon-Jones and associates have shown that after the induction of an unpleasant emotion (after suffering an insult), the activity of the left frontal cortex increases, while on the right it decreases.

It is believed that amygdaloid nuclei are of particular importance in the creation and modulation of feelings of fear, anger and disgust. Amygdala are anatomically composed of the basolateral complex, a medial nucleus, the medial nucleus, the cortical nucleus, and the intercalated cell clusters. It is still not known whether any of these structures is responsible for specific emotions. It is possible that there are significant differences between the amygdala on the left and the right. According to some authors, the right amigdaloid core is primarily responsible for negative emotions. Amygdala are closely related to other parts of the limbic system, and in particular to the structures responsible for the learning and memory process. The relationship with the hippocampus ensures that amygdaloid nuclei have a potentially important role in information selection and storage in long term memory. Such emotional learning is considered to be the key for the development and normal functioning of interpersonal relationships and connections. The latest research suggests that the amygdala is also significant in the modulation of positive emotions (Albert, Vahid-Ansari, & Luckhart, 2014; Haller, 2018; Mohammadi, Haghir, Fazel, & Vafaei, 2013; Young et al., 2018).

Central nucleus of the amygdale may be responsible for the changes in sympathicus resulting from emotions. This is one of the most important output structures within amygdala and connects them with regions of brain stem involved in internal organ functions. The major neurotransmitter participating in this connection is dopamine. Also an important projection of his nucleus goes to hypothalamus which serves as the higher autonomic nervous centre. This way, amygdala may influence blood pressure, heart frequency, as well as the rate of respiration. It is possible that, this way, particularly information on present or past experiences including pain and discomfort, may cause changes in autonomic nervous system activity (Haller, 2018; Mohammadi et al., 2013; Young et al., 2018).

Neuronal circuits in amygdala can be activated in both the circumstances that are related to happiness and sadness. This has been indicated in various neuroimaging studies trying to assess the function of specific brain regions as the result of emotions induced by external factors. In patients suffering from depression, it is possible that reactivity of these neurons in amygdala is increased for sadness-related factors, whereas the reactivity for happiness-inducing factors is reduced. Whether this is an inherited or acquired trait of this brain structure is unclear.

Cingulate cortex, or cingulate gyrus, is another structure that plays a very important role in the formation and alteration of emotions and mood. The front cingulate cortex is located below the genu of corpus callosum, closely related to the thalamus and other parts of the limbic system, and actively participates in the flow of information through the Papez circuit. It is considered to be important in the detection of errors and conflicts of information in the limbic system. The posterior cingulate cortex is closely related to the hippocampus and therefore has a certain function in emotional memory. It is possible that this structure participates in attaching emotional coloration to autobiographical data, or events from personal history. The posterior cingulate cortex is active in the modulation of both positive and negative emotions (Berlim, McGirr, Van den Eynde, Fleck, & Giacobbe, 2014; Bersani et al., 2014; Pauc & Young, 2010; Pecina et al., 2013; Rogers et al., 2004).

The role of hippocampus in emotions is particularly important and complex. The hippocampus belongs to the limbic system and has certain functions in approach-avoidance conflict processing. Approach-avoidance conflicts basically occur when the same situation/process can result in both a positive and negative outcome, and the prediction of outcome is difficult or impossible. For example, an experimental an experimental animal that presses a lever sometimes receives a reward (food), and sometimes a punishment electric shock). The animal does not know outcome, and is basically in a conflict regarding whether to apply approach avoidance – based behavior. Ventral regions of hippocampus have particularly been implicated to participate in emotional regulation during this conflict. Lesions in ventral hippocampus may be related with the reduction of anxiety and increase of exploratory (risk analysis) behavior (Andersen, 2007; R. C. Cannon, Wheal, & Turner, 1999; Hayman et al., 1998; Nicholson & Geinisman, 2009; Pantic et al., 2015).

JAMES-LANGE, CANNON-BARD AND SCHACHTER'S THEORIES OF NEUROPHYSIOLOGICAL BASIS OF EMOTIONS

In the past, there have been various theories that tried to elaborate the association between emotions and physiological changes in organ/tissue functions. Some of the most prominent include James-Lange, Cannon-Bard and Schachter's theories. William James (1842-1910) and Carl G. Lange (1834-1900) focused on the relationship between peripheral stimuli and emotions. They assumed that peripheral stimuli in the body (emotion-producing stimuli) are causing a specific physiological response that is perceived in a way that can be explained as having an emotion. Physiological response may be the activation of the autonomic nervous system. In other words, the peripheral sensation is crucial for emotional life. There were some researchers in the past who supported this theory by emphasizing the role of spinal cord and afferent neural pathways in mood. Destruction or damage of afferent pathways and sensory imput to the brain may lead to the decrease of intensity of certain emotions and affects. In this view, thalamus has one of the most important roles in this process. However, James-Lange theory failed to receive significant support from academic community (W. B. Cannon, 1987).

Another theory was suggested by Philip Bard (1898-1977) and Walter Cannon (1871-1945) with an emphasis to the brain functions, rather than the functions of the autonomic nervous system as curtail for emotion occurrence. Cannon became famous for his concept of Fight-or-flight response (hyperarousal, the acute stress response) in which a perceived danger (to physical or mental health) leads to a physiological response that manifests as an activation of the sympathetic nervous system. The brain makes a decision if the threat is sufficiently big to cause the response. In other words, the autonomic nervous system reaction is the effect (not the cause) of the emotion. The emotion predates the autonomic activity, which takes much more time to develop.

Finally, Schachter and Singer (1962) proposed another theory, in which the emotional response is a resultant of the cognitive functioning on one hand, and physiological arousal on the other. Cognitive functioning and interpretation of the emotional state, depends not only on internal factors, but also on a wider social context and environment. Physiological arousal (i.e. sympathetic activation, or adrenalin injection) provides a basis which is further upgraded by cognitive system and influenced by external context (Schachter, 2013).

DOPAMINE AND EMOTIONS

Dopamine is one of the most important regulatory neutransmitters in the central nervous system. It belongs to the group of catecholamine compounds, which also includes other neurotransmitters, norepinephrine and epinephrine. There are several dopaminergic pathways in the brain, some of which are important for motor functions, while others are directly or indirectly included in limbic system regulation. Dopamine is vital for emotional responses and mood, but also for other aspect of psychic functioning. Apart from depression, many mental disorders such as schizophrenia and other psychoses have in their pathogenesis alterations in dopamine transmission in different brain regions.

Dopamine receptors can be divided to 2 distinct families: D1-like family (D1 and D5), and D2-like family (D2, D3 and D4). These G protein-coupled receptors are spread throughout the brain and play important roles in cognition, arousal, reward-related functions, craving mechanisms, memory, learning, and even hormonal release. The receptors can be also found outside the central nervous system, the examples being heart, blood vessels and kidney (Besser, Ganor, & Levite, 2005; Bressan & Crippa, 2005; Lovheim, 2012; Pecina et al., 2013).

Adequate dopamine transmission is essential for reward-motivated behavior in both humans and animals. Brain reward circuit is rich in dopamine receptors, and probably the most important part of this dopamine-related reward system includes the mesolimbic pathway connecting ventral tegmental area and nucleus accumbens. Mesolimbic pathway is thought to play a major role in incentive salience, a process that is responsible for formation of desire towards reward stimuli. The desire is the essence behind the development of motivation, and the motivation results in appetitive behavioral. Apart from incentive salience positive reinforcement as a form of behavior is also regulated by this pathway. During positive reinforcement, an event or stimulus that causes pleasure is associated with a preceding behavioral pattern, resulting in a the behavioral pattern to take place more often. Positive reinforcement plays a vital role in the development of addiction to psychoactive substances. Also, aversion-related cognition is thought to be, at least indirectly related to the function of mesolimbic pathway (Bressan & Crippa, 2005; Pecina et al., 2013).

Another important dopaminergic pathway with impact on emotional functioning is a mesocortical pathway. It associates ventral tegmental area with the prefrontal cortex. Prefrontal cortex is not a homogenous region of the brain, but it is rather functionally divided into smaller units. Dorsolateral prefrontal cortex may have role in cognitive functioning both physiologically and during various mental disorders. On the other hand, ventromedial prefrontal cortex may have a substantial modulatory effects on mood and affective responses. For example, in schizophrenia, affective symptoms such as reduced emotional responsiveness, reduced interest and reduced social drive, may be the consequence of the dopamine-related dysfunction of the ventromedial prefrontal cortex (Stahl, 2013).

It is possible that the main role of dopamine in mood regulation is providing the capacity of the brain to feel and adequately interpret pleasurable stimuli. In other words, feelings of happiness, joy, as well as self-confidence and enthusiasm for everyday activities may be at least partially associated to dopamine transmission. Reduced positive affect which includes inability to experiance pleasure (anhedonia), loss of joy, reduced alertness and energy frequently occurs during depression. In these cases administration of antidepressive medications which increase dopamine transmission might be a good strategy, however this assumption needs confirmation in future research (Stahl, 2013).

Indeed, there are medications that exhibit their activity, at least partially, through the increase of dopamine transmission. The example could include bupropion (marketed as Wellbutrin and Zyban) which is a commonly prescribed antidepressant. Bupropion is a norepinephrine-dopamine reuptake inhibitor (NDRI) and acts by inhibiting dopamine transporter and norepinephrine transporter on the cell membrane consequently increasing the concentrations of both neurotransmitters in the synaptic cleft. There are indications that bupropion may be effective in treating the depression-related reduction of positive affect in cases when conventional antidepressants (selective serotonin reuptake inhibitors SSRIs) fail to do so (Demyttenaere & Jaspers, 2008; Dhillon, Yang, & Curran, 2008; Patel et al., 2016).

Some selective serotonin reuptake inhibitors may also have an effect on dopamine transmission as well. The example would include sertraline (commonly marketed as Zoloft), which in some countries is one of the most frequently prescribed antidepressants. To which extent sertraline is effective in positive affect enhancement remains unclear. The issue is further complicated knowing that serotonin and dopamine transmissions are often interrelated, so one neurotransmitter can influence the level of the other and vice versa in different regions of the brain.

MOOD, EMOTIONS AND BRAIN SEROTONERGIC TRANSMISSION

Serotonin (5-hydroxytryptamine, 5-HT) chemically belongs to the group of monoamine neurotransmitters and, according to some authors, might play a key role in regulation of affective responses and mood. Serotonin receptors are numerous and are distributed throughout the central nervous system as well as other tissues and organs. Serotonin is able to activate and regulate numerous intracellular signaling pathways such as the one via adenylyl cyclase and cyclic AMP. The resulting intracellular second messenger cascade influences membrane ion channel activity, gene expression and other aspects of cellular function (Albert et al., 2014; Cipriani, 2003; Drevets et al., 2007; D. R. Kim, Snell, Ewing, & O'Reardon, 2015; S. K. Kim & Jeon, 2012).

The main source of serotonin in the central nervous system are the raphe nuclei which are located in the brain stem and closely associated with reticular formation. Axons of the neurons of the raphe nuclei reach the majority of brain regions. The raphe nuclei can be divided into two major groups: the caudal (raphe pallidus nucleus, raphe obscurus nucleus, lateral medullary reticular formation, and nucleus raphe magnus) and the rostral group (the dorsal raphe nuclei, the median raphe nuclei and the caudal linear nuclei). The exact impact of each of the mentioned nuclei on mood and emotions is unclear.

Most of the evidence for the role of serotonin in mood and emotions, is centered around the drugs that increase serotonergic transmission and their effectiveness in the treatment of depression. Selective serotonin reuptake inhibitors, as previously mentioned, inhibit the protein pump (serotonin transporter) that evacuates the neurotransmitter from the synaptic cleft. This way, serotonin stays longer in the cleft and exhibits its activity on the receptors located on postsynaptic membrane. Some commonly used antidepressants with this dominant mechanism of action include Citalopram (Celexa), Escitalopram (Lexapro), Paroxetine (Paxil), Sertraline (Zoloft), Fluoxetine (Prozac) and Fluvoxamine (Luvox).These are currently ones of the most commonly used medications for the treatment of not only major depression, but also various anxiety disorders (generalized anxiety disorder, panic disorder etc). Many other medications applied in contemporary psychiatry for the treatment of affective and anxiety disorders, although not officially belonging to the SSRI group, also may increase serotonergic brain transmission, sometimes by blocking the serotonin transporter, and sometimes by some other molecular mechanism (Stahl, 2013).

However, it should be noted that many issues regarding the molecular activity and pharmacodynamics of SSRIs remain unclear. For example, SSRIs do not exhibit their action only on serotonin transported. As mentioned before, sertraline also blocks dopamine reuptake. Fluoxetine is also (a relatively weak) norepinephrine reuptake inhibitor (blocks norepinephrine transporter). Paroxetine also has certain anticholinergic activity (blocks M1 receptor) and also inhibits the enzyme nitric oxide synthetase.

It is possible that serotonin action (and dysfunction) is related to the features (and symptoms) of negative affect. Dysphoric mood during depression, fear and anxiety as symptoms of some depressed patients, as well as irritability, hostility and other negative experiences may be related to serotonin receptor/neurotransmitter dysfunction. The same goes to the feeling of loneliness that occurs (often without an obvious reason) during depression. This characteristic of serotonin as a neurotransmitter is contrary to dopamine, whose lack is connected to the reduced positive affect, as mentioned earlier. Therefore, it may be possible that in depressed patients with the predominant symptoms of increased negative affect, SSRIs might be more effective than dopamine reuptake inhibitors. Nevertheless, this is only an assumption and needs to be further investigated and confirmed (Cipriani, 2003; Padovan, 2013).

The most important metabolite of serotonin is 5-Hydroxyindoleacetic acid (5-HIAA). Its creation is catalyzed by Monoamine oxidases (MAO) and aldehyde dehydrogenase. It can be measured in urine (24-hour urine samples) and is a valuable indicator of serotonin concentrations in the human/animal organism. This compound is also present and can be measured in cerebrospinal fluid. Both in bipolar and unipolar depression patients, there are indications that cerebrospinal levels of 5-HIAA are decreased, however, some authors failed to reach this conclusion. Thus, it is still unknown if this metabolite can be used as an effective biological marker of depression. Reduction of 5-HIAA in cerebrospinal fluid has also been associated with suicidal behavior, as well as aggression (Stahl, 2013).

Increasing or decreasing brain serotonin levels does not necessarily lead to changes in affective behavior. The same goes to the levels of serotonin outside the central nervous system. This is a recently developed hypothesis, and it is contrary to the previous belief that serotonergic system is the main contributor to mood and emotions. For example, a study by Mariana Angoa-Pérez and associates, published in 2014 in ACS Chem Neurosci described the experiments on mice lacking the gene for tryptophan hydroxylase 2, a rate-limiting enzyme in the serotonin synthesis in the brain. Behavioral tests done on these animals (i.e. forced swim test, sucrose preference test, or tail suspension test) produced very similar results as in wild-type controls. The same was the case with responses to unpredictable chronic mild stress. This study, along with others challenged the established paradigm of serotonin as the main factor in emotional regulation and depression pathogenesis(Angoa-Perez et al., 2014).

Normal levels of serotonin in prefrontal cortex may be important for developing and sustaining behavioural self-control. This is particularly the case with orbitofrontal cortex. Serotonergic dysfunction (low levels of serotonin) in this part of the central nervous system has been linked to aggressive behavior. The aggression could be the result of the loss of impulse control. However, the studies on the connection between serotonin and impulsive (and non-impulsive) aggression have been done a relatively low samples without reaching the definite conclusions, so additional research on this subject will be needed in the future.

There is a common belief that diet rich in serotonin and its precursor, amino acid tryptophan, can have a positive impact on emotions and mood. Some such foods include bananas, turkey, nuts, seeds and dairy. However, there is little evidence that increasing serotonin intake through food can increase the its brain levels since it is doubtful that serotonin can pass through the blood-brain barrier. Also, increasing tryptophan in plasma (by food intake) is doubtful to be a significant contributor to the serotonin synthesis in the brain tissue.

It is suggested that physical activity and exercise have beneficiary role in depressed subjects, and the main mechanism of this effect may be the increase in brain serotonin transmission. Motor activation may have the positive effect on both the impulse frequencies in serotonergic neurons, and on the rate of serotonin synthesis. However, it is still unknown if this effect is the result of the direct influence of motor activation on serotonergic system, or if this is done indirectly, through the activity of noradrenergic, or even dopaminergic pathways.

Norepinephrine, Mood and Emotions

Norepinephrine (noradrenaline) belongs to the family of catecholamines (the family also includes epinephrine and dopamine), and is both a neurotransmitter and a hormone. Apart from brain transmission and regulation of neurological functions, outside of brain, it is also vital for blood pressure regulation, gastrointestinal motility, metabolism, and immune system functioning. It also plays a major role in sympathetic nervous system (Bradley & Lenox-Smith, 2013; Leonard, 1997; Lovheim, 2012).

In the central nervous system, probably the location with the highest concentration of norepinephrine is pons and its locus coeruleus nucleus which is responsible for the majority of norepinephrine production in the brain. Locus coeruleus is located close to the lateral floor of the fourth ventricle in rostral part of the pons. Its projections are numerous and reach other parts of the brain stem (including parts of the serotonergic system), thalamus, hypothalamus, corpus amygdaloideum, cerebellum, as well as various cortical areas. It gets inputs from hypothalamus, prefrontal cortex, nucleus paragigantocellularis, and other brain regions and nuclei. Locus coeruleus is an important part of reticular activating system which is responsible for regulating wakefulness and sleep-wake cycles. Alertness, attention, arousal and many other brain functions may be directly or indirectly regulated from the activity of locus coeruleus neurons (Bradley & Lenox-Smith, 2013; Leonard, 1997; Lovheim, 2012).

The (adrenergic) receptors for norepinephrine are located on the surface of the cell membranes. They are grouped into 2 families: alpha and beta. Alpha family consists of alpha-1 (Gq-coupled, increases inositol triphosphate as the second messenger), alpha-2 (Gi/Go-coupled, decrease cyclic adenosine monophosphate as the second messenger). Beta family consists of beta-1, beta-2, and beta-3, they are all Gs-coupled, and increase intracellular cyclic adenosine monophosphate. In the central nervous system these receptors are mostly excitatory. Alpha-2 are often located on presynaptic membranes and act as a part of negative feedback loop in which the excess norepinephrine inhibits its own release. Dysfunction of norepinephrine receptors has been implicated as a potential contributing factor to many neurological and psychiatric diseases.

Serotonin–norepinephrine reuptake inhibitors (SNRIs) were shown to be particularly effective in mood disorders. Unlike classical SSRI medications, they also increase the levels of norepinephrine in the synaptic cleft by inhibiting norepinephrine transporter (NET). Today, the most commonly used SNRIs are Venlafaxine (Effexor), Duloxetine (Cymbalta), Milnacipran (Ixel, Savella, Impulsor) and Desvenlafaxine (Pristiq). The efficiency of these drugs is comparable to SSRIs, as are the potential side effects. Apart from treating major depression, they can also be applied as a therapeutic strategy for a variety of anxiety disorders, as well as attention-deficit hyperactivity disorder (Venlafaxine) and chronic neuropathic pain (Bradley & Lenox-Smith, 2013).

A specific class of medications with an impact on norepinephrine brain transmission includes noradrenergic and specific serotonergic antidepressants (NaSSAs), the common example being Mirtazapine, marketed under the brand name Remeron. Mirtazapine is a potent antidepressant which acts as an antagonist of serotonin 5-HT2A and 5-HT2C receptors. Apart from its serotonergic action, it antagonizes the α2-adrenergic receptor. As mentioned before, α2-adrenergic receptor is inhibitory in nature, it is located on a presynaptic membrane, and acts as a part of negative feedback loop that controls (inhibits) the excess release of norepinephrine. By blocking this receptor, a NaSSA drug indirectly increases norepinephrine system activity (Stahl, 2013).

Noradrenergic and serotonergic transmission systems in the brain are interrelated on many levels, and many facts on these interactions are unknown. For example increasing the activity of α1 adrenoceptors can increase the serotonergic activity. Also, blocking α2-adrenergic receptors can increase the rate of firing in serotonergic neurons. So, in essence the effectiveness of NaSSAs and SNRIs in depression treatment does not necessarily mean that depression is (even partially) the result of dysfunction of noradrenergic pathways in limbic system or other brain regions.

CONCLUDING REMARKS

The neurophysiological basis of mood and emotions is today a focus of many research efforts often with conflicting results. The precise physiological mechanisms of emotional regulation remain elusive and unclear. Neurotransmitters such as dopamine, serotonin and norepinephrine have been suggested as one of the most important modulators of emotional responses and their dysfunction may be a contributing factor in the pathogenesis of mood disorders. However, it is doubtful that a complex psychic function such as emotions, or a mental disorder such as depression, can be explained merely based on a chemical interaction of mediators/neurotransmitters and their receptors. In the future, additional research is needed to provide us with a more detailed scientific insight on these issues.

ACKNOWLEDGMENT

The author is grateful to the project 92018 of the Mediterranean Society for Metabolic Syndrome, Diabetes and Hypertension in Pregnancy DEGU (Dr. Igor V. Pantic, principal author of this manuscript, is the Head of the project), as well as to the projects of the Ministry of Education and Science, Republic of Serbia (projects 175059 and 41027). Prof. Igor V. Pantic is also grateful to National Science Foundation's Center for Advanced Knowledge Enablement, Miami, FL, USA (I. Pantic is an external research associate). The authors are also grateful to Tatijana D. Paunovic, MA from University of Craiova, for her valuable help for English translation proof reading and writing of manuscript.

REFERENCES

Albert, P. R., Vahid-Ansari, F., & Luckhart, C. (2014). Serotonin-prefrontal cortical circuitry in anxiety and depression phenotypes: Pivotal role of pre- and post-synaptic 5-HT1A receptor expression. *Frontiers in Behavioral Neuroscience*, *8*, 199. doi:10.3389/fnbeh.2014.00199 PMID:24936175

Andersen, P. (2007). *The Hippocampus Book*. London, UK: Oxford University Press.

Angoa-Perez, M., Kane, M. J., Briggs, D. I., Herrera-Mundo, N., Sykes, C. E., Francescutti, D. M., & Kuhn, D. M. (2014). Mice genetically depleted of brain serotonin do not display a depression-like behavioral phenotype. *ACS Chemical Neuroscience*, *5*(10), 908–919. doi:10.1021/cn500096g PMID:25089765

Berlim, M. T., McGirr, A., Van den Eynde, F., Fleck, M. P., & Giacobbe, P. (2014). Effectiveness and acceptability of deep brain stimulation (DBS) of the subgenual cingulate cortex for treatment-resistant depression: A systematic review and exploratory meta-analysis. *Journal of Affective Disorders*, *159*, 31–38. doi:10.1016/j.jad.2014.02.016 PMID:24679386

Bersani, F. S., Minichino, A., Fojanesi, M., Gallo, M., Maglio, G., Valeriani, G., ... Fitzgerald, P. B. (2014). Cingulate Cortex in Schizophrenia: Its relation with negative symptoms and psychotic onset. A review study. *European Review for Medical and Pharmacological Sciences*, *18*(22), 3354–3367. PMID:25491609

Besser, M. J., Ganor, Y., & Levite, M. (2005). Dopamine by itself activates either D2, D3 or D1/D5 dopaminergic receptors in normal human T-cells and triggers the selective secretion of either IL-10, TNFalpha or both. *Journal of Neuroimmunology*, *169*(1-2), 161–171. doi:10.1016/j.jneuroim.2005.07.013 PMID:16150496

Bradley, A. J., & Lenox-Smith, A. J. (2013). Does adding noradrenaline reuptake inhibition to selective serotonin reuptake inhibition improve efficacy in patients with depression? A systematic review of meta-analyses and large randomised pragmatic trials. *Journal of Psychopharmacology (Oxford, England)*, *27*(8), 740–758. doi:10.1177/0269881113494937 PMID:23832963

Bressan, R. A., & Crippa, J. A. (2005). The role of dopamine in reward and pleasure behaviour--review of data from preclinical research. *Acta Psychiatrica Scandinavica. Supplementum*, *111*(427), 14–21. doi:10.1111/j.1600-0447.2005.00540.x PMID:15877719

Cannon, R. C., Wheal, H. V., & Turner, D. A. (1999). Dendrites of classes of hippocampal neurons differ in structural complexity and branching patterns. *The Journal of Comparative Neurology*, *413*(4), 619–633. doi:10.1002/(SICI)1096-9861(19991101)413:4<619::AID-CNE10>3.0.CO;2-B PMID:10495447

Cannon, W. B. (1987). The James-Lange theory of emotions: A critical examination and an alternative theory. By Walter B. Cannon, 1927. *The American Journal of Psychology*, *100*(3-4), 567–586. doi:10.2307/1422695 PMID:3322057

Cipriani, A. (2003). Review: Selective serotonin reuptake inhibitors as effective as tricyclic antidepressants for major depression, and may have fewer adverse effects. *Evidence-Based Mental Health*, *6*(4), 117. doi:10.1136/ebmh.6.4.117 PMID:14585790

Demyttenaere, K., & Jaspers, L. (2008). Review: Bupropion and SSRI-induced side effects. *Journal of Psychopharmacology (Oxford, England)*, *22*(7), 792–804. doi:10.1177/0269881107083798 PMID:18308785

Dhillon, S., Yang, L. P., & Curran, M. P. (2008). Bupropion: A review of its use in the management of major depressive disorder. *Drugs*, *68*(5), 653–689. doi:10.2165/00003495-200868050-00011 PMID:18370448

Drevets, W. C., Thase, M. E., Moses-Kolko, E. L., Price, J., Frank, E., Kupfer, D. J., & Mathis, C. (2007). Serotonin-1A receptor imaging in recurrent depression: Replication and literature review. *Nuclear Medicine and Biology*, *34*(7), 865–877. doi:10.1016/j.nucmedbio.2007.06.008 PMID:17921037

Haller, J. (2018). The role of central and medial amygdala in normal and abnormal aggression: A review of classical approaches. *Neuroscience and Biobehavioral Reviews*, *85*, 34–43. doi:10.1016/j.neubiorev.2017.09.017 PMID:28918358

Hayman, L. A., Fuller, G. N., Cavazos, J. E., Pfleger, M. J., Meyers, C. A., & Jackson, E. F. (1998). The hippocampus: Normal anatomy and pathology. *AJR. American Journal of Roentgenology, 171*(4), 1139–1146. doi:10.2214/ajr.171.4.9763010 PMID:9763010

Kim, D. R., Snell, J. L., Ewing, G. C., & O'Reardon, J. (2015). Neuromodulation and antenatal depression: A review. *Neuropsychiatric Disease and Treatment, 11*, 975–982. doi:10.2147/NDT.S80480 PMID:25897234

Kim, S. K., & Jeon, S. (2012). Simultaneous determination of serotonin and dopamine at the PEDOP/MWCNTs-Pd nanoparticle modified glassy carbon electrode. *Journal of Nanoscience and Nanotechnology, 12*(3), 1903–1909. doi:10.1166/jnn.2012.5169 PMID:22754997

Leonard, B. E. (1997). The role of noradrenaline in depression: A review. *Journal of Psychopharmacology (Oxford, England), 11*(4Suppl), S39–S47. PMID:9438232

Lovheim, H. (2012). A new three-dimensional model for emotions and monoamine neurotransmitters. *Medical Hypotheses, 78*(2), 341–348. doi:10.1016/j.mehy.2011.11.016 PMID:22153577

Mohammadi, S., Haghir, H., Fazel, A. R., & Vafaei, A. (2013). Analysis of Amygdala Nucleus in the Rat Brain: A review study. *Electronic Physician, 5*(2), 639–642. doi:10.14661/2013.639-642 PMID:26120396

Nicholson, D. A., & Geinisman, Y. (2009). Axospinous synaptic subtype-specific differences in structure, size, ionotropic receptor expression, and connectivity in apical dendritic regions of rat hippocampal CA1 pyramidal neurons. *The Journal of Comparative Neurology, 512*(3), 399–418. doi:10.1002/cne.21896 PMID:19006199

Padovan, C. M. (2013). Serotonin in anxiety and depression. *Journal of Psychopharmacology (Oxford, England), 27*(12), 1083. doi:10.1177/0269881113508831 PMID:24227796

Pantic, I., Dacic, S., Brkic, P., Lavrnja, I., Jovanovic, T., Pantic, S., & Pekovic, S. (2015). Discriminatory ability of fractal and grey level co-occurrence matrix methods in structural analysis of hippocampus layers. *Journal of Theoretical Biology, 370*, 151–156. doi:10.1016/j.jtbi.2015.01.035 PMID:25665716

Patel, K., Allen, S., Haque, M. N., Angelescu, I., Baumeister, D., & Tracy, D. K. (2016). Bupropion: A systematic review and meta-analysis of effectiveness as an antidepressant. *Therapeutic Advances in Psychopharmacology*, *6*(2), 99–144. doi:10.1177/2045125316629071 PMID:27141292

Pauc, R., & Young, A. (2010). Little-known neurons of the medial wall: A literature review of pyramidal cells of the cingulate gyrus. *Journal of Chiropractic Medicine*, *9*(3), 115–120. doi:10.1016/j.jcm.2010.05.001 PMID:22027033

Pecina, M., Mickey, B. J., Love, T., Wang, H., Langenecker, S. A., Hodgkinson, C., ... Zubieta, J. K. (2013). DRD2 polymorphisms modulate reward and emotion processing, dopamine neurotransmission and openness to experience. *Cortex*, *49*(3), 877–890. doi:10.1016/j.cortex.2012.01.010 PMID:22424959

Rogers, M. A., Kasai, K., Koji, M., Fukuda, R., Iwanami, A., Nakagome, K., ... Kato, N. (2004). Executive and prefrontal dysfunction in unipolar depression: A review of neuropsychological and imaging evidence. *Neuroscience Research*, *50*(1), 1–11. doi:10.1016/j.neures.2004.05.003 PMID:15288493

Schachter, D. (2013). *The source of toxicity in CTAB and CTAB/stabilized gold nanorods: Rutgers*. New Brunswick, NJ: The State University of New Jersey.

Stahl, S. M. (2013). *Stahl's Essential Psychopharmacology: Neuroscientific Basis and Practical Applications*. New York: Cambridge University Press.

Young, K. D., Zotev, V., Phillips, R., Misaki, M., Drevets, W. C., & Bodurka, J. (2018). Amygdala Real-Time fMRI Neurofeedback for Major Depressive Disorder: A Review. *Psychiatry and Clinical Neurosciences*. doi:10.1111/pcn.12665

Chapter 4
Chronic Stress and Chronic Pain:
Disability After Trauma and Global Trends

Branislav Starcevic
Clinic for Orthopaedic Surgery and Traumatology, Clinical Center of Serbia, Serbia

ABSTRACT

Pain and stress basically overlap in conceptual and physiological perceptions. Chronic stress and chronic pain share a common behavioral model of failure to extinguish negative memories as one of psychological and physiological mechanisms of defense. They also have discrepancies such that the final brain endophenotype of posttraumatic stress disorder (PTSD), depression, and chronic pain appears to be different among the three conditions, and the role of the hypothalamic-pituitary-adrenal axis remains unclear in the physiology of pain. Persistence of either stress or pain is maladaptive and could lead to compromised homeostasis. The effectiveness of interventions that may increase return to work and patient satisfaction in trauma victims should be a future directive of research.

DOI: 10.4018/978-1-5225-7513-9.ch004

INTRODUCTION

The concept of pain has remained a topic of long debate since its emergence in ancient times. It is considered that the initial ideas about pain as a new entity were defined before 1800. Since then, different theories of pain have emerged and become central topics of debate. The existing theories of pain may be appropriate for the interpretation of some aspects of pain, but the history of pain problems is as long as that of human beings and the understanding of pain mechanisms is still far from very well defined and requires extensive research.

Modern theories sought a consensus definition for pain, and in 1975, the International Association for the Study of Pain defined the pain as "an unpleasant sensory and emotional experience associated with actual or potential tissue damage, or described in terms of such damage".(IASP,2011)

As a physical phenomenon, the emotional state of a person, as well as the context or situation associated with the pain also impacts the perception of the nociceptive or noxious event. For example, if a human experiences a painful event associated with any form of trauma a reoccurrence of similar physical pain will not only inflict physical trauma but also the emotional and mental trauma first associated with the painful event. That was a basic hypothesis primarily for defining the concept of posttraumatic stress disorder (PTSD). Research has shown that should a similar injury occur to two people, one person who associates large emotional consequence to the pain and the other person who does not, the person who associates a large consequence on the pain event will feel a more intense physical pain that the person who does not associate a large emotional consequence with the pain.

Acute pain with its unpleasant features plays an important role in protecting the body from potential injury and represents the characteristic evolutionarily created with the aim of survival. Painful sensation promotes a change in actions and behavior which could stop any further injury. On the other hand, chronic pain represents a pathologic condition which neither serves the defense of the organism nor is it harmless. By the International Association for the Study of Pain (IASP), the pain is considered to be chronic when it lasts or recurs for more than 3 to 6 months(Chadi,2017)

It is estimated that chronic pain affects about 20% of people worldwide3-6 and its treatment is considered to be a significant unmet therapeutic need.

The link between stress and chronic pain is a well known but this interaction still demands further investigation. It is possible that there are common central mechanisms that facilitate both stress and nociception. Investigation of this relationship that exist between stress and nociception could possibly lead us to the atypical approach in pain treatment (Ponsford,2008).

In this text the author aimed to give the overview of pain pathways and pain matrix, discuss the potential mechanisms that underlies transformation of pain from acute to chronic form and to point out the key site of action of the currently available medications. Special attention will be devoted to the reports of so far conducted investigations supporting and explaining potential synergistic mechanisms of stress and chronic pain, pointing out the direction for further investigations in search of more effective drugs or treatments for chronic pain.

Pain is a multidimensional sensation comprising sensory information, affective processing and a cognitive-evaluative component. Furthermore, pain leads to changes in autonomic body functions such as blood pressure, heart frequency. Pain perception can be substantially altered in different psychiatric disorders.

Experimental studies have described different mechanisms for altered pain perception and processing in several psychiatric disorders. Pain and stress basically overlap in conceptual and physiological perceptions. Chronic stress and chronic pain share a common behavioral model of failure to extinguish negative memories as one of psychological and physiological mechanisms of defense. They also have discrepancies such that the final brain endophenotype of posttraumatic stress disorder (PTSD), depression, and chronic pain appears to be different among the three conditions, and the role of the hypothalamic-pituitary-adrenal axis remains unclear in the physiology of pain. Persistence of either stress or pain is maladaptive and could lead to compromised homeostasis.(Chadi, 2017)

Neuroanatomical morphological supstrate assumed to be involved in pain processing and perception id dorsolateral prefrontal cortex(DLPFC). As previously mentioned, depression presents the final endophenotype of posttraumatic stress disorder. Depression is suppose to be overlapping in a majority of times when it is difficult to distinguish between PTSD and depression differentially in final diagnostic. Patients psychological characteristics induce the prevalence of PTSD morbidity as well as coping mechanisms. Neurophysiologically, in depression, reduced activity of the dorsolateral prefrontal cortex is found to be involved in psychomotoric slowdown and attention and memory deficit. Also a positive correlation is found to exist with the severity of trauma and pain perception.

The explanation of the reduced pain perception in depression lies in cognitive deficit of pain processing stimuli, and manages the visualisation of the hyperstimulation of this brain area.

Amygdala presents grey matter which activity is increased in depression, but decreased activity is shown in healthy patients when experiencing pain.

Stress is often described as a feeling of being overwhelmed. Stress can affect people of all ages, genders and circumstances and can lead to both physical and psychological health issues. Stress presents any uncomfortable emotional experience accompanied by predictable biochemical, physiological and behavioral changes.(Baum, 1990; Anderson, 2003)

Chronic stress can occur in response to everyday stressors that are ignored or poorly managed, as well as to exposure to traumatic events. The consequences of chronic stress could be very serious, particularly if it induces to anxiety and depression.

Chronic or ongoing pain includes several symptoms and conditions, including acute posttraumatic pain, depression, hostility, anxiety, sleep and rest disturbances (Castillo, 2006). In a study of Duivenvoorden et al., they found a high prevalence of anxiety and depressive symptoms in a population with end-stage hip and knee Osteoarthritis. After surgery a significant decrease of the prevalence of anxiety and depressive symptoms for both hip and knee patients was seen. In hip as well as knee patients, preoperative depressive symptoms predicted a lower Patient Reported Outcomes after surgery. Hip and knee patients with preoperative anxiety or depressive symptoms were less satisfied postoperatively. Because of the close relationship between psychological symptoms and pain and disability, the prevalence of psychological symptoms would be high in end-stage hip and knee Osteoarthritis patients. Preoperatively higher prevalence of depressive symptoms was found in hip than in knee Osteoarthritis patients. And that might be a result of the difference in ability to perform their activities of daily living preoperatively (Duivenvoorden,2103). Many trauma patients suffer from long term impairments, disabilities and handicaps, and at least half of all major trauma patients are left with one or more residual problems. Therefore, understanding the determinants of long-term functional consequences following trauma is important in order to improve the chances of a patient's recovery (Ponsord,2008). Trauma has been proposed as a causal factor or trigger of chronic or persistent pain.

Work disability due to chronic pain is estimated to be four times more than productivity lost due to lost workdays alone (Castillo, 2006). The results of the prevalence and early predictors of chronic pain of major lower extremity trauma patients, present that more than a quarter of the study group reported that their pain highly interfered with daily activities (Clay et al., 2010). Pain also has other consequences for its victims, including psychological regression (Clay et al, 2010). Those who suffer from chronic pain also use five times more health services than the general population (Castillo, 2006). As surgeons, we know that pain is an inevitable result of traumatic injury and the accompanying healing process. However, why do patients continue to endure pain long after they have been treated?

CONCLUSION

The biomedical model of health focuses on pain as the result of a physical injury (Clay et al., 2010). This makes it difficult to clinically explain the presence of disability after the pathology related to the injury has healed . Studies focusing on trauma populations suggest that factors during the course of recovery other than the injury are critical to the development of persistent pain and associated functional impairment. Such factors include high initial pain intensity, PTSD, worker's compensation status, education, low recovery expectations and depression (Clay et al., 2010). In the aforementioned study by Castillo et al. (Castillo, 2006), several early predictors of chronic pain were identified at baseline, including having less than a high school education, having less than a college education, low self efficacy for return to daily activities, and high levels of alcohol consumption. In addition, high reported acute pain intensity, sleep and rest dysfunction, depression and anxiety at 3 months post discharge were found to be predictors of chronic pain at 7 years (Castillo,2006).

Return to work is defined as a complete or almost complete return to pre-injury state. Return to work may represent the level of appropriate successful social reintegration after minor or major trauma and therefore coming back to work surrounding may indicate the level of personal fulfilment and sense of self-worth. The effectiveness of interventions that may increase return to work and patient satisfaction in trauma victims should be a future directive of research.

REFERENCES

Abdallah & Geha. (2017). Chronic Pain and Chronic Stress: Two Sides of the Same Coin? *Chronic Stress (Thousand Oaks), 1*. doi:10.1177/2470547017704763

Anderson, N. B., & Anderson, P. E. (2003). *Emotional Longevity: what really determines how long you live*. New York: Viking.

Baum, A. (1990). Stress, Intrusive Imagery, and Chronic Distress. *Health Psychology, 6*(6), 653–675. doi:10.1037/0278-6133.9.6.653 PMID:2286178

Castillo, R. C., MacKenzie, E. J., Wegener, S. T., & Bosse, M. J. (2006). Prevalence of chronic pain seven years following limb threatening lower extremity trauma. *Pain, 124*(3), 321–329. doi:10.1016/j.pain.2006.04.020 PMID:16781066

Clay, F. J., Newstead, S. V., Watson, W. L., Ozanne-Smith, J., Guy, J., & McClure, R. J. (2010). Bio-psychosocial determinants of persistent pain 6 months after non-life-threatening acute orthopaedic trauma. *The Journal of Pain, 11*(5), 420–423. doi:10.1016/j.jpain.2009.12.002 PMID:20439055

Duivenvoorden, T. (2013). Anxiety and depressive symptoms before and after total hip and knee arthroplasty: a prospective multicentre study. *Osteoarthritis and Cartilage, 21*, 1834-1840.

International Association for the Study of Pain. (2011). *IASP Taxonomy*. International Association for the Study of Pain.

MacKenzie, E. J., Morris, J. A. Jr, Jurkovich, G. J., Yasui, Y., Cushing, B. M., Burgess, A. R., ... Swiontkowski, M. F. (1998). Return to work following injury: The role of economic, social, and job- related factors. *American Journal of Public Health, 88*(11), 1630–1637. doi:10.2105/AJPH.88.11.1630 PMID:9807528

Ponsford, J., Hill, B., Karamitsios, M., & Bahar-Fuchs, A. (2008). Factors infl uencing outcome after orthopedic trauma. *The Journal of Trauma, 64*(4), 1001–1009. doi:10.1097/TA.0b013e31809fec16 PMID:18404068

Chapter 5
Orthopedic Trauma and Post-Traumatic Stress Disorder:
Stress Disorder Associated With Trauma Injuries

Branislav Starcevic
Clinic for Orthopaedic Surgery and Traumatology, Clinical Center of Serbia, Serbia

ABSTRACT

Little is known about the clinical consequences of psychological morbidity associated with orthopedic trauma. Anxiety disorders, depression, bipolar disorder, schizophrenia, and personality disorders may all occur during the postoperative period. There are no currently clearly defined relations between orthopedic injuries and PTSD, but undoubtedly, we can say that, depending on the personality traits, one can develop PTSD if the orthopedics trauma triggers and induce PTSD in individuals, and that should be one of the main future perspectives and goals of investigative studies. The effectiveness of prevention strategies that could be developed through psychiatrists and orthopedic surgeon cooperation strategies as well as developing strategies when PTSD occur postoperatively should also be one of the main targets in the near future, as PTSD as an entity presents one of the greatest disability factors in society producibility nowadays, which is also very important from the economy perspective.

DOI: 10.4018/978-1-5225-7513-9.ch005

INTRODUCTION

Posttraumatic stress disorder (PTSD) is also common after surgery, especially after traumatic injuries, but most important very often underrecognized and undertreated and orthopaedic surgeon must remain aware of their possible effect. McCarthy further identified a high correlation between the Brief Symptom Inventory (a measure of psychological distress) and the Sickness Impact Profile (a measure of patient function). A high index of suspicion for the presence of psychiatric disorders is important in treating the orthopaedic patient with multiple trauma, chronic disease, factitious disorder, or suspected malingering or who fails to improve with recognized treatment. Recognition of a psychiatric problem should be part of preoperative planning in orthopaedic practice, and a formal psychiatric referral for diagnosis and treatment should be made for the patient with significant psychiatric involvement. When associated psychiatric disease is diagnosed and controlled before orthopaedic treatment, the patient is more likely to comply with the treatment regimen, which may lead to better results and less incidence of bad postoperative time. It is of a great importance to have a rapid screening for psychiatric disorders as part of the health assessment. And all that as a precaution in aim for patients to attain maximal functional recovery. Presence of a positive psychiatric history or a current psychiatric disorder should present a sign for a professional both orthopaedist and psychiatrist to treat these patients in an appropriate way with adequate emotional and therapeutic approach and treatment.

Not only most commonly connected with military combat, post-traumatic stress disorder can occur in civilians with consequences that are just as serious. Posttraumatic stress disorder is a type of anxiety disorder that occurs after a person experiences a traumatic event involving physical injury, and occurs in patients with an orthopedic injury. According to Daniel Aaron, MD, clinical instructor in the department of orthopedics at Brown University, PTSD occurs with a significant frequency in civilian patients who have sustained an orthopedic trauma and it can hinder their emotional, physical and functional recovery following orthopedic treatment. He also said that higher-energy mechanisms are most commonly associated with PTSD, but no specific type of fracture or injury has been identified for itself, so any type of musculoskeletal injury that results from significant trauma may be associated with PTSD. Many types of accidents can cause PTSD, including car or motorcycle accidents, gunshot wounds, vehicle-pedestrian accidents and falls from height. PTSD can have a significant impact on a patient's ability to perform simple, daily chores and can slow the rehabilitation process, even affecting how the patient experiences pain and perceives his or her recovery. A diagnosis of PTSD relies on the presence of specific behaviors or symptoms, including traumatic event reexperiencing, avoidance reminiscent of trauma origins, irritability, agitation, insomnia. There are no currently clearly defined relations between orthopedic injuries and PTSD, but undoubtedly, we can say that depend on the personality traits one can develop PTSD or not if the orthopedic trauma triggers and induces PTSD in individual and that should be one of the main future perspectives and goals of our investigation studies. The effectiveness of prevention strategies which could be develop through psychiatrists and orthopedic surgeons cooperation strategies as well as developing strategies when PTSD occur postoperatively should also be one of the main targets in the near future, as PTSD as an entity presents one of the greatest disability factors in society producibility nowadays, which is also very important from the economy perspective.

Psychological condition of the patient is among the most important parameters that predict one's good postoperative period and well being of the patient. Early recognition and treatment of possible psychological morbidity is significant due to prevention of long term disabilities in orthopedic patients. As one of the representations of the previous mentioned is an alteration in an individual's body image set up a series of emotional, perceptual and psychological reactions.

Stress is recognized as an important factor affecting any kind of performance and activity. Little is known about the clinical consequences of psychological morbidity associated with orthopedic trauma. Anxiety disorders, depression, bipolar disorder, schizophrenia, and personality disorders may all occur during the postoperative period. Other common postoperative issues include complications related to alcohol abuse, dependence, and withdrawal; pain management, personality disorders as one of the causes of lack of cooperation and very common postoperative delirium.(Tudo et al., 2017)

A high index of suspicion for the presence of psychiatric disorders is important in treating the orthopedic patient with multiple trauma, chronic disease, factitious disorder, or suspected malingering or who fails to improve with recognized treatment. Recognition of a psychiatric problem should be part of preoperative planning in orthopedic practice, and a formal psychiatric referral for diagnosis and treatment should be made for the patient with significant psychiatric involvement.(Rosenberg et al,2009) When associated psychiatric disease is diagnosed and controlled before orthopedic treatment, the patient is more likely to comply with the treatment regimen, which may lead to better results and less incidence of bad postoperative time. It is of a great importance to have a rapid screening for psychiatric disorders as part of the health assessment. And all that as a precaution in aim for patients to attain maximal functional recovery. Presence of a positive psychiatric history or a current psychiatric disorder should present a sign for a professional both orthopedist and psychiatrist to treat these patients in an appropriate way with adequate emotional and therapeutic approach and treatment.

Not only most commonly connected with military combat, post-traumatic stress disorder can occur in civilians with consequences that are just as serious. Posttraumatic stress disorder is a type of anxiety disorder that occurs after a person experiences a traumatic event involving physical injury, and occurs in patients with an orthopedic injury. According to Daniel Aaron, MD, clinical instructor in the department of orthopedics at Brown University, PTSD occurs with a significant frequency in civilian patients who have sustained an orthopedic trauma and it can hinder their emotional, physical and functional recovery following orthopedic treatment. He also said that higher-energy mechanisms are most commonly associated with PTSD, but no specific type of fracture or injury has been identified for itself, so any type of musculoskeletal injury that results from significant trauma may be associated with PTSD. Many types of accidents can cause PTSD, including car or motorcycle accidents, gunshot wounds, vehicle-pedestrian accidents and falls from height. PTSD can have a significant impact on a patient's ability to perform simple, daily chores and can slow the rehabilitation process, even affecting how the patient experiences pain and perceives his or her recovery.(Weiss, 2004) A diagnosis of PTSD relies on the presence of specific behaviors or symptoms, including traumatic event reexperiencing, avoidance reminiscent of trauma origins, irritability, agitation, insomnia. There are no currently clearly defined relations between orthopaedic injuries and PTSD, but undoubtedly we can say that depend on the personality traits one can develop PTSD or not if the orthopadic trauma triggers and induces PTSD in individual and that should be one of the main future perspectives and goals of our investigation studies.

POSTTRAUMATIC STRESS DISORDER

Posttraumatic stress disorder PTSD presents chronic, disabling anxiety disorder which can be triggered by exposure to psychological traumatic event. But, not everyone develops posttraumatic stress disorder. There could be explanation described as trauma characteristics of the individual-genetics and epigenetics, psychological skeleton of the individual and coping mechanisms.

PTSD is defined as a cluster of symptoms like reexperiencing, avoidance and hyperarousal in an individual who had undergone a traumatic event. Re-experiencing symptoms include intrusive, uncontrollable and involuntary instances of re-living the traumatic event with strong feeling of panic and fear which are followed by palpitation, sweating and muscle tension. Such intrusive experiences often occur upon exposure to cues that remind the individual of the stress event, but they can also show spontaneously as during nightmares and relaxation time as well. Avoidance presents phobic avoidance and numbing, followed by restricted range of affects, vanished interests in previously very significant activities for the individual, psychological encapsulation or estrangement from others and family.(Bremner,2016) Chronic condition leads to depression which can be overlapped with PTSD.

All these symptoms can be very determent in both preoperative and postoperative period and plan for treatment in orthopaedic surgery.

We can say that surgical expertise is very complex because it includes an interdisciplinary approach.

Posttraumatic Stress Disorder Associated With Orthopaedic Trauma Injuries

The prevalence of PTSD in civilian population is also very significant not only within the population of combat population as was defied at first. But, many previous studies have shown the incoherence and variations in methodologic factors and inhomogeneous selection of the patients such as including both man and women with a range of ages, education levels, injury severities or location and psychological variables as well. There are also very little amount of studies that were conducted and investigated the link between the PTSD and orthopaedic injuries.

One of the studies that was conducted to determine the prevalence of posttraumatic stress disorder in a group of male military with low extremity long bone fractures and to connect injury level in the mentioned group and its association with the development of PTSD, was by Chang Hoon Lee at al., and they showed that lower extremity fracture and multiple extremity fractures as well as the higher pain visual analog scale scores are related to PTSD occurrence.(Chang,2015)

Amputation of a limb affects almost all aspect of patients life and also affects in a major way the intrafamiliar relations and family dynamics and quality of life. Overall, psychological issues make a significant factor for adjustment with the disability. (Srivistava,2010)

In a manner of a previous state, there was a study conducted by Srivastava et al., in which they investigated fifty male patients from Artificial Limb Center. They comprised baseline and posttherapy assessment on HADS (Hospital Anxiety and depression scale) and used Trauma Symptom Inventory(TSI) along with Millon Index of personality styles (MIPS). They concluded significant differences in scores on HADS before and after the therapy was conducted and personality dimension very significant factor which was significant after therapy and associated with depression probably as a result of a poor coping mechanisms and adjustment to the newly situation.(Srivistava,2010)

Posttraumatic stress disorder (PTSD) is also common after surgery, especially after traumatic injuries, but most important very often underrecognized and undertreated and orthopaedic surgeon must remain aware of their possible effect. The prevalence of psychological illness following traumatic injuries varies according to the diagnostic criteria used in studies, the timing of the assessment and definitions of trauma, with psychological symptoms following musculoskeletal trauma have ranged from 6.5% to 51.0%.

A recent study of patients with severe lower limb injuries found a 42% prevalence of psychological disorder at 24-month follow-up and that only 22% of such patients reported receiving mental health services. No relation was found between injury severity and psychological distress; however, the authors suggested that low variability in injury severity might have obscured this result.(Chang,2015)

Another similar study was conducted by McCarthy et al, in which was shown that psychological distress was associated with severe lower limb injury. They enrolled 569 patients which completed Brief Symptom Inventory (BSI), self-reported measure of psychological distress and their results showed that two years after injury one fifth of the examined patients had severe phobic anxiety and depression which lead to conclusion that more attention should be paid to psychological health of patients who sustained a limb devastating injury.(McCarthy et al,2003)

Beside coping mechanisms of the patients and the psychological dimension of the personality of the patient, big roll plays support of the family and environment. There could be find a lot of data from different investigations interdisciplinary and multicentric which mention social support as one of the most important parameters in adjustment and acclimatization of the newly formed situation in a patients life. There are many comorbidities that can occur, but we can say that depression is one of them. Also, substance abuse presents one of the major risks for greater psychological distress after injury, but also, for some of the patients avoidant strategy within the coping stress mechanisms that prevent from stressful event.

CONCLUSION

Although as previously mentioned, there are not much studies that investigate the direct link between the stress as provoke factor of many comorbidity conditions after minor or major orthopedic trauma and surgery, we tried to highlight the importance of increasing the reasons for expanding the future investigations in this direction. There are no currently clearly defined relations between orthopaedic injuries and PTSD, but undoubtedly we can say that depend on the personality traits one can develop PTSD or not if the orthopadic trauma triggers and induces PTSD in individual and that should be one of the main future perspectives and goals of our investigation studies. The effectiveness of prevention strategies which could be develop through psychiatrists and orthopaedic surgeons cooperation strategies as well as developing strategies when PTSD occur postoperatively should also be one of the main targets in the near future, as PTSD as a entity presents one of the greatest disability factors in society producibility nowadays, which is also very important from the economy perspective.

REFERENCES

Bremner, J. D. (2016). Posttraumatic stress disorder from neurobiology to treatment. Wiley Blackwell.

Lee, C. H., Choi, C. H., Yoon, S.-Y., & Lee, J. K. (2015). Posttraumatic Stress Disorder Associated With Orthopaedic Trauma: A Study in Patients With Extremity Fractures. *Journal of Orthopaedic Trauma*, *29*(6), e198–e202. doi:10.1097/BOT.0000000000000255 PMID:25463428

McCarthy, M., MacKenzie, E. J., Edwin, D., Bosse, M. J., Castillo, R. C., & Starr, A. (2003). Psychological distress associated with severe lower limb injury. *JBJS*, *85-A*(9), 1689–1697. doi:10.2106/00004623-200309000-00006 PMID:12954826

Rosenberger, P. H., Ickovics, J. R., Epel, E., Nadler, E., Jokl, P., Fulkerson, J. P., ... Dhabhar, F. S. (2009). Surgical Stress-Induced Immune Cell Redistribution Profiles Predict Short-Term and Long-Term Postsurgical Recovery A Prospective Study. *The Journal of Bone and Joint Surgery. American Volume*, *91*(12), 2783–2794. doi:10.2106/JBJS.H.00989 PMID:19952239

Srivistava, K. (2010). A study of Psychological correlates after amputation. *MJAFI*, *66*, 367–373. PMID:27365745

Tudo, R. (2017). Psychological Morbidity Associated with Orthopedic Trauma. *American Journal of Psychiatry and Neuroscience*, *5*(6), 22.

Weiss, J. M., & Grunert, B. K. (2004). Posttraumatic stress disorder following traumatic injuries in adult. *Wisconsin Medical Journal*, *103*(6).

Chapter 6
Changing the Quality of Life After Therapy of Orthodontic Irregularities:
Quality of Life and Orthodontics

Mirka Stojanovic
Independent Researcher, Serbia

ABSTRACT

The effect of orthodontic therapy of different orthodontic anomalies on life quality referred to one's personality. Congenital or acquired orthodontic anomalies are a great problem of today's children and youth. Fast way of life, young mothers urging to be in top form after giving birth to a child, neglecting breastfeeding as a presumption to be the most important for the proper development of the orofacial system leads to numerous irregularities in the teeth development. Maternal deprivation and closeness deprivation, warmth deprivation, present the majority of proper children's development and their psycho-physical development. Any anomaly is evident on the face, either asymmetry, open bite with interlacing the tongue between the teeth, whether in the disorder of the face, the lowered jaw, the incongruous profile and speech disorder, breathing, etc. From the previous, the negative feelings of children and youth, depression, fall in the elimination of life, limitation of working abilities, etc. Solving them leads to joy, happiness, raising the quality of life.

DOI: 10.4018/978-1-5225-7513-9.ch006

INTRODUCTION

Since it is about growth and development and its errors, orthodontics present an important medical branch. Growth and life are synonymous and inseparable. It is a process that transforms zygote - one cell into a multicellular adult with about 12.5 trillion cells. It is a long period of time in the most vulnerable period of life. The skeleton of the head develops from the mesoderm which envelopes the brain during the development. It consists of a skeleton of neurocranium and viscerogranium. Neurocranium or chondrocranium initially consists of a cartilaginous base that is formed by merging the following cartilage: parachordal cartilage, occipital somite, hypophyseal cartilage, trabecule cranii, ala orbitalis, nasal capsules, etc. The membrane part of the neurocranium develops by intramembranosal ossification of the bone of the skull of the skull. Early basis of viscerocranium also makes cartilage tissue. Bone growth of the viscerocranium in the intrauterine period takes place in the processes of apposition and resorption, which are always associated with bone remodeling (Moss,1963)

That is why it is very important that the dynamics and proportions of the skeleton skull and face are in harmony. Like the relationship between the head and the whole body.

Movement of face height toward total body height by Krogman.

DIAGNOSTICS

Diagnostic approach is done prior to the therapy. The diagnosis is a set of symptoms and its purpose is to treat the disease or malformation causally. The main goal of orthodontic diagnostics is to recognize and evaluate morphological and functional deviations as well as deviations in the growth and development of the craniofacial complex.

The initial criterion for orthodontic diagnostics is eugnatia - the norm of occlusion. Functionally, in eugnatie, there is a dynamic balance between oral and vestibularly placed soft tissues that surround tooth jaws. Any deviation from normo-occlusion is called disgnathia or anomaly. In the diagnostic sense, we adhere to certain norms (Angle,1913).

Figure 1. Relationship of facial skull and skull size in newborn, five-year-olds and adults where the relationship between the skull and the face takes place in favor of the facial skeleton

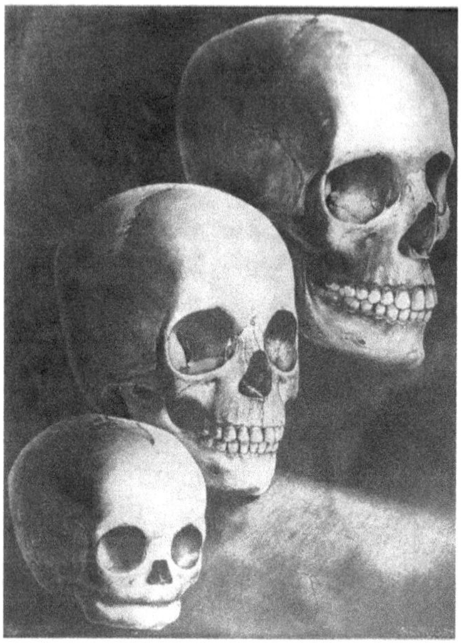

Figure 2. (A) Fourth month of fetal age, (B) Newborn, (C) Two years, (D) Five years, (E) Thirteen years, (F) Twenty-two years

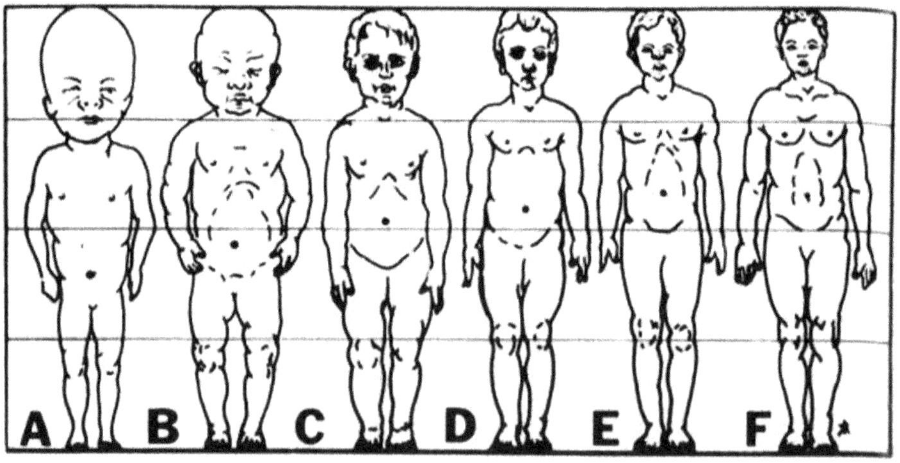

Figure 3. Angelo's classification of malocclusion

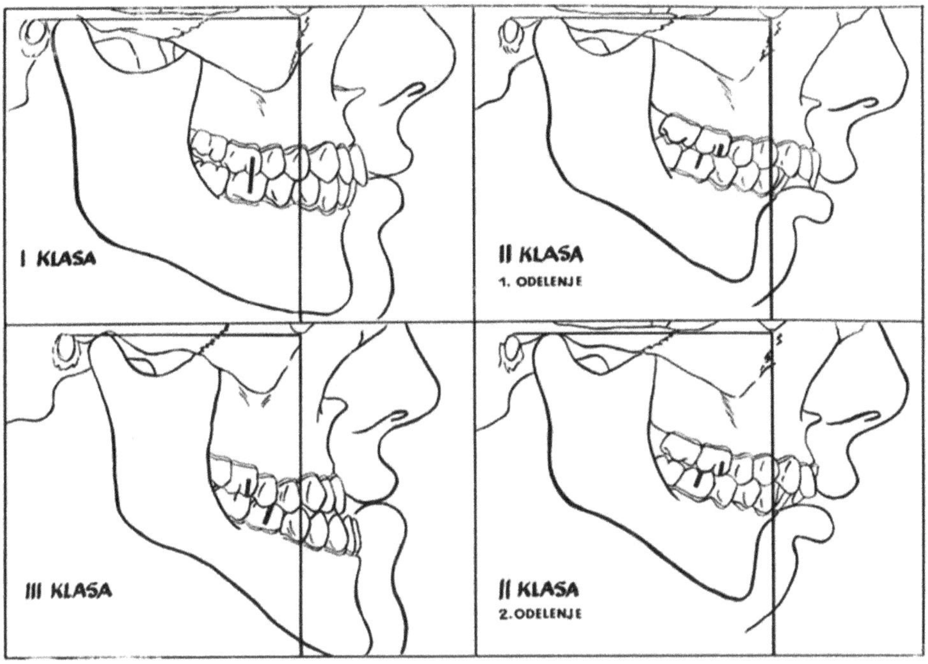

Figure 4. Dürer's performance of different face profiles: right (left), convex (middle) and concave (right)

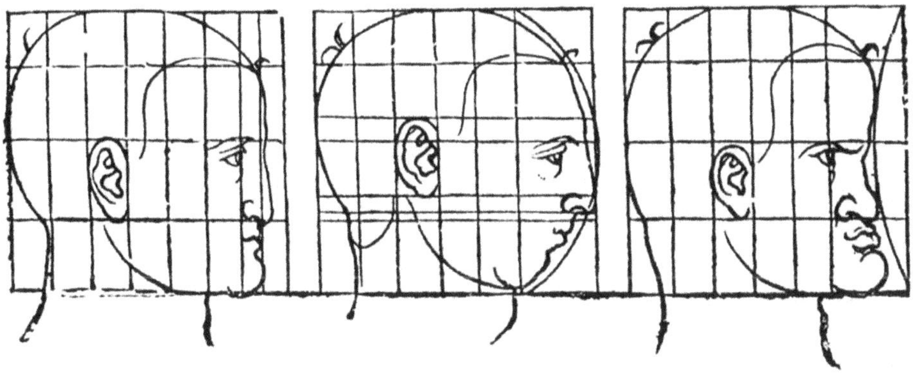

Figure 5. Facial features and appropriate shape and width of dental arches: brahikefal (levo), mezokephal (middle) and dolihokefal (right)

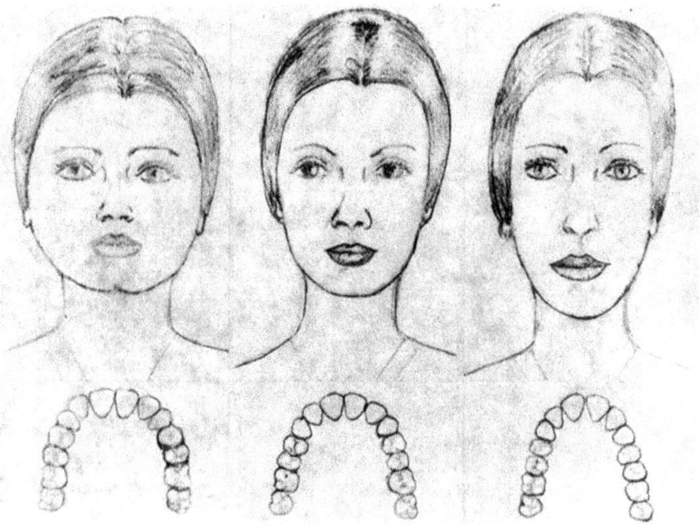

CLINICAL MANIFESTATION

It should be pointed out that there are great anomalies from the weak to the very serious. We will start with the most serious.

1. Pierre Robin's syndrome characterized by triad: macrognia of mandible, cleft palatalis, glossoptosis.
2. Ectodermal dysplasia syndrome characterized by triad: hypohidrosis, hypothyrosis, hypodontia. The syndrome is a hereditary nature.
3. Cleidocranialis dyzostozis syndrome: the lobes are short, brachyphalic, etc. It is of inherent nature.
4. Treacher Collins syndrome: characterized by hypoxia, abnormal hair growth towards the face, microstomy, dental disorder, open hips, mandibular hypoplasia
5. Down's syndrome

All syndromes are characterized by changes in cranium, face and body followed by mental retardation of varying degrees. Here our orthodontics domains are weaker.

Figure 6. Anomalies

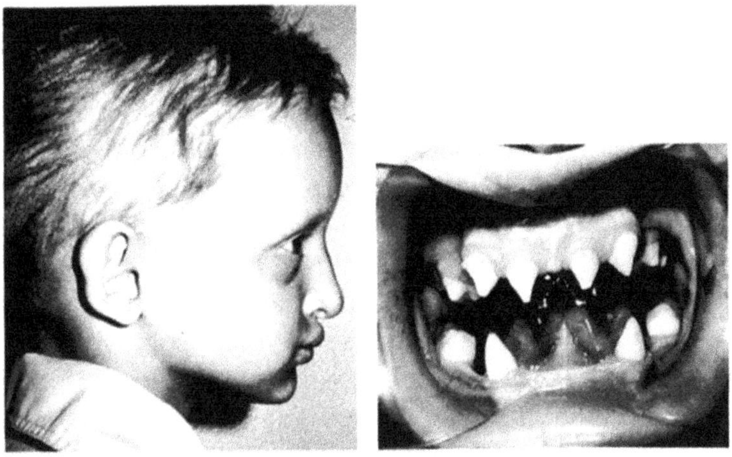

Figure 7. Severe head and neck anomalies in children

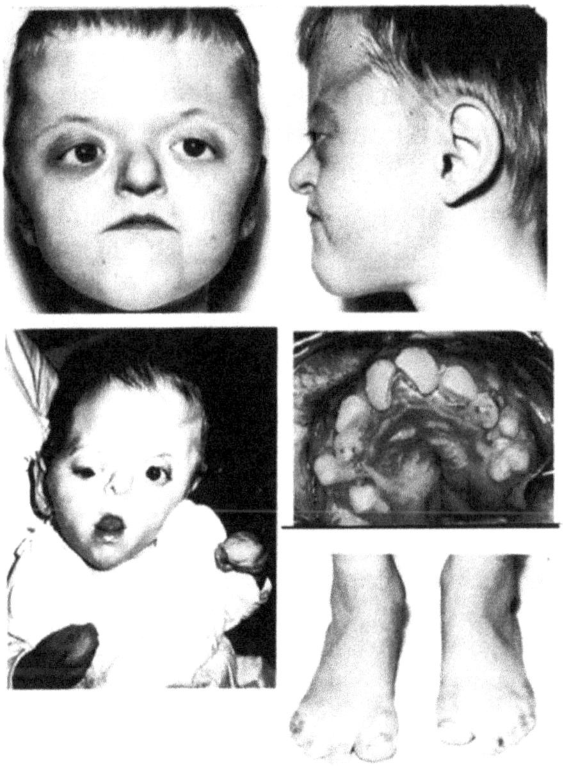

There is another group of serious deformations. These are distal and prone to bites.

Distal bites are characterized by the distal position of the mandible and the protrusion of the maxilla. They are divided into the second class by the first class and the second class by another department (Moss,1963).

The second class is characterized by the protrusion of the upper frontal teeth, the retruding of the lower, the deep bite, the large incisal staircase, the supraposition of the frontal and the infraposition of the lateral teeth, the incompetent lips and the position of the lower lip behind the upper incisors. Further, it is characterized by a very bad convex profile. Chewing is bad, infantile swallowing, pronunciation of some voices poor, swallowing leads to noticeable contraction of the musculus mentalis, the lower lip strengthens strongly behind the upper teeth, the tongue is pushed forward to make contact with the lower lip. If the pushing of the tongue is permanent in the long run, it is impossible to unable the growth of the lower incisors because of which an open bite develops and the speech is disturbed (interdental sigmatism). It can also reach the amphiloid of the joint.

At the end of the treatment we see the facial sensuality, raised the quality of life, optimism, happiness and working elan. This is an example of how to transform anomaly into a normal occlusion.

The second class second division or Dechbis is a dento-alveolo facial anomaly and is also called steep bite. In this anomaly, Spee's curves are highly blurred due to the supraposition of frontal and infra-lateral lateral teeth. There is the narrowness of incisors – due to their coronary retroclination. The

Figure 8. Serious deformation. Appearance of the face at the beginning of treatment: convex profile with incompetent lips and markedly visible upper central incisors, enlarged sulcus mentolabialis, and the lower lip is underlining behind the upper central incisors

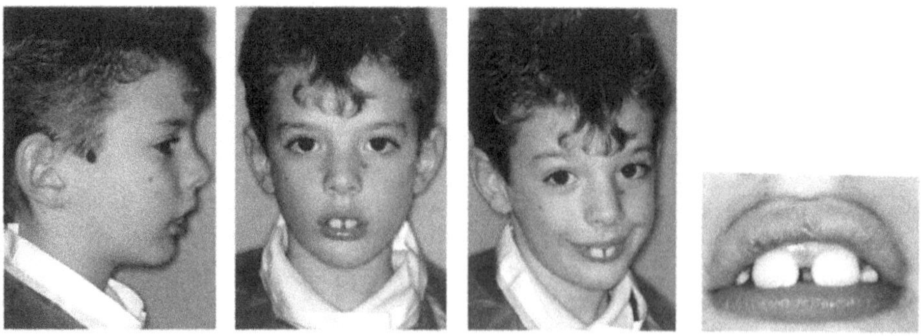

Figure 9. Condition in the mouth before the start of treatment: early mixed dentition (still non-lateral lateral incisors) with Class II 1st class and incision distance of 13mm; narrows the upper tooth in relation to the lower and pronounced deep bite with the traumatization of the palatinal mucosa

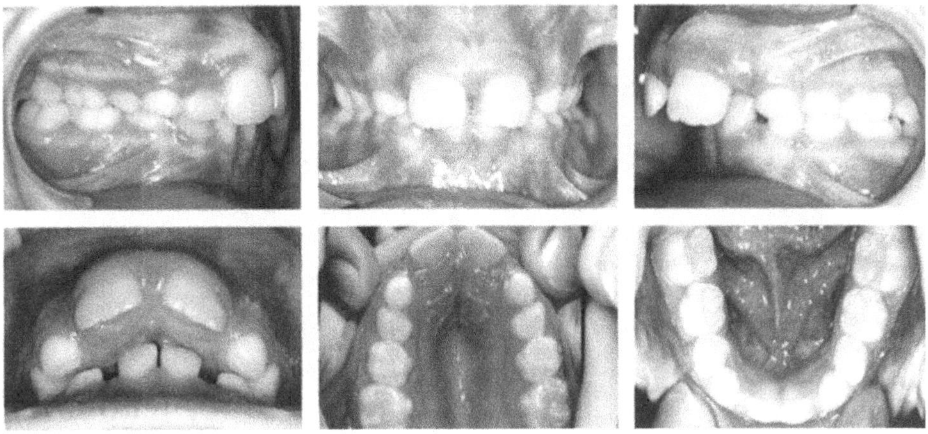

Figure 10. Comparative lateral telegenshots before (a), at the beginning of the second stage (b)and at the end of the treatment (c)

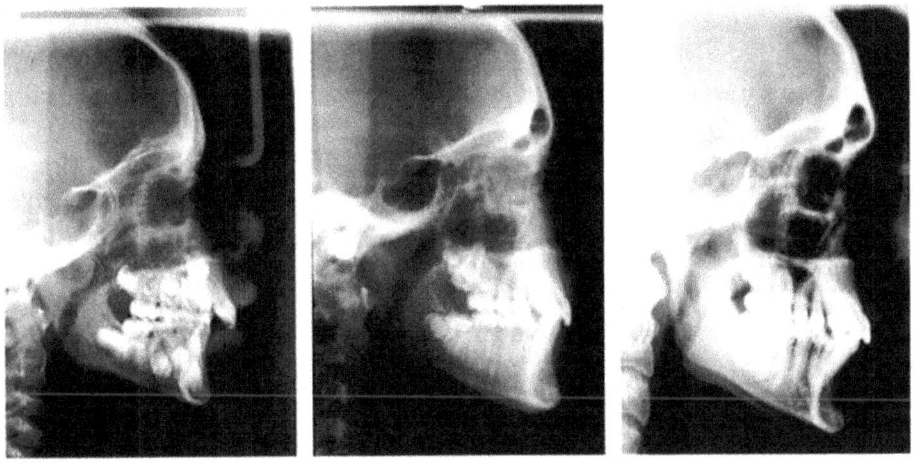

improper position of the upper frontal teeth is the most impressive feature of the maxillary line in persons with maloclusion (anomaly) of the second class, second division. Deep bite is a regular occurrence. The lower frontal teeth touch the palatal mucus, so they break over in time. Paradontic problems are expressed. The appearance and look of the face is quite distinct, with a more

Figure 11. Comparative face shots in the smile before the treatment at the end of the treatment

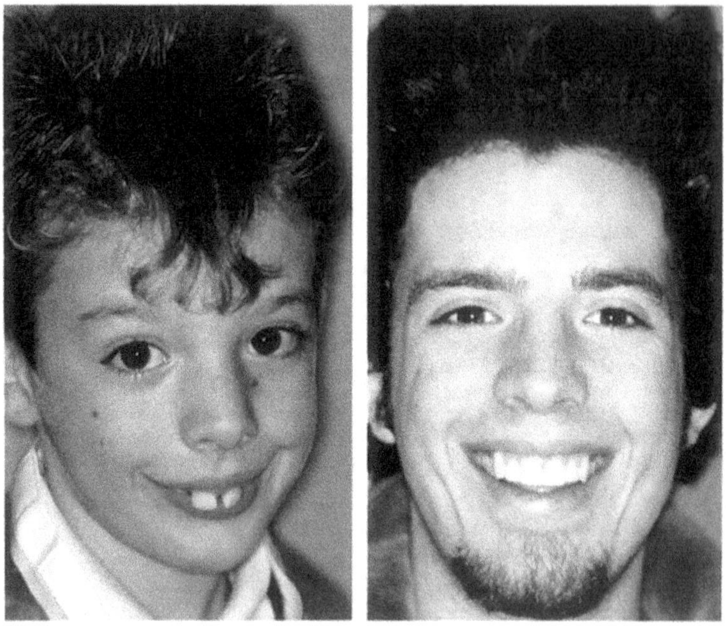

prominent nose, prominent anterior nasal spine, with a tendency of nose and chin joining together. This anomaly is very often hereditary. Its solution is to apply a fixed orthodontic device for a longer period of time and longer retention. The characteristic profile is also convex (Dascaloglannakis, 2000).

Mandibular prognosticism, mesioonclusion - the essence of malocclusion (anomalies) consists of a distinctive difference between the upper and lower jaw and in relation to the upper and lower incisors in the occlusion in the sagittal direction. Angle still noticed the consequence of third class malocclusion on "facial lines" that were very noticeable and unpleasant. Changes occur on teeth alveolar processes, forks and cranial base. Since the reverse shift of the incisors is the basic feature of these anomalies, it is logical to start the classification from there.

Hotz (1974) divided the third-class malocclusion into four groups: (1) a simple cross bite of the incisors, (2) the forced progeny bite, (3) pseudoprognatism, (4) real mandibular prognosticism. In the first group there are variations of the reversed switching. The forced progeny bite is characterized by the reversed switching of all the incisors but also the incisors and the eyelids, premature contact in the area of some of the frontal teeth,

Figure 12. Condition at the beginning of treatment: the profile is slightly convex with pronounced sulcus mentolabialis and pulled back lower back; in the smile of the lower lip, touches the edges of the upper incisors (a), the relationship between molars and furrows is in Class II with retrusions of the upper central incisors and deep bite (b), the upper lateral incisors are pushed over and overlapping the central (c)

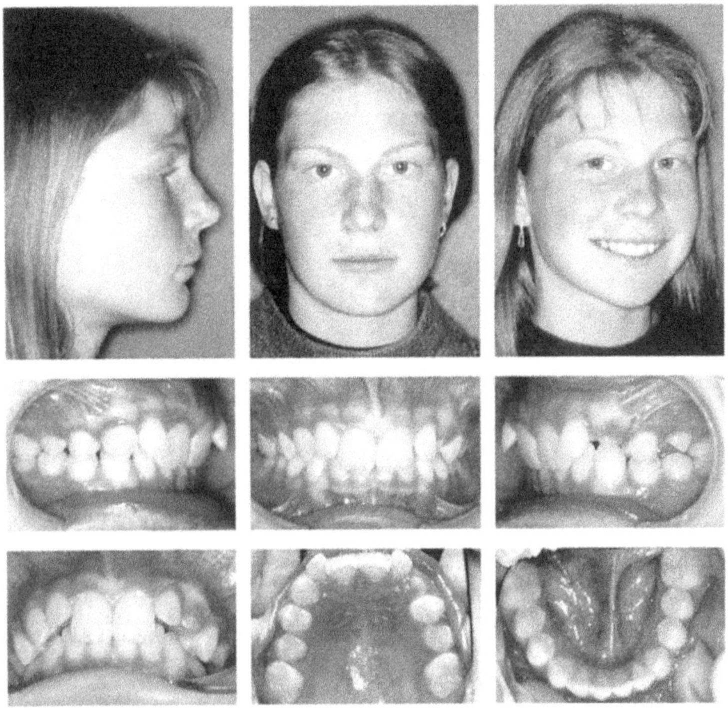

most often the central and natural loosening of the lower jaw in advance when bringing the lower teeth into the onculation with the upper. In most patients, the intercolation space in physiological sleep was increased. There are differences in the size of the fork, the bottom is overclocked. Pseudoprognatism denotes an underdeveloped maxilla while the mandible is normally developed. This anomaly is seen in syndrome and inherited in nature. Progeny of faith is the most difficult form of mesiooclock, the overdeveloped lower jaw and undeveloped or normally developed upper in all segments. Due to the overload of the mandible in the sagittal and transverse direction, the large angle of the mandible and the often insufficient development of maxillary, there is an open bite of varying degrees(Proffit,2000). There is often both sides crossing the bite. Face-to-face disturbances are intense and aggravated with age. Lower

Figure 13. Status at the end of treatment

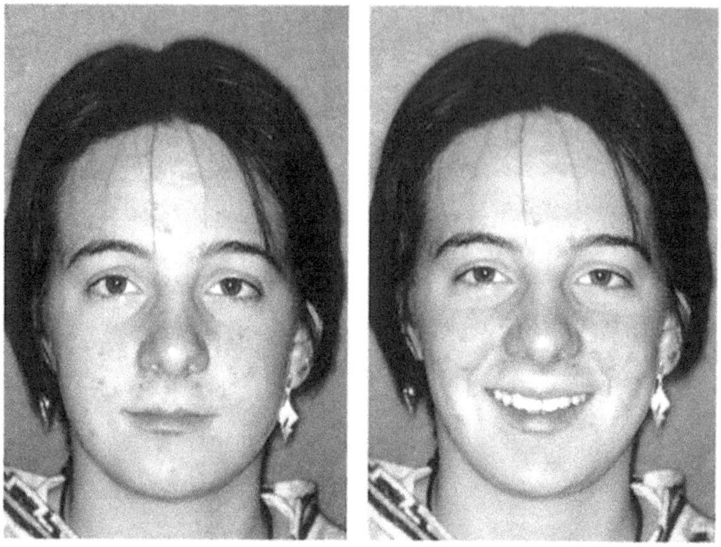

Figure 14. Condition in the oral cavity after the end of treatment

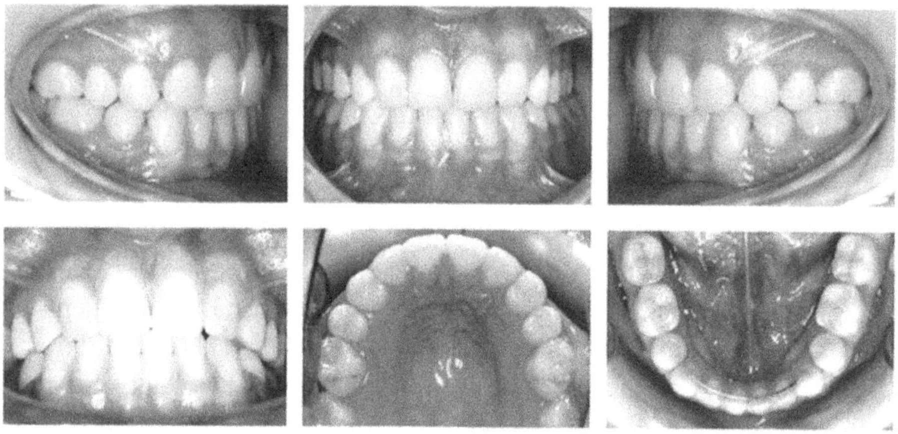

lips and chin are significantly protruded, there is an enlarged lower third of the face, the profile is concave, cephalometric X-ray examinations show that it is not only about the overload of the mandible, but also about the reduction of the angle of the cranial base (NSBa). The occurrence of macroglossia is common. If it is more pronounced, the tongue swims through the biting teeth of the teeth and with contact with the lower lip. In such cases there is infantile swallowing, and speech is disturbed. Anomaly is inherited, and there are known cases of the Habsburg dynasty (Habsburg jail). The therapy of these cases is performed by orthodontic surgical treatment. It must be pointed out that these patients are very depressed and with the solution of their cases from the fundamentals, their view of life changes, the faith and confidence are restored(Proffit,2000)

Transversal irregularity in occlusion is a crossbite where there is an irregular tooth ratio in the buccoral direction, and there are variations, but the most difficult form is the failure of the upper and lower lateral bites and the complete lingual cross-bite. A crossed bite can be unilateral and bilateral. There is often a disorder in the temporomandibular joint.

Bilateral cross-bite occurs as a result of disproportion in the width of the upper and lower dental portions.

Figure 15. Condition at the beginning of the treatment: the profile is convex with an unspoken beard and fuller and protruding lips; a pleasant smile with visible most of the maxillary gingiva. Tinnitus of the upper dental port compared to the lower with a cross-bite on the left side, deviation of mandibular left and middle edges of the lower incisors towards the upper left for 2mm.

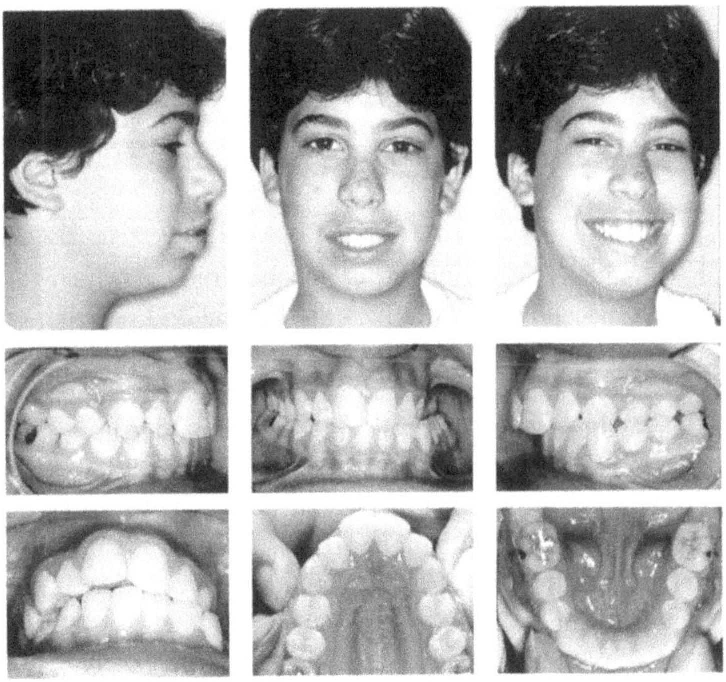

Figure 16. The situation after the removed apparatus: there is a convex profile, the incompetence of the lips is minimized, the smile is more attractive with the minimal visibility of the maxillary gingiva (a); correct tooth interkuspidation with I class of molar and hemorrhagic relationship on both sides, harmonized center of the incisor with the correct and harmonic shape of dental arrays - six keys of optimal occlusion (b).

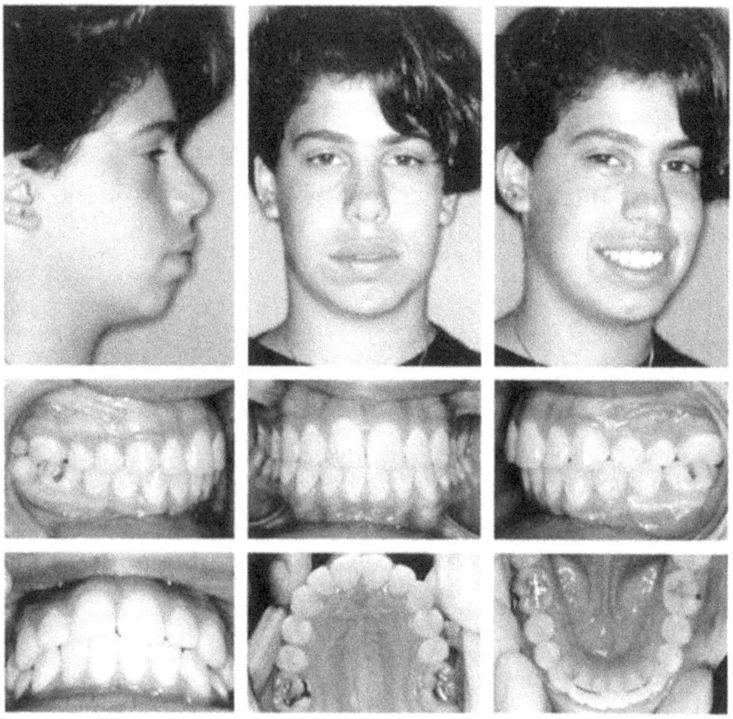

Vertical irregularity in occlusion is an open bite in which there is no contact between the antagonist teeth in the central and habitual occlusion. It most often occurs in the area of the frontal teeth and rarely in the lateral region. An open bite may occur due to finger sucking, language printing, due to inadequate therapeutic treatment of the patient, due to rachitis, or may be skeletal open bite as the most severe form of open bite resulting from disturbed growth of the skeleton of the face. (Graber,1972) Here heritage plays a role. In most patients, changes are observed on the cranial base: the angle of the base and the length of its back are reduced. The lower third of the face is enlarged. In the most difficult cases, contact is established at the last molars. In all patients, the chewing function is primarily disturbed, the food is brittle, and the chewing and destruction of complete teeth tissue that are out of function. The functions of perioral mastication and lingual muscles are regularly disrupted. Incompatibilities of the lips, breathing through the mouth, infantile swallowing, interdental sigmatism are clinical symptoms of disturbed function. By solving these cases, patients gain self-confidence and faith in life.

Figure 17. Open bite at the beginning of treatment. Patients are sad, isolated, unsafe, depressed and often sick

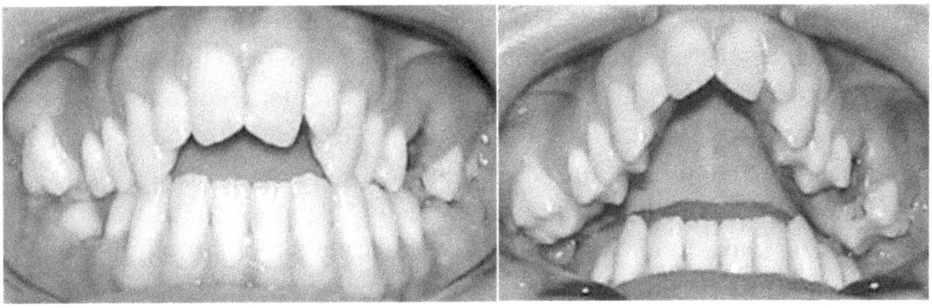

Figure 18. Open bite at the end of the treatment. A smile shows life-giving

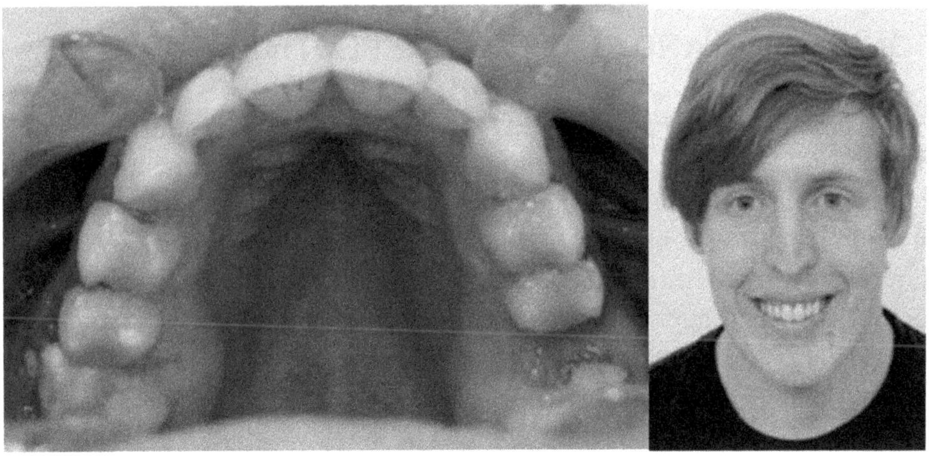

Vertical irregularity is a deep bite. The essence of a deep bite is reflected in the excessive appearance of the frontal teeth due to the distorted inclination of the said teeth. The lower teeth reach the palatinal mucosa and the upper touch the gingival margin of the mandible. The deep bite is associated in all occlusal anterioposterior relationships of the I, II and III classes. If the lower incisors fail the cingulum, the upper incisors form a deep bite. In the deep bite of the Svee's curve is strongly expressed in the lower row, especially in the second class of the second department of the degbis (Thailander,1985).

Gerlah deploys deep bite on hereditary and acquired ones. For hereditary deep bite, the fork bases overlap, and the teeth only overlap the teeth. (Bishara, 2001; AAOS, 2012)A deep bite occurs when the first molars are removed early. In occlusion gradients (anomalies) we have the largest number with less seriousness, although it all depends on the psychological type of personality, because for some it is a little rotated frontal tooth of catastrophes, especially in teenage years, and for some serious anomaly is acceptable in some way. What does all belong to the rest of the anomaly? Dentinogenesis imperfecta, anelogenezis imperfecta, Huchinson tooth, Turner's tooth, tooth dilatation, dysplasia of the dental arteries, delirium, dyspnoea, dyspnoea, hyperdonia, fusion, concordance, macrodontia., medial diastema, odontoma, irregularities in size and shape of dental arches.

CONCLUSION AND FUTURE PERSPECTIVES

When approaching the anomaly therapy, we always proceed from whether the anomalies of dentoalveolar nature or skeletal. Orthodontic treatment is planned to encourage the normal development of teeth and other facial structures. In adults, tissue response to the orthodontic forces is somewhat slower. The movement of the tooth is also slower. The forces for the need to shift the tooth must be stronger and the retention period longer. The psychologist's role is to analyze and monitor the mental development of the child, stimulate it and help him to overcome and successfully overcome psychological crises. The psychologist creates conditions that will enable optimal development of the total and specific potentials. It helps parents to overcome possible psychological trauma and provide them with relevant explanations important for the treatment and rehabilitation of the child and the prospect of further childbirth. Pediatrician takes care of the overall health of the child since birth. Special efforts are needed to understand the complexity of the physical and spiritual being of man, especially as the very diseases and abnormalities in the form and function of his organs and tissues are multidimensional. Orthopedic fork is one of the rare branches of dentistry that plays the role of an interdisciplinary discipline. Its domain extends from monitoring the resolution of the development of the organism from its conception to the completion of the growth process through preventive activity related to the occurrence of anomalies in the construction of tissue, organs and functions of the craniofacial complex until their correction and rehabilitation, which usually lasts until the end of the maturity of the organism and beyond. In therapeutic activity, the basic task of a speech therapist is to alleviate speech disorders and its consequences. It should be pointed out that orthodontic treatment should be carried out seriously, carefully and well planned.

REFERENCES

American Association of Orthodontics. (2012). *Glossary of Orthodontists*. AAO.

Angle, E. H. (1913). *Okklusions Anomalien der Zahne*. Veri.H.

Bishara ES Textbook of Orthodontics. (2001). WB Saunders Company.

Dascaloglannakis, J. (2000). *Glossary of Orthodontics Terms*. Ouintessence Publishing Co, Inc.

Graber, T. M. (1972). *Unfavorable sequelae of malocclusion*. Philadelphia: Orthodontics -Principles and Practice.

Moss, M.L. (n.d.). The functionalal matrix. *U Vistas in Orthodontics*.

Proffit, W. R., & Fields, H. W. (2000). *Contemporary Orthodontics* (3rd ed.). St. Louis, MO: Mosby.

Thilander, B. (1985). *Ronning O.Introduction to Orthodontics*. Tandiakastforlaget.

Chapter 7
Self-Determination Calibration for Cochlear Implant Rehabilitation

Dionysios Politis
Aristotle University of Thessaloniki, Greece

Sophia Aidona
Aristotle University of Thessaloniki, Greece

Petros Stagiopoulos
Aristotle University of Thessaloniki, Greece

Georgios Kyriafinis
Aristotle University of Thessaloniki, Greece

Jannis Constantinidis
Aristotle University of Thessaloniki, Greece

ABSTRACT

Cochlear implantation is a well-established therapeutic approach for deaf or hearing-impaired patients. After the medical intervention, which aims to restore hearing, subjects undergo rehabilitation procedures in order to cure instructional disadvantages, problematic schooling circumstances, or deficits in their sociability. Essential physical, mental, social, and cognitive skills are taken into perspective, as the prerequisite of a notable aptitude determines the suitability of a subject to get professional and communal roles. Quality of life, as an indicator, provides the metrics that demonstrate the level of adoption with established norms.

DOI: 10.4018/978-1-5225-7513-9.ch007

INTRODUCTION

For many years, cochlear implantation has served as a well-established therapeutic approach for patients with severe to profound sensorineural hearing loss. Cochlear implants are advanced electronic devices that work as an artificial ear, surpassing the outer and middle ear structures and stimulating directly the acoustic nerve.

The aim of this research is to investigate the impact of cochlear implantation on the Quality of Life in patients, and compare and correlate the above results to pure tone audiometry scores, speech recognition scores, and acoustic performance scores (Fletcher et al., 1992). Indeed, the disability for hearing sufficiently suppresses emotionally impaired in hearing subjects, as they are obviously deficient for sustaining adequate levels of human communication, depreciates significantly their learning efficiency and the continuity of their social interactions. As they experience a plodding degradation of their sensual awareness, they gradually loose their composure and self-possession for their emotional equilibrium. Drifting into a state of reduced excitational contact accompanied by a constantly limited promulgation of information to and from everything that exists outside themselves, they experience a deteriorating practical contact with facts and a limited observation of events that are crucial for acquiring knowledge and skills (Venail et al., 2010). Overall, they seemingly have deficient channels of communication for fully exerting their schooling potential, their social intelligence through time and their agility in performing tasks that are admonished for them in the general public's perception. In some occasions, this state may lead to agoraphobia and isolation.

Therefore, this research aims to measure the success of the rehabilitation procedures by introducing Quality of Life metrics. When a patient undergoes therapeutic treatment for his hearing disability, it is not given as a necessary or inevitable result that he will re-enter the schooling and social communities of normally hearing people without becoming annoyed or anxious (Baker et al., 2009). A series of mental faculties and cognitive phenomena take place that severely affect the psychological equilibrium of the person receiving treatment, not counting the implications with the group of people directly associated with him or her (Clarke – Stewart et al., 2003).

In this survey, pure tone audiometry scores, speech recognition scores, and acoustic performance scores were obtained for all patients after cochlear implantation. In addition, all patients were administered the Profile

Questionnaire for Rating Communicative Performance, proposed by Sanders (1975, 1982). The parents of the children evaluated the quality of life and the auditory performance of their offspring's before and after cochlear implantation.

The results showed significant improvements in pure tone audiometry scores, in speech recognition, in acoustic performance scores, and in Quality of Life scores as well.

IMPAIRED IN HEARING SUBJECTS AND THEIR THERAPEUTIC APPROACH

Hearing Impairments and Deafness

By the term impaired in hearing patients we characterize people with an evident reduction in their acoustic capacity. Depending on the localization of the damage, we can distinguish three types of hearing loss: conductive hearing loss, sensorineural hearing loss and mixed hearing loss (American Academy of Otolaryngology, 2015; Kyriafinis, 2005).

1. **Conductive Hearing Loss:** It can be caused by pathologies involving the external and middle ear (external auditory meatus, tympanic membrane, ossicular chain). Possible causes may be structural malformations and dysfunctions, traumatic injuries, the presence of foreign bodies, degeneration of stem cells. Conductive hearing loss is effectively amenable via surgical correction, or, in many milder cases, using pharmaceutical treatment.
2. **Sensorineural Hearing Loss:** It results as a consequence of disruption in the passage of sound beyond the oval window. Such pathologies can be located to the auditory receptor cells of the cochlea and the eighth cranial nerve. It is clearly the most common type of hearing loss, resulting from cochlear or retrocohlear pathology. Sensorineural hearing loss is discriminated in inherited or acquired. Inherited impairments may be caused due to genetic factors or viral infections of the mother during pregnancy, like rubella, cytomegalovirus (CMV), toxoplasmosis, disorders of the endocrine system, hypothyroidism, diabetes mellitus, preeclampsia, other infections like HIV (Human Immunodeficiency Virus), syphilis, impaired renal function, radiotherapy or chemotherapy,

and ototoxic drugs like antibiotics, loop diuretics, and some other 100 at least nonsteroidal antiinflammatory drugs and chemotherapeutic agents. On the other hand, acquired hearing impairment results from perinatal diseases and epidemiology, like prematurity, asphyxia neonatorum, hyperbilirubinaemia, and post-natal disorders, like malignant, virulent infections that may follow birth, meningitis, ototoxic drugs, autoimmune diseases, serious injuries or damages of the inner ear, and acute otitis or chronic otitis media as result of infections of the middle ear.

3. Mixed hearing loss, which represents a mixture of both conductive and sensorineural hearing loss.

Quantitative Assessment of Acoustic Ability and Their Impact for Language - Speech - Communication

The quantitative estimate of the acoustic capacity determined by tone audiometry and the hearing rate levels are set as follows (1 dB = deciBel, HL = Hearing Level):

- Hearing threshold between 0-20 dBHL: Normal hearing
- Hearing threshold between 21-40 dBHL: Low degree of hearing impairment
- Hearing threshold between 41-60 dBHL: Average hearing impairment
- Hearing threshold between 60-85 dBHL: High degree of hearing impairment
- Hearing threshold between 86-95 dBHL: Very high hearing impairment
- Hearing threshold above 95 dBHL: Residual hearing / deafness practically.

Pictorially these levels can be seen in Figure 1.

When a patient does not hear well, his ability to develop oral communication, language and social skills is seriously handicapped. To remedy this poignant situation, the patient's cognitive development, if he is young, is enhanced by amplifying and supplementing his residual acoustic basis and by inclusive education in his early settings or primary school education (Politis et al., 2016).

A subject is characterized as suffering from hearing impairment when a clear reduction in his ability to hear properly is traced. It can be congenital or acquired, unilateral or bilateral, and it varies within the range of 25-95

Figure 1. Hearing level curves for normal hearing, conductive hearing loss and sensorineural hearing loss.

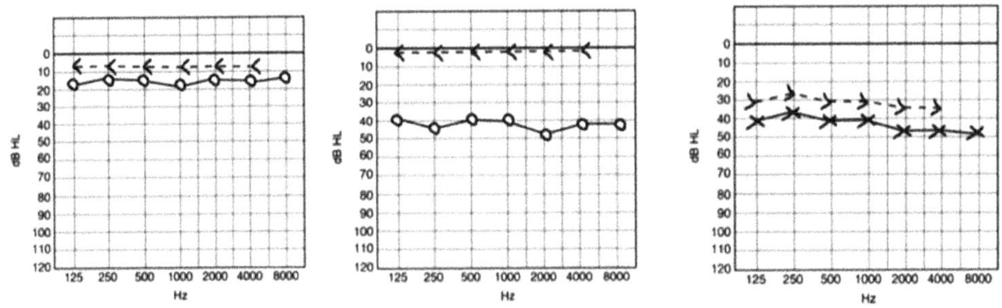

dBHL. Nearly all children with hearing loss experience have evident disorders in their language and speech development process.

People with hearing loss often experience problems in the fields of language, speech and communication. According to the literature the above fields are defined as follows:

- **Language:** Code or system of human communication, consisting of the use of words in a structured and conventional way, either spoken or written, that uses abstract symbols and has rules governing symbol combinations to portray ideas.
- **Speech:** Complex brain function, triggering the somatosensory-optical-acoustic and kinetic complex, aiming to express thoughts and feelings by articulate sounds, to which is added the ability to synthesize with previous experiences. It is influenced by heredity and is enriched, while it develops through the mechanisms of imitation and matching with the mother (Hytoglou - Antoniadou, 2003).
- **Communication:** A process by which individuals exchange information, news and transfer ideas (Owens, 2013). Communication requires the existence of a transmitter that encodes and forms a message, a receiver that receives and decodes the message and uses a code, that is, a common language.

In acoustic terms, the ability of the person to understand speech is evaluated with the help of spoken audiometry, which is also considered an important tool for hearing assessment. Its combination with tonic audiometry can help determine the degree and type of hearing loss of the patient, while its role in determining the appropriate signal gain that can provide the patient with hearing aids (Jerger & Hayes, 1977). Speech audiometry determines the speaker threshold (in dB HL) and the discretion of the subject in speech (in percent) with the ultimate goal of assessing the central auditory system of the brain. The peculiarity of the method is that the acoustic stimuli used are similar to those of everyday life, and that it can reveal the effect of an acoustic impairment that affects a person's communication capability as well as the ability to process the verbal signal.

CONSEQUENCES OF HEARING LOSS AND DEAFNESS

Hearing impaired or deaf people face difficulties to an extend that makes their every day living quite challenging. These difficulties relate to social interaction, language and communication, education, behavior, mental health, safety and work (Kochkin et al., 2007).

Social Interaction

The problems faced by impaired in hearing in the field of social interaction cover a wide range of relative issues. These individuals find it difficult to create and maintain relationships with normally hearing persons (Weisel & Cinamon, 2005). Also, the social skills of deaf or impaired in hearing are often inadequate, making their overall social development more difficult. Patients with a high to very high degree of sensorineural hearing loss usually have fewer relationships, participate less often in social activities, resulting in feelings of isolation, have limited social visibility (Nunes et al., 2001) and often report that they feel more loneliness than their listening peers (Kent, 2003). In addition, cases of depression and irritability are higher in this population compared to those of the normally hearing audience.

The difficulty in communicating often leads to experiencing degradable emotions, as the self-confidence and self-awareness degree of patients is often limited, affecting their relationship with peers and their own families as well. The difficulty in hearing reduces the chances of participation, even in recreation or play, leading to isolation. In addition, impaired in hearing people report that normally hearing people often do not devote them the time they need to understand and have lower expectations of social interaction with them because they consider them a prior less capable than their peers. Thus, deaf or impaired in hearing are led to a lower quality social interaction, thus limiting their opportunities to develop properly their language skills (Harris & Vanzandt, 1997). Indeed, many deaf children have limited social skills that are compulsory for adequate social interaction. The normally hearing population often misinterpret their call for more information as a sign of incompetence or lack of interest in the content of discussion.

The intrinsic need for deaf or hard in hearing people to draw the attention of others or to be in visual contact so to enhance their speech communication intelligibility is often considered non-socially acceptable and extends furthermore their isolation. Social relationships with peers prove particularly important for their school adaptation (Mc Elwain & Volling, 2005) and their subsequent academic evolution (Bohs et al., 2006). In addition, the education of impaired in hearing children plays an extremely important role in developing social interaction skills, as the first years of schooling are the period in which friendships are built through common interests, school activities and sport, making it particularly important for the hard in hearing pupils to communicate at all levels with their normally hearing classmates.

Language and Communication

Normally developing children learn the language of their environment without much education, as long as they are regularly exposed to it. The newborn's brain is structured to be able to master the language of his aural and oral communication channel. Children usually learn the language or languages used in their environment exclusively through continuous exposure to this one(s). The language(s) learned by a child in the first years of his/her life is called the first(s). Around the age of five years, the plasticity of the brain gradually begins to decrease. A child who has not been able for linguistic communication until that time, which is referred to as critical, is exposed to the danger of never becoming able to manipulate his speech communication with linguistic competence (Lenneberg, 1967; Kraashen, 1973).

This symptom is rarely reported in the case of normally hearing children exposed in the language of their environment. The first three years in a child's life are particularly important in terms of acquiring knowledge about the world, communicating with the family and developing the cognitive and linguistic foundations on which its future development will be based upon. When a child is able to acquire age-appropriate speech skills, he or she is more likely to successfully attend a normal schooling educational program, participate in its activities and interact socially with teachers and peers. Deaf or hard in hearing children, who lack qualitative language stimuli in their first years of life, are more likely to encounter difficulties in language development and in their academic performance (Hart & Risley, 1995). As expected, limited language skills combined with the deficient parent-child interaction in early life, due to insufficient aural communication, are associated with posterior socio-emotional and behavioral problems (Prizant & Meyer, 1993), with language development disorders (Rescorla, 2002) in addition to profound reading difficulties (Nathan et al., 2000).

Impaired in hearing or deaf subjects more frequently demonstrate a significant delay in speech development or poor speech communication quality that hinders their ability to communicate effectively and prevents their mental alertness. As they do not have the pre-requisites to ask questions or ask for clarification, even to ask for help, their surroundings are often forced to guess what meets their needs rather than what complies with their actual need (Robbins et al., 1997). This serious delay in the acquisition of adequate linguistic or speech communication skills may affect the need for exchanging information, and even further, proper for the circumstances and age cognitive and social development.

It may also affect self-esteem and socio- emotional adaptation (Percy - Smith et al., 2008; Grenberg and Krusche, 1993). Dyslexia in speech impedes in the long run their school performance, vocational training and opportunities for professional rehabilitation (Snowling et al., 2001). In addition, impaired in hearing develop lower linguistic intelligence than their properly hearing peers (Hart & Risley, 1995). Obviously deaf or hard of hearing children do not have the same experiences as normally hearing children. Limited or no exposure to linguistic communication is associated with a range of problems, which extend beyond language pathology. Cognitive activities, which require a minimum level of language knowledge, such as mathematics or the organization of memory, are also affected (Ronnenberg, 2003).

They also experience problems with their metacognitive processes, such as is problem solving (Beer et al., 2009). Their limited exposure to linguistic communication reduces the chances for educational and professional success as well (MacSweeney, 1998), leading to psychosocial problems due to the isolation and desolation experienced by the impaired in hearing subjects due to their reduced linguistic and cognitive ability (Leigh et al., 2008).

Deaf or impaired in hearing subjects demonstrate higher illiteracy rates, (Stewart and Clarke 2003), frequent more than their normally hearing counterparts in penal institutions (Tucker, 1988; National Association of the Deaf, 2002) and have higher unemployment (Yuwen & Goldscmidt, 2009).

Illiteracy is closely linked to higher unemployment, poverty and poor health indicators (Humphries et al., 2012). Moreover, impaired in hearing people, due to their limited communication with the surrounding, become more often victims of abuse (Sullivan & Knutson, 2000; Knutson et al., 2004). The development of linguistic skill, instead of using a sigh language for the deaf (Figure 2) greatly influences their social interaction, as it allows them to communicate, create relationships and develop a positive identity (Stinson & Whitmire, 2000). Conversely, deaf or impaired subjects with reduced speech output and limited speech comprehension, find it difficult to comprehend what others feel or think about them (Remmel & Peters, 2009).

Education

Child hearing impairment is a major public health problem as it is associated with long-term academic and communicative difficulties (Davis, 1997). 1 to 6 children in 1000 have moderate to very severe sensorineural or conductive hearing deficiency (Sokol & Hyde, 2002).

When a deaf child is enrolled in a school destined for the general public, he or she needs to be able to make good use of oral and written speech. But many of these students have not developed the prerequisite communication skills to the extent that their listening classmates have acquired them. Aural perception, of any grade, adversely affects psycho-educational development, leading

Figure 2. A sign language for the deaf communication scheme in American English, as used by the "HD Deaf Newspaper" TV channel.

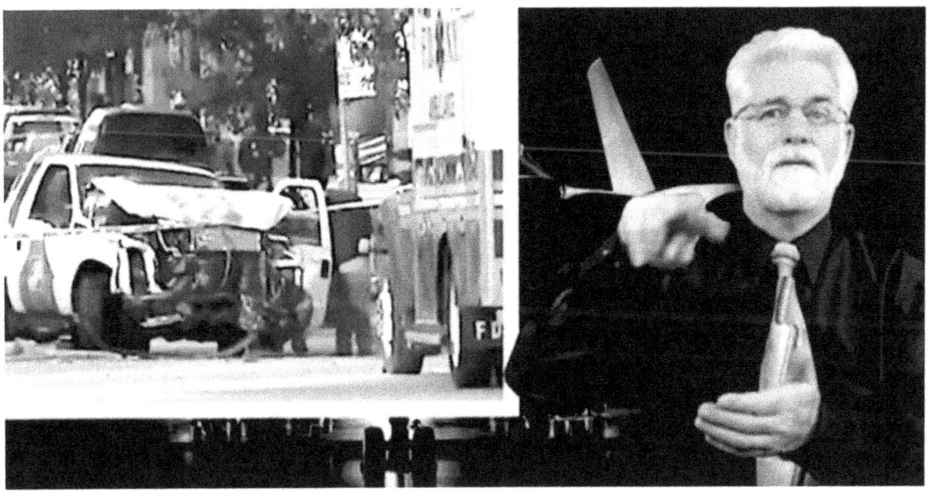

these students to the high-risk group of language and learning deficiencies. One of these mental faculties which is severely affected is attention, which appears limited when compared to normally hearing populations (Mitchell & Quittner, 1996).

As expected, their academic performance and average grades are usually lower than those scored by normally hearing students. Hard of hearing subjects demonstrate reduced ability in reading, writing and mathematics (Hindley& VanGent, 2004) and one in three needs special educational help at school. This may commence by his placement on a front desk, the provision of sign language interpreter or a person who helps by taking notes (Schirk et al., 2006). Many of these students abandon school earlier than their listening classmates and, as they received a degraded in quality education, are finally led to limited professional choices (Venail et al., 2010).

Behavior

Speech disorders are often associated with behavioral disorders. However, it is not clear whether speech disorders lead to behavioral problems, if they are generated by them or if merely they are two independent manifestations of a wider developmental process, since it is rather difficult to isolate these two components (Beitchman et al., 2001). Children with sensorineural hearing deficiency have higher rates of extrovert behavioral problems (e.g. aggression, violation of social norms) compared to normally hearing groups of people (Van Eldik et al., 2004).

These difficulties are often caused by the feeling of despair a handicapped child experiences when interacting with his / her group of healthy peers, resulting to one-third of them developing behaviors associated with breakdown and disintegration (Smith et al., 1998). When behavioral problems are introverted (e.g. anxiety, withdrawal, depression) it is difficult to be diagnosed by the suffering children themselves and as they are not as disturbing as other groups of deviant behaviors, such as the cases of extrovert conduct, they often pass unnoticed by parents and teachers (Clarke - Stewart et et al., 2003).

Unfortunately, the internalization of behavioral problems is associated with future mood and communication disorders, as well as cognitive and academic problems (Kovacs & Devlin, 1998). Language plays an important role in the child's development. It is the primary means of social exchange and helps to internalize social norms as well as to develop behavioral control (Luria, 1961). The speech disorders encountered by the hard of hearing lead to behavioral problems, constraining the understanding capacity for the desires and needs of others, while reducing the communication potential and the ability to control their feelings and behavior (Schick et al., 2007). Parent-child communication is particularly important for child development and socialization. Impaired in hearing or deaf children have difficulty in communicating with their listening parents, resulting in negative emotions. Parents, for their part, tend to be more instructive and develop more controlling interactions with their children (Vaccan & Marshark, 1997). Communication problems between deaf and dumb children and their parents make it more difficult to connect with each other and hamper children's psychological development. Parents who are unable to accept their child's hearing disability exacerbate the sense of rejection and withdrawal experienced by the child, which often leads to problematic behaviors. Hard of hearing children children often have difficulty in communicating their needs and wishes while conforming to parenting and social rules. This weakness may be the cause of the increased behavioral problems observed in this study group. On the other hand, parents do not understand the behavior of their children and misinterpret them as problematic (Baker et al., 2009).

Maintaining adequate levels of attention is another important factor in controlling one's behavior. Children need to be able to monitor important social and environmental notions in order to successfully control their behavior and meet their needs (Murphy et al., 2007). Surveys highlight the link between limited attention control and behavioral problems, as well as between delayed linguistic development and attention control (Beitchman et al., 2001). The visual attention of impaired in hearing children, which usually focuses on maintaining contact, can play an extremely important role in the occurrence of behavioral problems due to hearing loss (Ruff & Rothbart, 1996). Deaf children, if they can not control the environment in which they live, are limited to communication within visual control range, thus reducing their overall ability to sustain adequate attention levels (Quittner et al., 2007).

Mental Health

The mental health of impaired in hearing people is affected, as these individuals persistently feel different from others. The need to rely on others for what they can not hear reduces their sense of independence. The discouragement they experience when they cannot be understood, as well as the distress or anger, when they cannot have a comprehensive assessment of the incoming acoustic stimuli, disturbs their mental health and leads to reduced self-confidence and low self-esteem (Freeman et al., 1975).

This sub group of the impaired in hearing people exhibits noteworthy psychiatric disorders (Toppelberg & Shapiro, 2000). In addition, emotional adjustment problems are 3 to 6 times more common in deaf children than in children with normal hearing capabilities (Meadow & Trybus, 1979).

Pathological neurological findings associated with the causes of hearing loss adversely affect the mental health of the impaired in hearing. When deafness is the result of cerebral palsy, it is likely that speech or writing problems will coexist. Additionally, concurrence of epilepsy limits self-esteem and can cause overprotective behaviors towards deaf or hard of hearing subjects (Du Feu & Fergusson, 2003).

People with disabilities face more often than other practical and / or social problems in their lives that considerably limit their activity. These problems can trigger the development of mental health problems (Chwalisz & Vaux, 2000). Deaf or impaired in hearing are more likely to be victims of physical, emotional and sexual violence than normally hearing persons (Knutson et al., 2004), risking mental health problems at some point in their lives (Dows & Harrison, 1998). Patients with hearing loss, who suffer from psychoses, experience auditory and visual hallucinations as well (Haskins, 2004).

Hearing loss and limited communication ability cause feelings of despair, and there is a close link between hearing impairment or deafness and depression (La forge et al., 1992), which is not associated with specific age and socio-economic groups (Herbst & Humphrey, 1980). Also, hearing loss often leads to social isolation, low self-esteem, and functional disability (Uhlmann et al., 1989).

The greater the loss of hearing, the more common the appearance is of mental health problems (Eide & Roysamb, 2002), while those who suffer from such complications are often characterized as psychologically healthy, as experts attribute their symptoms merely to hearing loss and their limited language skills (Pollard, 1994).

Safety

Deaf and hard of hearing citizens are more likely to face security problems than their normal hearing counterparts. Both deaf and impaired in hearing children and their parents feel that they are not absolutely safe. Hearing loss may mean that even alert alarms or sirens in public places cannot be detected (Kochkin et al., 2007).

Employment Conditions

Work and family play a key role in the lives of Western societies. People with disabilities experience difficulties in different fields of their professional development (Szymanski & Hershenson, 2005). Adults with such disabilities face dramatically higher rates of unemployment and underemployment (Burkhauser & Heutenville, 2010), which have a negative impact on their social and economic level, as well as on their self-esteem. Surveys in Australia, Sweden, USA and Finland argue that despite the normal distribution of deaf and impaired in hearing as far as their intelligence is concerned, these people face more problems in higher education and their professional rehabilitation than their normally hearing counterparts do (Ruben, 2000).

The lack of satisfaction from vocational opportunities and choices is attributed to limited academic skills, low educational levels, but also to social and environmental barriers (e.g., noise in the workplace, see Bowe et al., 2005). In addition, deaf or impaired in hearing workers earn less money than the normally hearing people do (Ruben, 2000), resulting in increased social costs mainly for those with severe or very severe hearing loss (Mohr, et al., 2000). People with hearing loss as well as speech disorders often experience communication problems. Over the last few decades, there has been a decline in the availability of manual jobs and a shift to professions requiring increased communication skills and academic qualifications. This change affects those who have difficulty in communicating and leads them to a lower level socio-economic status compared to those who do not have such problems (Ruben, 2000). In addition, deaf and hard of hearing subjects demonstrate lower professional expectations than the normally hearing ones (Schroedel, 1992). They think they can perform better on manual jobs and believe that the professions of increased prestige do not fit them at all (Weisel & Cinamon, 2005). Hearing and speech communication disorders are combined with unemployment rates of 41.9% compared to 29.5% for workers of the same age group without disabilities in the United States (Kruse, 1997).

Also, communication disorders often lead to a lower social class positioning and a lower income. As speech is the dominant means of social interaction in society, communication disorders are basic causes or consequences of poverty (Elwan, 1999). The low income of the hard of hearing subjects is related to their academic, social and economic background. In many Western countries, pre-linguistic deaf people do not enjoy the same academic opportunities as the rest of the population. In Denmark, for example, they are more likely to be trained in a manual job than going to a University (Parving & Christensen, 1993).

Although deaf or impaired in hearing do not fall short in cognitive abilities and skills compared to the normally hearing population, they face an increased risk of not being able to complete secondary education (Stinson & Walter, 1997), resulting in higher unemployment and / or underemployment rates (Blanchfield et al., 2001). Obstacles to professional careers are defined as mere "events or situations involving a person or his / her environment that make his / her professional development challenging" (Swanson & Woitke, 1997). Frequently, deaf or impaired in hearing experience racist attitudes while confronted with a lack of public or private help systems. These difficulties arise in their working environment and reflect the attitude of contemporary societies, characterized by social stigmatization and discrete behavior.

Due to all the previously mentioned reasons, a number of deaf or hard of hearing subjects face problems in promoting their professional activity (Foster & Mcleod, 2003). The difficulties that they usually encounter in their working environment are noise, the need to use the telephone, sound alarms, and situations where group hearing is required, such as staff gatherings (Laroche et al., 2000). The deaf or severely impaired in hearing constantly signify that they feel socially isolated in work and are often excluded from social interactions during breaks (Steinberg et al., 1999). They also have fewer demands from their employers because they fear they will be denounced or appear less able to work (Hallberg & Carlsson, 1993).

ASSESING PERFORMANCE OF COCHLEAR IMPLANTATION REHABILITATION PROCESSES WITH QUALITY OF LIFE INDICES

Quality of Life

World Health Organizations define more or less health as "a state of absolute physical, mental and social well-being, and not simply the absence of disease or weakness." On the contrary, Quality of Life is defined as a composite indicator that reflects subjective and objective findings concerning all aspects of human existence, including health, economy, politics, cultural, environmental, aesthetic and intellectual aspects (Gold et al., 1996).

The notion for Quality of Life has been described and measured in many ways in the relative literature. Haas (1999) proposes the following definition in order to differentiate it from related concepts such as well-being, satisfaction with life and functionality. Thus, Quality of Life is considered to be multidimensional in construct including physical, emotional, mental, social, and behavioral components. Health-related definitions are part of a wider range that starts with those who give holistic emphasis to the social, emotional and physical well-being of patients, after medical intervention, up to those who focus on the health impact of the patients' ability to lead a satisfactory life afterwards (Bullinger et al., 1993). It is a broad field that deals with whether illness or disability limits a person's potential to assume a normal role (Carr & Higginson, 2001).

It is important for the scientific community to use objective descriptions for the mechanisms through which illness, health and medical practices affect Quality of Life, as there are patients with serious illnesses who feel that they dissipate their lives under poor quality circumstances. The concept in perspective involves everything a person can do, including access to resources and opportunities to use assets, to enjoy his or her interests and to have an overall sense of good living conditions. The first two elements are often referred to as objective Quality of Life, while the latter, i.e. the sense of well being as subjective Quality of Life (Attkisson et al., 1992).

In the field of health care provision, Quality of Life research focuses on the overall context that is associated with a particular disease. Research is intended to highlight the social aspect of how groups of people subsist, and to evaluate how well the rehabilitation process revives a patient's functionality, improves access to resources and opportunities, as well as how the sense of well-being is experienced in a multitude of areas that may not be directly affected by the health services provided (e.g. housing, employment, etc., see Lehman, 1988).

Finally, the Quality of Life area associated with a particular disease should be evaluated with specialized tools. Some basic tools can be used in every occasion, regardless of the disease that a patient is undergoing, but most tools are only suitable for specific patients and illnesses (Oerger, 1989). In addition, such measurements, as associated to health in general, make it possible to make comparisons between groups of different subjects and lead to improvements, as far as therapeutic processes are concerned (Wells et al., 1989).

Quality of Life Assessment Tools and Cochlear Implantation

In recent years there has been an increasing interest in using more holistic evaluations for the therapeutic effect of cochlear implantation. This need arises because traditional evaluation criteria, such as speech perception or economic evaluation are unable to capture the full range of influence that cochlear implantation has on the daily life of individuals.

A special interest group consists of children who have undergone cochlear implantation. Research on children's Quality of Life after surgical intervention studies the effect of cochlear implantation, compares these children with their normally hearing peers and monitors the relationship between Quality of Life indices and other relevant parameters. There are various tools that evaluate the results of medical interventions. Some of them are health-oriented, which do not target a specific group of patients and can be used with a variety of other groups (Torrance & Feeny, 1989).

The use of generic methodologies for cochlear implant users has lead to some complications, as these metrics are less sensitive to the identification of hearing and communication difficulties (Bess, 2000). As a result, new practices have been proposed.

For example, the Glasgow Benefit Inventory (G. B. I.) is a questionnaire created to evaluate the results of otorhinolaryngological interventions. It examines whether therapeutic treatment improves the patient's state of health, as well as his psychological, social and physical well being (Robinson et al., 1996). It is adequately sensitive in detecting changes in health and it is patient-oriented. It evaluates Quality of Life in three areas: social, general and physical. It includes some 18 questions, 12 of which express concern in general improvement of Quality of Life, 3 in social improvement and 3 in health improvement. Each question has five possible answers.

SF -36 (Short Form 36 General Health Survey) is a generic questionnaire, which is not addressed to any particular disease patients. It consists of 36 questions related to physical activities, social activities, limitations diagnosed due to physical problems, vitality, longevity, physical pain, health acceptance, mental state and health status changes (Stansfeld et al., 1997).

In 1975 Sanders proposed three scales for evaluating communication at home, at work and within the social environment. By using these methods of measurement, it is possible to examine the attitudes of deaf or hard of hearing patients and to highlight their communication difficulties. When the scales are administered before and after treatment, they help the rehabilitation team to arrange the treatment plan, and to evaluate success of the rehabilitation strategy for each patient separately (Sanders, 1975). By using the Sanders scales, the rehabilitation program can focus on each patient individually, be multifaceted and oriented towards his needs, not only with lip-reading and acoustic training (Sanders, 1982; Sanders & Jutai, 2004).

Another similar test, he Nijmegen Cochlear Implant Questionnaire (NCIQ) was created to evaluate the Quality of Life of deaf or severely impaired in hearing subjects after cochlear implantation. It includes questions about communication, the psychological state of the implanted person and other areas of its sociality (Krabbe et al., 2000).

Results From the Rehabilitation Processes

The research described in this chapter was carried out in collaboration with two major Cochlear Implantation Centers in Greece. In Athens it was the 2nd Academic ENT Clinic of the ATTIKON General Hospital, while in Thessaloniki it was the 1st Academic ENT Clinic of the AHEPA General Hospital. 123 randomized patients (57 men and 66 women), aged from 6 to 82 years were examined between 2011 and 2015. The research excluded subjects less than 6 years of age and patients who had operated less than 2 years from the date of examination. Subjects were divided into four major categories:

1. Adults postlingually deaf or impaired in hearing, aged 17 and over
2. Children aged 6 to 17 years
3. Children aged 6 to 17 with associated neurological problems
4. Adults prelingually deaf or impaired in hearing aged 17 or more, who used some kind of hearing aid before undergoing cochlear implantation. They were using oral communication prior to their surgery in the cochlea.

From the participants in this survey

- 43 patients were adults, of which:
    - 15 were suffering from sensorineural hearing loss of idiopathic etiology
    - 14 were suffering from related sensorineural hearing loss, worsening as time passed by
    - 4 were suffering from sensorineural hearing loss after meningitis

- 2 were suffering of sensorineural hearing after bacterial infection of the middle ear
- 2 were suffering from sensorineural hearing loss after virus infection of varicella
- 2 were suffering of sensorineural hearing loss due to the Ménière disease
- 2 of sensorineural hearing loss following traumatic brain injury and fracture of the temporal bone
- 1 was suffering from of sensorineural hearing loss due to cochlear otosclerosis
- 1 was suffering from sensorineural hearing loss due to taking ototoxic drugs

- 80 patients were children, of which:
    - 71 were suffering from associated or related sensorineural hearing loss
    - 4 were suffering from sensorineural hearing loss after meningitis
    - 3 were suffering of sensorineural hearing loss due to taking ototoxic drugs
    - 1 was suffering from of sensorineural hearing loss due to due to prematurity < 32 weeks and prolonged hospitalization in the intensive care unit
    - 1 due to perinatal asphyxia (APGAR score <5)

89 subjects were operated on the right ear and 34 on the left. 74 patients used the external processor Nucleus FreedomTM, 19 the ESPrit 3GTM and 17 the Nucleus CP810TM of the COCHLEAR company, while 13 patients were using the Opus IITM processor of the MEDEL company.

The average use of the cochlear implant by the time they were examined during this research was 8.7 years.

Pure Tone and Speech Audiometry

Throughout the study, each of the participants was examined by the speech therapist himself / herself as well as by the rest of the counseling team at the Cochlear Implantation Center. The equipment used for the measurements was the Grason - Stadler GSI 61 clinical audiometer, mod. 1761, using as basic speakers (90 dB) the GSI Madison WI 53711-4495 kit and as input source the Compact Disk player Techniks SLPG 200A.

The tests were carried out in an acoustically insulated chamber. The subject was seated in the middle of the room. The two GSI loudspeakers were calibrated to an amplification level of 65 dBHL, which corresponds to the hearing level of a normal conversation (American National Standards Institute, 2009). They were placed each 1m away from the center with an azimuth of 0° (Byrne & Noble, 1998).

All subjects were assessed with pure tone audiometry, acoustic performance and speech audiometry. The most important for the Quality of Life metrics are the speech recognition scores.

In this assessment, the ability to recognize words and sentences is quantified, by means of a verbal audiometry discrimination test (measured on % scale). The subject was asked to repeat the sentence or the word he heard and had no choice between different possible answers (open type test). During the process, the subject was given via the aural communication channel of the speaker system, in intensity equal to 65 dBHL, a series of sentences and words in Greek. The test used is the well-known Bamford-Kowal-Bench examination (Bench et al., 1979) translated and adapted to the Greek language by P. Nikolopoulos, Professor at the University of Athens.

This assessment is considered to be the most classical and easy-to-use in the English literature. The words to be recognized were embedded in 16 different sentences. Each sentence contained between 4 and 7 words. The target words that each subject had to repeat correctly were 50. They included one-syllable, two-and three-syllable words. Before the beginning of the procedure explanatory instructions were given. The subject listened to each sentence separately and was expected to reproduce it. Even if he was not sure about the content of each word separately, he was encouraged to answer and complete on his own what he did not hear clearly. The subject had to reproduce the sentence he had just heard within the 20-second interval between two consecutive sentences (confirmation time). The speech therapist recorded the answers.

The results for all 123 participants are shown in Figure 3.

It becomes evident, out of this assessment, that the groups of patients which have undergone special education (as is the case of children) during their rehabilitation, or have a remnant in their long term memory of acquired speech communication (as is the case of postlingually deafened adults) excel. On the contrary, for problematic groups, like that of children with associated and related problems, or adults that were prelingually deafened and did not have the chance to undergo special education, the results are rather disheartening.

Figure 3. Speech audiometry results demonstrating the performance of four characteristic groups

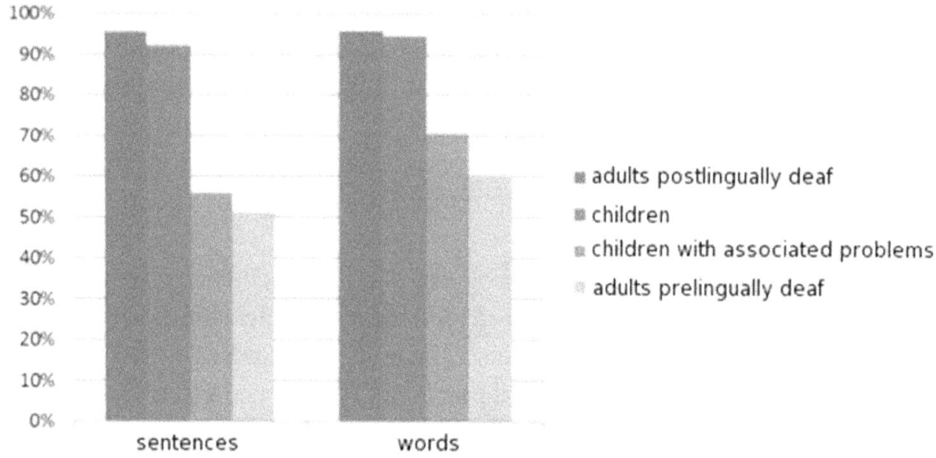

It seems that the lack of special counseling is indeed destructive for building up proper speech communication and may lead to all the stressing patterns of behavior mentioned in the previous section.

Quality of Life Questionnaires: The Sanders Test

After having undergone cochlear implantation, all adult cochlear implant users were given the Sanders psychometric questionnaires (at home, at work, at social events), which were completed by themselves.

In the case of unemployed or retired people, the questionnaires relating to the work were not provided. In addition, the children who had been implanted were also provided with the questionnaires relating to the child's home communication levels, which were completed by both parents (except for single-parent families). In addition, questionnaires were sent about the child's communication to the school, with instructions on how to fill them up, which were completed by the responsible teachers and returned to the Center of Cochlear Implantation. All patients were evaluated preoperatively and post-operatively.

The first questionnaire on the adult's home communication potential includes 9 questions, which evaluate the ability to communicate in different listening situations everyday at home. Each answer includes the choices: "without difficulty", "with little difficulty", "with enough difficulty" and "very difficult" and is calibrated with +2, +1, -1, -2 points respectively. It is also combined with the preferences: "very few times", "often", "very often" which correspond to 1, 2 and 3 points respectively. Each patient completes both selection series for each answer, the grades of which multiply. Each answer can be rated by -6 indicating great difficulty, up to +6 suggesting no difficulty. Thus this questionnaire can gather from -54 points highlighting major difficulties in home communication, up to +54 degrees in cases where the patient does not face any difficulty at all, as if he were a very fit normally hearing person.

The second questionnaire decodes how the adult subject manages communication in his / her work and includes 6 questions that reflect different conditions and communication frameworks. Each answer contains the same selection series as described in the previous questionnaire and is rated the very same way.

The third questionnaire relates to adult communication in social events and includes 7 questions that decode a number of different communication conditions met in the social events of each subject. Each answer includes the same options as described for the adult's home and work communication questionnaires and is calibrated more or less the same way.

The results for this test are shown in Figure 4.

Figure 4. Sanders Quality of Life metrics (%) for adults at home, at work, at social events before and after cochlear implantation

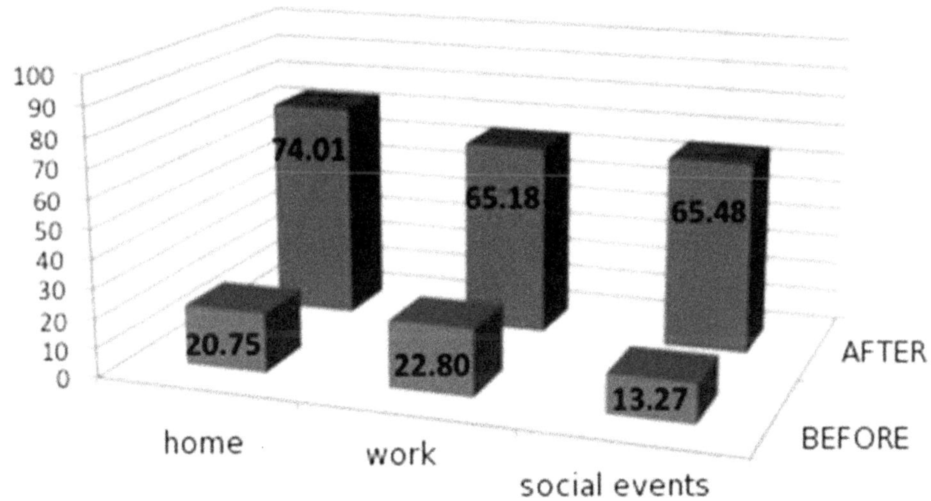

It is apparent in Figure 4, that cochlear implantation is a game changer for adults, as far as their communication in the environments they frequent is concerned. However, there is room for further improvement.

All the children who participated in this research were provided with the psychometric questionnaires for a "Sanders" style assessment. Children where mainly evaluated on their communication at home levels. The questionnaires were completed by the parents of the implanted subjects. Where this was possible, they were completed by both parents. This questionnaire included 9 questions about the different communication conditions the child is expected to face in his living habitat. In Figure 5 is depicted how children control their self-determination when their communication with their parents is taken into consideration.

Unfortunately, many children that have undergone cochlear implantation are burdened by side effects caused by related or associated with their hearing deficit problems. The performance of this group is considerably lower than that of the group of children that cope with hearing impairment only (Figure 5).

Figure 5. Sanders Quality of Life metrics (%) for children at home, before and after cochlear implantation. Left, the group of children with no other problems apart from hearing impairment. Right, the group of children with related and associated mental or physical problems, apart from their hearing impairment.

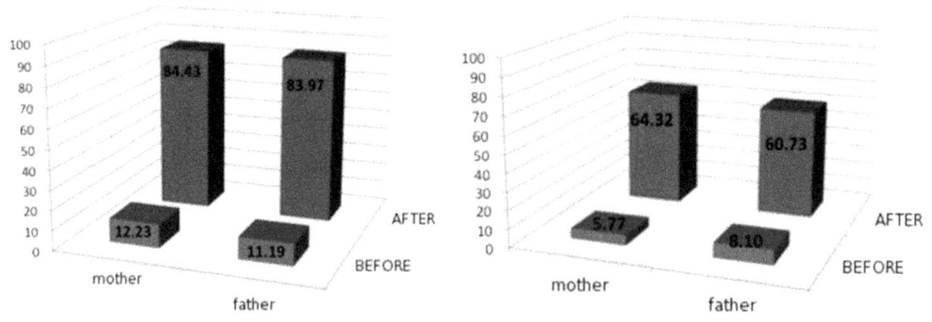

CONCLUSION

Cochlear implantation is a game changer for impaired in hearing patients or totally deaf persons. For many years such subjects had limited possibilities in joining their physically fit counterparts in their everyday activities, as is schooling, work and social reunions.

As technology offers an increased potential for future development in the field of bionics, prosthetics and augmentation, it becomes evident that the improvement of Quality of Life interactions and indices will become the center of the rehabilitation process.

REFERENCES

American Academy of Otolaryngology — Head and Neck Surgery portal. (2018). *Cochlear Implants*. Retrieved from http://www.entnet.org/content/cochlearimplants

Attkisson, C., Cook, J., Karno, M., Lehman, A., McGlashan, T. H., Meltzer, H. Y., ... Hohmann, A. A. (1992). Clinical services research. *Schizophrenia Bulletin*, *18*(4), 561–626. doi:10.1093chbul/18.4.561 PMID:1439613

Baker, D. H., Quittner, A. L., Fink, N. E., Eisenberg, L. S., Tobey, E. A., & Niparko, J. K. (2009). Predicting behavior problems in deaf and hearing children: The influences of language, attention, and parent-child communication. *Development and Psychopathology*, *21*(2), 373–392. doi:10.1017/S0954579409000212 PMID:19338689

Beer, J., Pisoni, D. B., & Kronenberger, W. (2009). Executive function in children with cochlear implants: The role of organizational integrative processes. *Volta Voices*, *16*, 18–23. PMID:23687425

Beitchman, J. H., Wilson, B., Atkinson, L., Young, A., & Adalf, E. (2001). Fourteen year follow up of speech impaired and control children: Psychiatric outcome. *Journal of the American Academy of Child and Adolescent Psychiatry*, *40*(1), 75–82. doi:10.1097/00004583-200101000-00019 PMID:11195567

Bench, J., Kowal, A., & Bamford, J. (1979). The BKB (Bamford-Kowal-Bench) sentence lists for partially-hearing children. *British Journal of Audiology*, *13*(3), 108–112. doi:10.3109/03005367909078884 PMID:486816

Bess, F. H. (2000). The role of generic health-related quality of life measures in establishing audiological rehabilitation outcomes. *Ear and Hearing*, *21*(Supplement), 74S–79S. doi:10.1097/00003446-200008001-00009 PMID:10981596

Blanchfield, B. B., Feldman, J. J., Dunbar, J. L., & Gardner, E. N. (2001). The severely to profoundly hearing-impaired population in the United States: Prevalence estimates and demographics. *Journal of the American Academy of Audiology*, *12*, 183–189. PMID:11332518

Bohs, E. S., Ladd, G. W., & Herald, S. L. (2006). Peer exclusion and victimization: Processes that mediate the relation between peer group rejection and children's classroom engagement and achievement? *Journal of Educational Psychology, 98*(1), 1–13. doi:10.1037/0022-0663.98.1.1

Bowe, F. G., McMahon, B. T., Chang, T., & Louvi, J. (2005). Workplace discrimination, deafness and learning impairment the national, EEEC ADA research project. *Work (Reading, Mass.), 25*, 19–25. PMID:16006672

Bullinger, M., Anderson, R., Cella, D., & Aaronson, N. (1993). Developing and evaluating cross- cultural instruments from minimum requirements to optimal models. *Quality of Life Research: An International Journal of Quality of Life Aspects of Treatment, Care and Rehabilitation, 2*(6), 451–459. doi:10.1007/BF00422219 PMID:8161979

Burkhauser, R. V., & Heutenville, A. J. (2010). Employment among working-age people with disabilities: What current data can tell us. In R. Parker & E. M. Szymanski (Eds.), *Work and disability: Contexts, issues, and strategies for enhancing employment outcomes for people with disabilities* (3rd ed.; pp. 49–86). Austin, TX: Pro-Ed.

Byrne, D., & Noble, W. (1998). Optimising sound localisation with hearing aids. *Trends in Amplification, 3*(2), 51–73. doi:10.1177/108471389800300202 PMID:25425879

Carr, H. J., & Higginson, I. J. (2001). Are quality of life measures patient centered? *BMJ (Clinical Research Ed.).*

Chwalisz, K., & Vaux, A. (2000). Psychology, Social support and adjustment to disability. In Handbook of rehabilitation psychology. American Psychological Association.

Clarke-Stewart, K. A., Allhusen, V. D., McDowell, D. J., Thelen, L., & Call, J. D. (2003). Identifying psychological problems in young children: How do mothers compare with child psychologists? *Journal of Applied Developmental Psychology, 23*(6), 589–624. doi:10.1016/S0193-3973(03)00006-6

Davis, A. (1997). Epidemiology of hearing impairment. In A. G. Kerr & D. Stephens (Eds.), *Scott Brownis Otolaryngology* (6th ed.; Vol. 4, pp. 18–19). Oxford, UK: Butterworth Heiremann.

Dows, W. R., & Harrison, L. (1998). Childhood maltreatment and the risk of substance problems in later life. *Health & Social Care in the Community*, *6*(1), 35–46. doi:10.1046/j.1365-2524.1998.00097.x PMID:11560575

Du Feu, M., & Fergusson, K. (2003). Sensory impairment and mental health. *Advances in Psychiatric Treatment*, *9*(02), 95–103. doi:10.1192/apt.9.2.95

Eide, A. H., & Roysamb, E. (2002). The relationship between level of disability, psychological problems, social activity and social networks. *Rehabilitation Psychology*, *47*(2), 165–183. doi:10.1037/0090-5550.47.2.165

Elwan, A. (1999). *Poverty and Disability: A Survey of the Literature*. Washington, DC: World Bank.

Fletcher, A., Gore, S., Jones, D., Fitzpatrick, R., Spiegelhalter, D., & Cox, D. (1992). Quality of life measures in health care: Design, analysis and interpretation. *BMJ (Clinical Research Ed.)*, *305*(6862), 1145–1148. doi:10.1136/bmj.305.6862.1145 PMID:1463954

Foster, S., & Macleod, J. (2003). Deaf people at work: Assessment of communication among deaf and hearing persons in work settings. *International Journal of Audiology*, *42*(sup1), S128–S139. doi:10.3109/14992020309074634 PMID:12918620

Freeman, R. D., Malkin, S. F., & Hastings, J. O. (1975). Psychosocial problems of deaf children and their families: A comparative study. *American Annals of the Deaf*, *120*, 391–405. PMID:1163401

Gold, M. R., Siegel, J. E., Russell, L. B., & Weinstein, M. C. (1996). *Cost effectiveness in Health and Medicine*. New York: Oxford University Press.

Grenberg, M. T., & Krusche, C. A. (1993). *Promoting social and emotional development in deaf children*. Seattle, WA: The PATHS Project U of Washington Press.

Haas, B. K. (1999). Clarification and integration of similar quality of life concepts. *Image--the Journal of Nursing Scholarship*, *31*(9), 215–220. doi:10.1111/j.1547-5069.1999.tb00483.x PMID:10528449

Hallberg, L. R., & Carlsson, S. G. (1993). A qualitative study of situations turning a hearing disability into a handicap. *Disability, Handicap & Society*, *8*(1), 71–85. doi:10.1080/02674649366780051

Harris, L. K., & Vanzandt, C. E. (1997). Counseling needs of students who are deaf and hard of hearing. *The School Counselor, 44*, 271.

Hart, B., & Risley, T. R. (1995). *Meaningful differences in the everyday experience of young American children. Paul H.* Baltimore, MD: Brookes Publishing Co.

Haskins, B. G. (2004). Serving Deaf Adult Psychiatric Impairments. *Psychiatric Services (Washington, D.C.), 55*(4), 439–441. doi:10.1176/appi.ps.55.4.439 PMID:15067159

Herbst, K. G., & Humphrey, C. (1980). Hearing impairment and mental state in the elderly living at home. *British Medical Journal, 281*(6245), 903–905. doi:10.1136/bmj.281.6245.903 PMID:7427503

Higginson, I. (1994). Clinical teams, general practice, audit and outcomes. In *Outcomes into clinical practice*. London: BMJ Books.

Hindley, P., & VanGent, T. (2004). Psychiatric aspects of specific sensory impairments. In M. Rytter & E. Taylor (Eds.), *Child and Adolescent Psychiatry* (4th ed.; pp. 842–857). Blackwell.

Humphries, T., Kushalnagar, P., Mathur, G., Napoli, D. J., Padden, C., Rathmann, C., & Smith, S. R. (2012). Language acquisition for deaf children: Reducing the harms of zero tolerance to the use of alternative approaches. *Harm Reduction Journal, 9*(16). PMID:22472091

Hytoglou-Antoniadou. M. (2003). The Social Cerebrum. Thessaloniki, Greece: Publish City. (in Greek)

Jerger, J., & Hayes, D. (1977). Diagnostic speech audiometry. *Archives of Otolaryngology (Chicago, Ill.), 103*(4), 216–222. doi:10.1001/archotol.1977.00780210072008 PMID:849199

Kent, K.A. (2003). Identity issues for hard of hearing adolescents ages 11, 13 and 15 in mainstream settings. *Journal of Deaf Studies and Deaf Education, 8*, 315-324.

Knutson, J. F., Johnson, C. R., & Sullivan, P. M. (2004). Disciplinary choices of mothers of deaf children and mothers of normally hearing children. *Child Abuse & Neglect, 28*(9), 925–937. doi:10.1016/j.chiabu.2004.04.005 PMID:15450759

Kochkin, S., Luxford, W., Northern, J., Mason, P., & Tharpe, A. M. (2007). Are a million dependents with hearing loss in America being left behind? *Hearing Review*. Retrieved from http://www.betterhearing.org/sites/default/files/hearingpedia-resources/M7_children_hearing_loss_left_behind.pdf

Kovacs, M., & Devlin, B. (1998). Internalizing disorders in childhood. *Journal of Child Psychology and Psychiatry, and Allied Disciplines*, *39*(1), 47–63. doi:10.1017/S0021963097001765 PMID:9534086

Kraashen, S. (1973). Lateralization, language learning, and the critical period. Some new evidence. *Language Learning*, *26*(1), 63–71. doi:10.1111/j.1467-1770.1973.tb00097.x

Krabbe, P. F. M., Hinderink, J. B., & Vanden Broek, P. (2000). The effect of cochlear implant use in postlingually deaf results. *International Journal of Technology Assessment in Health Care*, *16*(03), 864–873. doi:10.1017/S0266462300102132 PMID:11028141

Kruse, D. (1997). *Employment and Disability: Characteristics of Employed and Non-Employed People with Disabilities*. Washington, DC: US Department of Labor.

Kyriafinis, G. (2005). *Cochlear implantation*. Thessaloniki, Greece: Publish City. (in Greek)

La forge, R.G., Spector, W.D., & Sternberg, J. (1992). The relationship of vision and hearing impairment to one-year mortality and functional decline. *J. Aging Health, 4*, 126-148.

Laroche, C., Garcia, L. J., & Barrette, J. (2000). Perceptions by persons with hearing impairment, audiologists and employers of the obstacles to work integration. *Journal of the Academy of Rehabilitative Audiology*, *33*, 63–90.

Lehman, A. F. (1988). A Quality of Life Interview for the Chronically Mentally Ill. *Evaluation and Program Planning*, *II*(1), 51–62. doi:10.1016/0149-7189(88)90033-X

Leigh, J., Dettman, S., Holland, J., Dowell, R., & Briggs, R. J. (2008). Long-term language, speech production and speech perception outcomes for children who received a cochlear implant at or before 12 months of age. Reflecting Connections: A Joint Conference Between New Zealand Speech-Language Therapists Association and Speech Pathology Australia, Auckland, New Zealand.

Lenneberg, E. (1967). *Biological Foundations of Language*. New York: Willey.

Luria, A. R. (1961). *The role of speech in normal and abnormal behavior*. New York: Liveright.

MacSweeney, M. (1998). Cognition and Deafness. In S. Gregory, P. Knight, W. MacCracken, S. Powers, & L. Watson (Eds.), *Issues in Deaf Education* (pp. 20–27). London: David Fulton Publishers.

Mc Elwain, N. L., & Volling, B. L. (2005). Preschool children's interactions with friends and older siblings: Relationship specificity and joint contributions to problem behavior. *Journal of Family Psychology*, *19*(4), 486–496. doi:10.1037/0893-3200.19.4.486 PMID:16402863

Meadow, K. P., & Trybus, R. J. (1979). Behavioral and emotional problems of deaf children: an overview In Hearing and Hearing Impairment. Grune and Stratton.

Mitchell, T., & Quittner, A. (1996). Multimethod study of attention and behavior problems in hearing impaired children. *Journal of Clinical Child Psychology*, *25*(1), 83–96. doi:10.120715374424jccp2501_10

Murphy, M. B., Laurie-Rose, C., Brinkman, T. M., & McNamara, K. A. (2007). Sustained attention and social competence in typically developing preschool-aged children. *Early Child Development and Care*, *177*(2), 133–149. doi:10.1080/03004430500349559

Nathan, L., Goulandris, N., & Snowling, M. J. (2000). The development of early literacy skills among children with speech difficulties: A test of the critical age hypothesis. *Journal of Speech, Language, and Hearing Research: JSLHR*, *43*, 380–394. PMID:10757691

Nunes, T., Pretzlik, U., & Olson, J. (2001). Deaf children's social relationships in mainstream schools. *Deafness & Education International*, *3*(3), 123–136. doi:10.1179/146431501790560972

Oerger, M. (1989). Quality of Life, Health Status, and Clinical Research. *Medical Care*, (Supplement), S148–S156. PMID:2646487

Owens, R. (2013). *Language Disorders: A Functional Approach to Assessment and Intervention* (6th ed.). Pearson.

Parving, A., & Christensen, B. (1993). Training and employment in hearing-impaired subjects at 20-35 years of age. *Scandinavian Audiology*, 22133–22139. PMID:8321998

Percy-Smith, L., Caye-Thomasen, P., Gudman, M., Jensen, J., & Thomsen, J. (2008). Self-esteem and social well-being of children with cochlear implant compared to normal hearing children. *International Journal of Pediatric Otorhinolaryngology*, *72*(7), 1113–1120. doi:10.1016/j.ijporl.2008.03.028 PMID:18501436

Pollard, R. Q. (1994). Public mental health service and diagnostic trends regarding individuals who are deaf or hard-of-hearing. *Rehabilitation Psychology*, *39*(3), 147–160. doi:10.1037/h0080318

Prizant, B., & Meyer, E. (1993). Socioemotional aspects of language and social-communication disorders in young children. *American Journal of Speech-Language Pathology*, *2*(3), 56–71. doi:10.1044/1058-0360.0203.56

Quittner, A. L., Barker, D. H., Snell, C., Cruz, I., McDonald, L., & Grimley, M. E. (2007). Improvements in visual attention after cochlear implantation. *Audiological Medicine*, *5*, 242–249. doi:10.1080/16513860701745401

Remmel, E., & Peters, K. (2009). Theory of mind and language in children with cochlear implants. *Journal of Deaf Studies and Deaf Education*, *14*(2), 218–237. doi:10.1093/deafed/enn036 PMID:18796736

Rescorla, L. (2002). Language and reading outcomes to age 9 I late-talking toddlers. *Journal of Speech, Language, and Hearing Research: JSLHR*, *45*(2), 360–371. doi:10.1044/1092-4388(2002/028) PMID:12003517

Robbins, A.M., Svirsky, M., & Kirk, K.I. (1997). Children with implants can speak but can they communicate? *Otolaryngol. Head Neck Surg.*, *117*(ph I), 155-160.

Robinson, K., Gatchouse, S., & Browning, G. G. (1996). Measuring benefit from otorhinolaryngological surgery and therapy. *The Annals of Otology, Rhinology, and Laryngology*, *105*(6), 415–422. doi:10.1177/000348949610500601 PMID:8638891

Ronnenberg, J. (2003). *Working memory, neuroscience, and language: Evidence from deaf and hard-of-hearing individuals.* In M. Marschark & P. Spencer (Eds.), *Handbook of Deaf Studies, Language, and Education* (pp. 478–490). Oxford University Press.

Ruben, R. J. (2000). Redefining the survival of the fittest. Communication disorders in the 21st century. *Laryngoscope, 110*(2), 241–245. doi:10.1097/00005537-200002010-00010 PMID:10680923

Ruff, H. A., & Rothbart, M. K. (1996). *Attention in early development: Themes and Variations.* New York: Oxford University Press.

Sanders, D. A. (1975). Hearing aid orientation and counseling. In M. C. Pollack (Ed.), *Amplification for the Hearing-Impaired.* New York: Grune and Stratton.

Sanders, D. A. (1982). *Aural Rehabilitation: A Management Model* (2nd ed.). Englewood Cliffs, NJ: Prentice-Hall.

Sanders, G. H., & Jutai, J. W. (2004). Hearing specific and generic measures of the psychosocial impact of hearing aids. S. *Am Acad Audiol., 15*(3), 238–248. doi:10.3766/jaaa.15.3.6

Schick, B., de Villiers, P., de Villiers, J., & Hoffmeister, R. (2007). Language and Theory of Mind: A study of deaf children. *Child Development, 78*(2), 376–396. doi:10.1111/j.1467-8624.2007.01004.x PMID:17381779

Schirk, B., Williams, K., & Kupermintz, H. (2006). Look who's being left behind? Educational interpreters and access to education for deaf and hard of hearing students. *Journal of Deaf Studies and Deaf Education, 11*, 3–20. PMID:16192404

Schroedel, J. (1992). Helping adolescents and young adults who are deaf make career decisions. *The Volta Review, 94*, 37–46.

Smith, L. B., Quittner, A. I., Osberger, M. J., & Miyamoto, R. (1998). Audition and Visual Attention the developmental trajectory in deaf and hearing populations. *Developmental Psychology, 34*(5), 840–850. doi:10.1037/0012-1649.34.5.840 PMID:9779732

Snowling, M. J., Adams, J. W., Bishop, D. V. M., & Stohard, S. E. (2001). Educational attainments of school leavers with a preschool history of speech-language impairments. *International Journal of Language & Communication Disorders*, *36*(2), 173–183. doi:10.1080/13682820010019892 PMID:11344593

Sokol, J., & Hyde, M. (2002). Hearing Screening. *Pediatrics*, *23*, 155–161. PMID:11986491

Stansfeld, S., Roberts, R., & Foot, S. (1997). Assessing the validity of the SF-36 General Health Survey. *Quality of Life Research: An International Journal of Quality of Life Aspects of Treatment, Care and Rehabilitation*, *6*(3), 217–224. doi:10.1023/A:1026406620756 PMID:9226979

Steinberg, A. G., Sullivan, V. J., & Montoya, L. A. (1999). Loneliness and social isolation in the work place for deaf individuals during the transition years: A preliminary investigation. *Journal of Applied Rehabilitation Counseling*, *30*(1), 22–30.

Stewart, D. A., & Clarke, B. R. (2003). *Literacy and Your Deaf Child: What Every Parent Should Know*. Washington, DC: Gallaudet University Press.

Stinson, M., & Walter, G. (1997). Improving retention for deaf and hard of hearing students: What the research tells us. *Journal of the American Deafness and Rehabilitation Association*, *30*(4), 14–23.

Stinson, M. S., & Whitmire, K. A. (2000). Adolescents who are deaf or hard of hearing: A Communication Perspective on educational placement. *Topics in Language Disorders*, *20*(2), 58–72. doi:10.1097/00011363-200020020-00006

Sullivan, P. M., & Knutson, J. F. (2000). Maltreatment and disabilities: A population-based epidemiological study. *Child Abuse & Neglect*, *24*(10), 1257–1273. doi:10.1016/S0145-2134(00)00190-3 PMID:11075694

Swanson, J. L., & Woitke, M. B. (1997). Theory into practice in career assessment for women: Assessment and interventions regarding perceived career barriers. *Journal of Career Assessment*, *5*(4), 443–462. doi:10.1177/106907279700500405

Szymanski, E. M., & Hershenson, D. B. (2005). An ecological approach to vocational behavior and career development of people with disabilities. In R. Parker, E. M. Szymanski, & J. B. Pattersson (Eds.), *Rehabilitation Counseling: Basics and beyond* (4th ed.; pp. 225–280). Austin, TX: PRO-ED.

Toppelberg, C. O., & Shapiro, T. (2000). Language disorders: A 10-year research update review. *Journal of the American Academy of Child and Adolescent Psychiatry, 39*(2), 143–152. doi:10.1097/00004583-200002000-00011 PMID:10673823

Torrance, G. W., & Feeny, D. (1989). Utilities and quality- adjusted life years. *International Journal of Technology Assessment in Health Care, 5*(04), 559–575. doi:10.1017/S0266462300008461 PMID:2634630

Tucker, B. (1988). Deaf Prison Inmates. Los Angeles, CA: Loyola of Los Angeles School of Law.

Uhlmann, R. F., Larson, E. B., Rees, T. S., Koepsell, T. D., & Duckert, L. G. (1989). Relation of hearing impairment to dementia and cognitive dysfunction in older adults. *Journal of the American Medical Association, 261*(13), 1916–1919. doi:10.1001/jama.1989.03420130084028 PMID:2926927

Vaccan, C., & Marshark, M. (1997). Communication between parents and deaf children: Implications for social-emotional development. *Journal of Child Psychology and Psychiatry, and Allied Disciplines, 38*(7), 793–801. doi:10.1111/j.1469-7610.1997.tb01597.x PMID:9363578

Van Eldik, T., Trefferes, P. D. A., Veerman, J. W., & Verhulst, F. C. (2004). Mental health problems of deaf Dutch children as indicated by parents responses to the Child Behavior Checklist. *American Annals of the Deaf, 148*(5), 390–395. doi:10.1353/aad.2004.0002 PMID:15132019

Venail, I., Vieu, A., Artieres, F., Mondain, M., & Uziel, A. (2010). Educational and Employment Achievements in Prelingually Deaf Children who receive cochlear implants. *Archives of Otolaryngology--Head & Neck Surgery, 136*(4), 366–372. doi:10.1001/archoto.2010.31 PMID:20403853

Weisel, A., & Cinamon, G. C. (2005). Hearing, deaf and HH Israeli adolescents' evaluation of deaf men and deaf women's occupational competence. *Journal of Deaf Studies and Deaf Education*, *10*(4), 376–389. doi:10.1093/deafed/eni045 PMID:16037482

Wells, K. B. (1989). The functioning and well-being of Depressed Patients: Results from the Medical Outcomes Study. *Journal of the American Medical Association*, *262*(7), 914–919. doi:10.1001/jama.1989.03430070062031 PMID:2754791

Yuwen, L., & Goldscmidt, J.E. (2009). *Taking Employment Discrimination Seriously. Chinese and European Perspectives*. Leiden: Martinus Nijhoff Publishers.

Chapter 8
Quantum Cognition and Its Influence on Decrease of Global Stress Level Related With Job Improvement Strategies:
Quantum Brain and Global Stress

Aleksandar Stojanovic
Federal University of Ceara, Brazil

Ana Starcevic
University of Belgrade, Serbia

ABSTRACT

The quantum mind or quantum consciousness group of hypotheses propose that classical mechanics cannot explain consciousness. Quantum theory is used to insert models of cognition that target to be more innovative than models based on traditional classical probability theory, which includes cognitive modeling phenomena in science. At the moment we can say that there is no clearly defined neurophysiological mechanisms of creation of the quantum-like representation of information in the brain, but we can mention the hypothesis of matching the information processing in the brain with quantum information and probability with contextuality as the key word. Using limited cognitive resources, incompatibility provides humans the means for answering an unlimited number of questions, thus promoting parsimony and cognitive economy.

DOI: 10.4018/978-1-5225-7513-9.ch008

INTRODUCTION

The idea that quantum mechanics has something to do with the workings of the mind was proposed by Eugene Wigner who suggested that wave function collapses due to its interaction with consciousness. Freeman Dyson argued that "mind, as manifested by the capacity to make choices, is to some extent inherent in every electron." ("Quantum Approaches to Consciousness", 2011; Dyson, 2004).

Many scientists considered this option as unprobable describing it as a myth with no scientific basis.

David Chalmers argued against quantum consciousness. He instead discussed how quantum mechanics may relate to dualistic consciousness. Chalmers is skeptical of the ability of any new physics to resolve the hard problem of consciousness.

The main argument against the quantum mind hypothesis was the assertion that quantum states in the brain would lose coherency before they reached a scale where they could be useful for neural processing, which was elaborated by Tegmark, who made calculation in which quantum systems in the brain decohere at sub-picosecond timescales, which are considered to be too short to control brain function. If there is no brain-mind identity, mind-states could be in an abstract space that is not affected by decoherence.(Khrennikov,2009;Van den Noort,2016).

Quantum cognition represents an inovative field which applies the mathematical formalism of quantum theory to model of cognitive phenomena such as information processing by the human brain, language, decision making, human memory, concepts and conceptual reasoning, human judgment, and perception. This field makes a great difference from the quantum mind as it is not reliant on the hypothesis that there is something micro-physical quantum mechanical about the brain as it is based on the quantum structure paradigm. The main mechanism or concept is based on a information processing by complex systems such as brain structures. It is hypothesised that contextual dependence of information and probabilistic reasoning could be mathematically described in the framework of quantum information and quantum probability theory ()Caves, 2002;Tversky, 1992; Savage, 1954).

Quantum theory is used to insert models of cognition that target to be more inovative than models based on traditional classical probability theory which includes cognitive modeling phenomena in science. Since the use of a quantum-theoretic framework is for modeling purposes, the identification of quantum structures in cognitive phenomena does not presuppose the existence of microscopic quantum processes in the human brain (Pothos, 2009).

We can observe the brain as macroscopic physical system operating on the scales (of time, space, temperature) which differ crucially from the corresponding quantum scales. But as alive organ it hold some temperature and is simply too hot to be able perform the real quantum information processing, and use the quantum carriers of information such as photons, ions, electrons. Neuron is by definition a morphological unit of central nervous system and the brain as well. From this perspective we can say that neuron presents also basic unit of information processing. Neuron couldn't be in the superposition of two states: firing and non-firing. Hence, it cannot produce superposition playing the basic role in the quantum information processing. Superpositions of mental states are created by complex neural networks of neurons. The activity of such neural networks can produce effects which are formally described as interference and entanglement (Khrenikov,2009).

The quantum cognition project is based on the observation that various cognitive phenomena are more adequately described by quantum information theory and quantum probability than by the corresponding classical theories.

At the moment we can say that there is no clearly defined neurophysiological mechanisms of creation of the quantum-like representation of information in the brain, but we can mention the hypothesis of matching the information processing in the brain with quantum information and probability with contextuality as the key word. Quantum systems do not have objective properties which can be defined independently of measurement context as contextuality implies existence of incompatible mental variables, violation of the classical law of total probability and interference effects, so we can summarize that quantum cognition approach can be considered as an attempt to formalize contextuality of mental processes by using the mathematical apparatus of quantum mechanics.

Consciousness and Quantum Brain

The quantum mind or quantum consciousness group of hypotheses propose that classical mechanics cannot explain consciousness. It posits that quantum mechanical phenomena, such as quantum entanglement and superposition, may play an important part in the brain's function and could form the basis of an explanation of consciousness (Yukalov, 2011; Allis, 1953).

If we want to discuss about the highest of all psychological functions, consciousness, let it definiate it first. The widest definition includes the state or quality of awareness the executive control system of the mind. Despite the difficulty in definition, many philosophers believe that there is a broadly shared underlying intuition about what consciousness is. As Max Velmans and Susan Schneider wrote in The Blackwell Companion to Consciousness: "Anything that we are aware of at a given moment forms part of our consciousness, making conscious experience at once the most familiar and most mysterious aspect of our lives.

Many philosophers tried to comprehend the nature of consciousness and identify its essential properties. Issues of concern in the philosophy of consciousness include whether the concept is fundamentally coherent; whether consciousness can ever be explained mechanistically; whether non-human consciousness exists and if so how can it be recognized; how consciousness relates to language; whether consciousness can be understood in a way that does not require a dualistic distinction between mental and physical states or properties; and whether it may ever be possible for computing machines like computers or robots to be conscious, a topic studied in the field of artificial intelligence (Allais, 1953; Ellsberg, 1961).

The base of the very well coordinated connection between the consciousness and brain physiological processes is seem to be separated in two very different kinds of processes.

Descartes and Pineal Gland

Descartes formulated the Cartesian dualism in which he proposed that consciousness resides within an immaterial domain he called the realm of thought, in contrast to the domain of material things, which he called the realm of extension. He suggested that the interaction between these two domains occurs inside the brain, perhaps in a small midline structure called the pineal gland.

Pineal gland is a midline, unpaired pine-cone shape brain structure. It is reddish-gray and about the size of a grain of rice (5–8 mm) in humans. The pineal gland, also called the pineal body, is part of the epithalamus, and lies between the laterally positioned thalamic bodies and behind the habenular commissure. It is located in the quadrigeminal cistern near to the corpora quadrigemina. It is also located behind the third ventricle and is bathed in cerebrospinal fluid supplied through a small pineal recess of the third ventricle which projects into the stalk of the gland.

Although it is widely accepted that Descartes considered the pineal gland as if it the heart of the soul and been supported by many philosophers of his age back than but no alternative solution has gained general acceptance. Proposed solutions can be divided broadly into two categories: dualist solutions that maintain Descartes' rigid distinction between the realm of consciousness and the realm of matter but give different answers for how the two realms relate to each other; and monist solutions that maintain that there is really only one realm of being, of which consciousness and matter are both aspects. Each of these categories itself contains numerous variants. The two main types of dualism are substance dualism (which holds that the mind is formed of a distinct type of substance not governed by the laws of physics) and property dualism (which holds that the laws of physics are universally valid but cannot be used to explain the mind). The three main types of monism are physicalism (which holds that the mind consists of matter organized in a particular way), idealism (which holds that only thought or experience truly exists, and matter is merely an illusion), and neutral monism (which holds that both mind and matter are aspects of a distinct essence that is itself identical to neither of them). There are also, however, a large number of idiosyncratic theories that cannot cleanly be assigned to any of these schools of thought (Machina, 2009).

A few theoretical physicists have argued that classical physics is intrinsically incapable of explaining the holistic aspects of consciousness, but that quantum theory may provide the missing ingredients. Several theorists have therefore proposed quantum mind (QM) theories of consciousness. Notable theories falling into this category include the holonomic brain theory of Karl Pribram and David Bohm, and the Orch-OR theory formulated by Stuart Hameroff and Roger Penrose. Some of these QM theories offer descriptions of phenomenal consciousness, as well as QM interpretations of access consciousness. None of the quantum mechanical theories has been confirmed by experiment. Recent publications by G. Guerreshi, J. Cia, S. Popescu, and H. Briege could falsify proposals such as those of Hameroff, which rely on quantum entanglement in protein. At the present time many scientists and philosophers consider the arguments for an important role of quantum phenomena to be unconvincing.

Apart from the general question of the "hard problem" of consciousness, roughly speaking, the question of how mental experience arises from a physical basis, a more specialized question is how to square the subjective notion that we are in control of our decisions (at least in some small measure) with the customary view of causality that subsequent events are caused by prior events. The topic of free will is the philosophical and scientific examination of this conundrum.

Quantum Mechanics, Mind-Different Theories

The idea that quantum mechanics has something to do with the workings of the mind was proposed by Eugene Wigner who suggested that wave function collapses due to its interaction with consciousness. Freeman Dyson argued that "mind, as manifested by the capacity to make choices, is to some extent inherent in every electron."

Many scientists considered this option as unprobable describing it as a myth with no scientific basis.

David Chalmers argued against quantum consciousness. He instead discussed how quantum mechanics may relate to dualistic consciousness. Chalmers is skeptical of the ability of any new physics to resolve the hard problem of consciousness.

The main argument against the quantum mind hypothesis was the assertion that quantum states in the brain would lose coherency before they reached a scale where they could be useful for neural processing, which was elaborated by Tegmark, who made calculation in which quantum systems in the brain decohere at sub-picosecond timescales, which are considered to be too short to control brain function. If there is no brain-mind identity, mind-states could be in an abstract space that is not affected by decoherence (Khrennikov, 2008).

Quantum Cognition

Quantum cognition represents an inovative field which applies the mathematical formalism ofquantum theory to model of cognitive phenomena such as information processing by the human brain, language, decision making, human memory, concepts and conceptual reasoning, human judgment, and perception. This field makes a great difference from the quantum mind as it is not reliant on the hypothesis that there is something micro-physical quantum mechanical about the brain as it is based on the quantum structure paradigm. The main mechanism or concept is based on a information processing by complex systems such as brain structures. It is hypothesised that contextual dependence of information and probabilistic reasoning could be mathematically described in the framework of quantum information and quantum probability theory.

Quantum theory is used to insert models of cognition that target to be more inovative than models based on traditional classical probability theorywhich includes cognitive modeling phenomena in science. Since the use of a quantum-theoretic framework is for modeling purposes, the identification of quantum structures in cognitive phenomena does not presuppose the existence of microscopic quantum processes in the human brain (Khrennikov, 2009).

Human Brain

Morhological supstrate for the soul and all the psychological functions that applied refer to „inner me" is generally refered to the brain with emphasis to specific brain structures that are parts of the telencephalon, their connections are coorelations with other important structures inside the body. We can here try to describe the human brain from the neuroanatomical point, non metaphysical. The shape and size of the brain varies greatly between species, and identifying common features is often difficult, mostly the ones that are the most included in higher functions. There are a number of principles of brain architecture that apply across a wide range of species and some aspects of brain structure are common to almost the entire range of animal species (like rats).

The simplest way to gain information about brain anatomy is by visual inspection, where we can see the brain tissue in its natural state is too soft to work with, but it can be hardened by immersion in fixative, such as formaline. Visually, the interior of the brain consists of areas of so-called grey matter, with a dark color, separated by areas of white matter, with a lighter color. Inner microscopic description of the different barin structures and regions can be gained by staining followed by mictroscopic analysis, slices of brain tissue with a variety of chemicals that bring out areas where specific types of molecules are present in high concentrations. As a side effect of the electrochemical processes used by neurons for signaling, brain tissue generates electric fields when it is active. When large numbers of neurons show synchronized activity, the electric fields that they generate can be large enough to detect outside the skull (Van den Noort, 2016).

Many brain structures are involved in current investigation as a possible morhological supstrates of consciousness, but the most examined are brain cortex, brainstem, diencephalon, amygdala and hippocampus.

These structures are also mantioned to be neuroanatomical markers involved in stress response and reaction both in acute and chronic state. However, stress can induce, if prolonged, chronic inflamation, or excitation state of the cell, and consequently volumetric changes as well.

We can observe the brain as macroscopic physical system operating on the scales (of time, space, temperature) which differ crucially from the corresponding quantum scales. But as alive organ it hold some temperature and is simply too hot to be able perform the real quantum information processing, and use the quantum carriers of information such as photons, ions, electrons. Neuron is by definition a morphological unit of central nervous system and the brain as well. From this perspective we can say that neuron presents also basic unit of information processing. Neuron couldn't be in the superposition of two states: firing and non-firing. Hence, it cannot produce superposition playing the basic role in the quantum information processing. Superpositions of mental states are created by complex neural networks of neurons. The activity of such neural networks can produce effects which are formally described as interference and entanglement. (Tversky, 1992)

The quantum cognition project is based on the observation that various cognitive phenomena are more adequately described by quantum information theory and quantum probability than by the corresponding classical theories.

At the moment we can say that there is no clearly defined neurophysiological mechanisms of creation of the quantum-like representation of information in the brain, but we can mention the hypothesis of matching the information processing in the brain with quantum information and probability with contextuality as the key word. Quantum systems do not have objective properties which can be defined independently of measurement context as contextuality implies existence of incompatible mental variables, violation of the classical law of total probability and interference effects, so we can summarize that quantum cognition approach can be considered as an attempt to formalize contextuality of mental processes by using the mathematical apparatus of quantum mechanics.

Stress and Work

Work stress refers to the process of job stressors, or stimuli in the workplace, leading to strains, or negative responses or reactions. Organizational development refers to a process in which problems or opportunities in the work environment are identified, plans are made to remediate or capitalize on the stimuli, action is taken, and subsequently the results of the plans and actions are evaluated. When organizational development strategies are used to assess work stress in the workplace, the actions employed are various stress management interventions. Two key factors tying work stress and organizational development are the role of the person and the role of the environment. In order to cope with work-related stressors and manage strains, organizations must be able to identify and differentiate between factors in the environment that are potential sources of stressors and how individuals perceive those factors. Primary stress management interventions focus on preventing stressors from even presenting, such as by clearly articulating workers' roles and providing necessary resources for employees to perform their job. Secondary stress management interventions focus on a person's appraisal of job stressors as a threat or challenge, and the person's ability to cope with the stressors (presuming sufficient internal resources, such as a sense of meaningfulness in life, or external resources, such as social support from a supervisor). When coping is not successful, strains may develop. Tertiary stress management interventions attempt to remediate strains, by addressing the consequence itself (e.g., diabetes management) and/or the source of the strain (e.g., reducing workload). The person and/or the organization may be the targets of the intervention. The ultimate goal of stress management interventions is to minimize problems in the work environment, intensify aspects of the work environment that create a sense of a quality work context, enable people to cope with stressors that might arise, and provide tools for employees and organizations to manage strains that might develop despite all best efforts to create a healthy workplace (Machina, 2009).

Why Quantum Cognition?

Rational models of cognition adhere to the laws of classical probability theories, although human thinking and decision making does not conform these laws. Quantum models present cognitive phenomena with proven recalcitrant with means of classical probability theory. This is all Refered to classical probabilty theory, Kolmogorov theory on which Bayesian model rests and it says that the Bayes rule is a simple theorem that follows from the classical probability definition of conditional probability. Suppose {H1, . . ., HN} is a set of hypotheses that you wish to evaluate, and D represents some data that provide evidence for or against each hypothesis. Then according to the definition of conditional probability, p(HijD) = p(Hi\D)/p(D). Bayes rule uses the classical definition of joint probability to rewrite the numerator on the right hand of the equation: p(Hi\D) = p(Hi)p(DjHi); and the Bayes rule uses the law of total probability to rewrite the denominator: P j p(Hj) p(DjHj). Bayesian models of cognition use these rules to construct models that predict how people make complex inferences from a set of observations. Why use quantum probability theory? After all, the preva-lence of the Bayesian models is testament to the success of classical probability theory in modeling cognition. Despite this success, however, there has been a steady accumulation of puzzling, even paradoxical, cognitive phenomena that violate the axioms upon which classical probability theory (and hence Bayesian inference) is based. Thus far, these violations have been explained using heuristic rules such as the representativeness heuristic and the anchoring-and- adjustment heuristic. Rather than resorting to heuristics, quantum cognition successfully accounts for these violations using a coherent, common set of principles. Although this review focuses on judgment and decision making, we briefly highlight the expressive power of quantum models by pointing out that they have already been applied to a broad range of cognitive phenomena, including perception, memory, conceptual combinations, attitudes, probability judgments, causal reasoning, decision making, and strategic games. It is not possible to survey the myriad of applications in this review. We will restrict our attention to a representative set of examples which intuitively illustrate the basic quantum principles introduced previously. Quantum cognition also raises many new questions for cognitive scientists and psychologists to address. One is about rationality. Classical probability theory may provide an upper bound that achieves optimal performance irrespective of computational costs and resource limitations. Quantum models may provide a more realistic bound that performs close to optimal but with fewer computational demands. Consider, for example, a strategic game involving yourself and n 1 other players, and each player can choose one of K actions. If human cognition directly implements classical probability theory (i.e., it treats all events as compatible), then Kn joint probabilities are required to represent your beliefs regarding the actions that could be taken by yourself and the other n 1 players, producing an exponential growth in dimensionality. If instead, human cognition applies a new incompatible perspective to each player, then all of the required probabilities can be assigned by using a single state vector that is evaluated with respect to different bases within a fixed K-dimensional space (Caves, 2002).

CONCLUSION

Using limited cognitive resources, incompatibility provides humans the means for answering an unlimited number of questions, thus promoting parsimony and cognitive economy. However, the use of incompatibility comes at the cost of introducing non-commutativity and sequential effects. Our view is that incompatibility of events provides an effective solution to bounded resources, which is the reason for bounded rationality.

REFERENCES

Allais, M. (1953). Le comportement de l'homme rationnel devant le risque: Critique des postulats et axiomes de l'ecole Americaine. *Econometrica, 21*(4), 503–546. doi:10.2307/1907921

Caves, C. M., Fuchs, C. A., & Schack, R. (2002). Quantum probabilities as Bayesian probabilities. *Physical Review A., 65*(2), 022305. doi:10.1103/PhysRevA.65.022305

Dyson, F. (2004). Infinite in All Directions: Gifford Lectures Given at Aberdeen, Scotland April--November 1985. New York: Perennial.

Ellsberg, D. (1961). Risk, ambiguity, and the Savage axioms. *The Quarterly Journal of Economics, 75*(4), 643–669. doi:10.2307/1884324

Khrennikov, A. (2008). The Quantum-Like Brain on the Cognitive and Subcognitive Time Scales. *Journal of Consciousness Studies, 15*(7).

Khrennikov, A. (2009). *Contextual Approach to Quantum Formalism (Fundamental Theories of Physics 160)*. Springer. doi:10.1007/978-1-4020-9593-1

Machina, M. J. (2009). Risk, ambiguity, and the dark-dependence axioms. *American Econonomical Review, 99*(1), 385–392. doi:10.1257/aer.99.1.385

Pothos, E. M., & Busemeyer, J. R. (2009). A quantum probability explanation for violations of 'rational'decision theory. *Proceedings of the Royal Society B: Biological Sciences, 276*(1665), 2171–2178.

Quantum Approaches to Consciousness. (2011). In Stanford Encyclopedia of Philosophy. Stanford University Press.

Savage, L. J. (1954). *The Foundations of Statistics*. John Wiley & Sons.

Tversky, A., & Shafir, E. (1992). The disjunction effect in choice under uncertainty. *Psychological Science, 3*(5), 305–309. doi:10.1111/j.1467-9280.1992.tb00678.x

Van den Noort, M., Lim, S., & Bosch, P. (2016). On the need to unify neuroscience and physics. *Neuroimmunology and Neuroinflammation*, *3*(12), 271–273. doi:10.20517/2347-8659.2016.55

Yukalov, V. I., & Sornette, D. (2011). Decision theory with prospect interference and entanglement. *Theory and Decision*, *70*(3), 283–328. doi:10.100711238-010-9202-y

Chapter 9
Digital Heath Interventions in Mental Health

Aleksandra Stanimirovic
University of Toronto, Canada

ABSTRACT

Technological renaissance of the last century stimulated the application of digital interventions in the healthcare domain. Digital healthcare interventions (DHIs) could be implemented through smartphone applications (apps), remote monitoring and tracking devices, and wearable computers. Technology is positioned to transform how mental healthcare is delivered and accessed. In fact, remote active and passive monitoring of parameters, such as mood, activity, and sleep, could be integrated with therapeutic interventions. However, the transformation entails combined conscription of science, regulation, and design. Implementation, adoption, and evaluation of DHI present special challenges. This chapter presents brief history of DHIs in mental health and frameworks an evaluation strategy in terms of the appropriate methods required for appraisal of DHIs.

DOI: 10.4018/978-1-5225-7513-9.ch009

INTRODUCTION

Defining Digital Health Interventions [DHIs]

Twenty years ago digital health interventions [DHIs] were nothing but a distant impossibility. The revolution of information technology [IT] in the last century means that technology can be utilized to confront pressing healthcare needs. The range and scope of DHIs and digitally delivered healthcare services have evolved rapidly since Eysenbach's (2001) initial description of Internet-enabled or computer-enabled interventions. (Hollis et al., 2017) Early DHIs in the mental health field were based on static content with limited interactivity and were 'fixed' in terms of access (e.g. via a PC or laptop, requiring a wired Internet connection), whereas users were required to be in a specific location to access the intervention. Examples of these DHIs include computerised cognitive behavioural therapy typically mimicking, face to face (FtF) delivered CBT sessions by providing a series of discrete modules that users complete (Hollis et al., 2017) Initial approaches are often referred to as 'tele-health', 'tele-medicine' or 'tele-psychiatry' and fall within the broad description of 'eHealth. (Hollis et al., 2017) Over the last decade, the increased popularity and availability of mobile digital technologies, such as smartphones and wearable technologies, has led to the development and evaluation of mobile DHIs, also known as 'mHealth' (see Table 1 below). (Hollis et al., 2017) mHealth DHIs include devices such as smartphone applications ('apps'), remote monitoring and tracking devices, and wearable computers (e.g. smartwatches, virtual reality headsets). Remote active and passive monitoring of parameters, such as mood, activity and sleep, are now being integrated with therapeutic interventions. Hence, the distinction between mHealth digital monitoring and interventions is likely to become increasingly blurred. (Hollis et al., 2017) (Murray et al., 2016) Mental health DHIs target a range of psychological disorders and differ in design and functionality. (Chandrashekar, 2018) National institute of mental health (NIMH) categorizes mental health DHIs into six categories based on: 1) functionality: 2) self-management; 3) cognition improvement; 4) skills-training; 4) social support; 5) symptom tracking; and 6) passive data collection. (Chandrashekar, 2018) Evidence indicates that technology present a tremendous opportunity for delivery of high-efficacy mental health interventions in domains of anxiety, depression; and schizophrenia. Considering scarcity of accessible mental health care professionals. and lack of mental health care access in rural and urban areas, DHIs have emerged as a practical tools that may bridge the mental health treatment gap. (Chandrashekar, 2018) Technology is well-poised to transform how mental health care is delivered and accessed, however the transformation requires the combined conscription of science, regulation, and design. (Chandrashekar, 2018)

Generally speaking, DHIs are complex interventions with multiple intertwined components, and typically have multiple aims, including; 1) enabling users to be more informed about their health; 2) share experiences with others in similar positions; 3) modify perceptions and comprehension around health, 4) remotely assess and monitor specified health states; 5) titrate medication; 6) realize health priorities and reach congruent treatment

Table 1. Glossary of common terms and abbreviations used in the field of digital healthcare

Term	Definition
Digital health intervention (DHI)	Interventions that provide information, support and therapy (emotional, decisional, behavioural and neurocognitive) for physical and/or mental health problems via a technological or digital platform (e.g. website, computer, mobile phone application (app), SMS, email, videoconferencing, wearable device)
eHealth (Electronic Health)	Internet-based healthcare delivery/anything health-related that uses information and communications technology (Blackwell et al.), incorporating computers or Internet in its delivery
Internet, online/web-based interventions	Computerised program or service delivered through the Internet (e.g. a website), designed to create a positive change in behaviour or health status with different levels of support (e.g. completely unguided, human-supported)
Computer-based/computer-delivered interventions	Similar to Internet-based interventions, but usually refers to a program delivered via a computer: the intervention may be via the Internet or an offline computerised program (e.g. CD-ROM, or installed software). Includes psychoeducation and psychotherapy packages, 'serious' games and neurocognitive 'brain training' interventions
Computer, Internet-based or mobile-based CBT	Delivery of Cognitive Behavioural Therapy (CBT) via computer (cCBT), Internet (iCBT) or mobile devices or applications (mCBT). Collectively may be referred to as electronically delivered CBT (eCBT)
mHealth (Mobile-delivered Health)	Subdivision of eHealth focusing on delivering healthcare-related information, interventions and monitoring through portable electronic/mobile devices and technologies, such as smartphones, tablets and wearable devices. Examples of mHealth for mental health include smartphone applications ('apps'), text/SMS-delivered interventions and patient monitoring devices
Telehealth, telepsychiatry and telemedicine	Delivery of health services and treatment via telecommunications technology (e.g. videoconferencing/SMS/email), including: online counselling and therapy that may be synchronous (e.g. real-time videoconferencing) or asynchronous (e.g. email /SMS).

*Note: Adapted from: (Hollis et al., 2017)

decisions; and 6) improve communication between patients and various healthcare professionals [HCPs]. (van Beugen et al., 2014) DHIs have been heralded as revolutionizing access and equity of care including the ways in which individuals monitor and improve their health behaviors by improving outcomes, reducing costs, and improving the patient experience and increasing patient engagement. DHIs vary widely with respect to clinical range, format, functionality and mode of delivery, including mechanisms through which they aim to change mental health and well-being.

Clinical Range

Devices and programs using digital technology to support behavior change are increasingly ubiquitous, being adopted for use in patient diagnosis and treatment, remote monitoring and self-management of chronic diseases. (Michie, Yardley, West, Patrick, & Greaves, 2017) In fact, DHIs have been utilized to: 1) promote healthy behaviors such as smoking cessation (Free et al., 2011); and physical activity (Vandelanotte, Spathonis, Eakin, & Owen, 2007); 2) improve outcomes in people with long-term conditions such as heart failure, (Hunting G, 2015) hypertension (McLean et al., 2016) and diabetes (Pal et al., 2014); 3) provide remote access to effective treatments (van Beugen et al.); 4) improve mental health conditions. (Zhuo et al., 2015)

Available DHIs vary in the breadth of psychopathology that they address. Typically, they tend to be disorder-specific but a few are even more precisely targeted such as one designed for people with suicidal thoughts. (van Spijker, van Straten, & Kerkhof, 2014) On the other hand, some are "transdiagnostic" in scope and have a broad clinical range indicating a great potential clinical effectiveness.(Craske et al., 2009; Titov et al., 2011) There are well established DHIs for depression; anxiety disorders and insomnia. Most have been designed as self-help programs that are meant to be used on their own or with some form of support. These treatments vary markedly in their content, clinical range, format, functionality and mode of delivery. (Andersson & Titov, 2014)

Format

DHIs designed to address mental health conditions vary in their format. Interventions can be designed as face-to-face treatment that may entail having regular weekly sessions. Others modify the format to match the way that websites or apps are meant to be used. (Ben-Zeev et al., 2015) Typically, modified format results in briefer, more frequent, sessions compared with face-to-face treatment, and often the overall length of treatment is shorter. (Ben-Zeev et al., 2015) Further, DHIs may vary in their structure. Some are linear, progressively leading users through the intervention step-by-step, whereas others have a variety of modules which may be applied with some flexibility. (Ben-Zeev et al., 2015)

These interventions often require some level of personalisation or so called "tailoring". Tailoring can imply little more than matching the text and clinical examples to the user's demographic group [e.g., gender specific - female]. meanwhile others go beyond by incorporating algorithms that generate a treatment which matches aspects of the user's psychopathology. (Abdullah et al., 2016) These algorithms may be acquired from strategy specific to the treatment or the recommendations of experienced clinicians. It is likely that, machine learning may be used for this in the future. (Abdullah et al., 2016) An alternate to tailoring is permitting end-users to pick out elements of the intervention that match their specific concerns. (Abdullah et al., 2016) Additional studies are required to evaluate which of the tailoring approaches lead to improved patient outcomes.

Functionality

During infancy DHIs compromised of text and thus resembled printed self-help programmes. This is changing. As technology matures, additional attention was devoted to their appearance, appeal and ease of navigation. Nowadays, most DHIs may embrace features such as: 1) learning exercises; 2) self-monitoring tools; 3) progress reports; 4) downloadable documents; 5) audio- and video-files; 6) audio- and video-feedback; 7) avatars; 8) quizzes and games. Currently there are multifaceted and technologically sophisticated DHIs to address social anxiety disorder (Stott et al., 2013) and post-traumatic disorder (Wild et al., 2016); meanwhile several interventions have been designed game format, a form that may particularly suit younger users (Merry et al., 2012). Further, novelties that may likely to gain ground in the near future are: 1) the use of virtual reality-based procedures as the equipment required is becoming more readily available; and 2) artificial intelligence-informed communication with the end-user.(Fairburn & Patel, 2017)

Mode of Delivery

DHIs in domain of mental health are provided via websites and can be accessed on a wide range of devices. However, some may not suitable for viewing on the small screen of the typical smartphone. (Donker, Petrie, et al., 2013) Others interventions are app-based and have been designed specifically with smartphones in mind. Whether interventions are website-based or app-based impacts the form that they can take and the functions that can be used. Some DHIs engage both modes of delivery; such as a website-based intervention with an accompanying app for purposes such as self-monitoring or planning ahead. (Donker, Petrie, et al., 2013)

The Promise and Challenges of DHIs in Psychiatry

Evidence suggests that DHIs are increasingly being adopted by individuals living with mental illnesses such as schizophrenia and bipolar disorder, as a means of better understanding and managing their condition.(Biagianti, Hidalgo-Mazzei, & Meyer, 2017) The portable, connected nature of wearable devices pragmatically supports remote and valid capture of clinical information in various settings—both actively, such as self-rated assessments, and passively, using instruments to size objective markers of social, emotive and cognitive states, meanwhile ensuring reduced user burden. (Biagianti et al., 2017) Information can be transferred back to the users and and clinical teams in real time, offering the opportunity to facilitate self-management, and ensure timely, preventative interventions. (Biagianti et al., 2017)

However, majority of DHIs in mental health have only been evaluated in small studies focused on short-term feasibility, albeit with mostly positive findings.(Firth & Torous, 2015) (Lewis & Wyatt, 2014) This has raised questions around interventions' long-term impact in more diverse patient groups. (Biagianti et al., 2017) It is imperative to accumulate scientific evidence on DHIs impact on mental health using rigorous evaluation frameworks meanwhile considering heterogeneous patient population and long term impact. (Lewis & Wyatt, 2014) (Chan, Torous, Hinton, & Yellowlees, 2015) (J. B. Torous, Chan, Yellowlees, & Boland, 2016) This will be required to ensure alleged benefits are realised, and to warrant that benefits outweigh potential harms such as breaches of security and privacy. (J. Torous & Roberts, 2017) At present, it is unclear as how: 1) to optimise the process of designing effective DHIs focused on mental health domain that are both timely and cost-effective;2) to select methods to ensure the optimal clinical dimensions to be targeted; creating interventions that may adapt to a shifting and ever-changing technological landscape, while retaining their core functionality; 3) to optimally determine as to what degree to integrate end users in the design process.

As suggested by Biagianti et al. [2017], the following dimensions should be considered when designing DHIs in arena of mental health: 1) Define the intervention based on unmet clinical need; 2) Develop meaningful partnership; 3) Ensure user-centered design; 4) Determine the appropriate software platforms; 5) Assess the use of appropriate grade devices. (Biagianti et al., 2017) Each one of these is described in substantial detail.

Define the Interventions

The first step is to define an intervention and mitigate the potential that technology is deployed solely for the purpose of implementing technology alone, rather than being applied to target specific clinical problems. (Biagianti et al., 2017) At the initial stage, it is vital to ensure that a specific clinical dimension and unmet need drive the research question; including definition of essential parameters and key variables. Clinical researchers are uniquely positioned to guide development of research questions and DHIs by learning from patients, recognising areas of unmet clinical need, and then considering which of the various properties of DHIs might be most appropriate. As the field develops further, tools should be merged into multidimensional, modular and more flexible platforms. (Biagianti et al., 2017)

Develop Partnerships

Interdisciplinary partnerships among clinicians, patients, big data scientists, software engineers and user experience designers are essential in ensuring that an intervention meets scientific and technical standards. (Biagianti et al., 2017) During this phase it is critical to apply 'team science' principles (Borner et al., 2010). The principle entails regularly scheduled meeting and initiatives that would promote interdisciplinary dialogue, and ultimately the formation of a collective knowledge base. Prior to any collective work, it is critical for agreement to be reached between collaborators on issues of payment/financial support, academic credit, authorship, intellectual property, and data ownership, storage and security. (Biagianti et al., 2017)

Ensure User-Centered Design

Evidence suggests that interventions are more likely to be adopted for long-term use when they provide inherent value for the 'user' in managing their condition, or improve critical aspects of their functioning and well-being. Bottom-up approach, involving end-users [i.e. patients/caregivers] in the co-development of DHIs has therefore become central to this goal. Yet, it is unclear as to how this should be implemented, as only a limited number of studies to date have reported user-involvement during the DHI development. (Killikelly, He, Reeder, & Wykes, 2017) End-users must remain integral to forming the research agenda, clinical focus and technology selection over the entirety of the development cycle. (Biagianti et al., 2017)

Native vs. Existing Software Platforms

Native software platofrm requires up-front expenditures of time, energy and capital. Yet, it allows adhoc modifications to address specific difficulties of people with mental conditions to be taken into account, including cognitive impairments, poor technology literacy and text reading level.(Rotondi, Eack, Hanusa, Spring, & Haas, 2015) Nonetheless, potential risks associated with building native technology such that rapid technological advances may make the prototype for the intervention already obsolete and uncompetitive by the time the development process is complete. This may have profund implications on the acceptability and scalability of the intervention. (Rotondi et al., 2015) This can be overcome by outsourcing design and development to established firms, so that the intervention is regularly maintained and enhanced. This may entail supplemental costs and such may be unaffordable to early stage researchers. (Rotondi et al., 2015)

An alternate is to capitalise on available solutions if these: 1) meet specific needs and goals; 2) are secure; and 3) adhere to current ethical and clinical governance structures. (Biagianti et al., 2017) Advantages include a significant reduction in costs and the possibility to promptly test the feasibility and acceptability of the technology in the clinical population. However, researchers may have limited control over design and development process. Further, they may need to adapt DHIs to the rapidly changing features of the tool, which may lead to difficulties associated with consistency of study procedures and replicability of findings. (Biagianti et al., 2017)

Regardless whether one opts for naïve versus existing platforms, allowing interoperability between mobile operating systems is desirable, particularly android and iOS systems, in order to maximise the reach and generalisability of the intervention. It is desirable to employ software that could be freely downloaded regardless of the device. (Biagianti et al., 2017)

Consumer vs. Clinical Grade Devices

A key objective is to design and develop DHIs that are affordable and acceptable for prolonged use. Devices are to be validated in clinical populations. In the case of wearable devices, data may be preprocessed on the device using unpublished algorithms, to which the research team may have access. The process may raise concerns regarding validation, data quality, replicability and scientific acceptability. (Naslund, Aschbrenner, & Bartels, 2016; J. Torous, Kiang, Lorme, & Onnela, 2016)

Albeit very useful, consumer devices convey some limitations. Although technology needs to be 'good enough' to address the clinical question, it may not represent the most innovative technological option. Although, one attempts to curtail variability between devices by ensuring all participants are equipped with standardised study devices, and by primarily examining longitudinal within-person variation. This may not always be possible. Considering swift development cycle of consumer devices, each platform should be designed as to integrate with novel technologies devices as they emerge, thus 'future-proofing' the intervention. (Biagianti et al., 2017)

As the technological landscape rapidly advances, new opportunities will arise for delivering DHIs for mental health. Strong collaboration between academic and industry partners are required to fuse the advantages of consumer and clinical grade technologies in the design and development of devices that assimilate into the users' lives, while delivering clinical-quality data. (Biagianti et al., 2017)

The Contribution of DHIs to Psychological/ Psychiatric Treatments

DHIs, including digital technology in general, have been heralded as presenting massive potential as scalable tools to improve outcomes, to widen access and meet the increasing demand on mental health services. As a result of the widespread availability of digital technology, treatments of mental health conditions has been undergoing momentous changes Most of DHIs are forms of cognitive behaviour therapy that have been modified from existing face-to-face treatments or from self-help books based upon them. (Andersson, Cuijpers, Carlbring, Riper, & Hedman, 2014) Some may represent a simplified versions of the original treatment and are little more than collections of "tools. Others preserve both the treatment's procedures and the strategies that govern their use. At large, DHIs in mental health domain seem to make more use of behavioural than cognitive procedures and contain a prominent educational component. It has been popular for DHIs to present themselves as educational programmes rather than treatments, and deliver the intervention in "lessons", instead of "sessions" (Andersson et al., 2014).

There are digital versions of psychotherapy including: acceptance and commitment therapy (Pots et al., 2016); behavioural activation (Ly et al., 2014); interpersonal psychotherapy (Donker, Bennett, et al., 2013); mindfulness interventions (Spijkerman, Pots, & Bohlmeijer, 2016); and problem-solving therapy (Kleiboer et al., 2015). However, these variations have received less research attention than the cognitive behavioural ones. Similar to cognitive behavioural interventions, they vary in the range to which they retain the strategies and procedures of the original treatment

Truly novel DHIs are few and far between. Examples include: positive cognitive bias modification to treat depression (Blackwell et al., 2015); virtual reality based exposure in the treatment of anxiety disorders (Valmaggia, Latif, Kempton, & Rus-Calafell, 2016) and persecutory delusions (Freeman et al., 2016); and the use of robotic technology to improve social interaction in autism spectrum disorders and dementia (Riek, 2016). The use of a computer game to block the reconsolidation of intrusive traumatic memories remains at the experimental stage (James et al., 2015).

THE APPLICATION OF DHIS IN PATIENT POPULATIONS

DHIs for Children and Young People With Mental Health Problems

Recent advances in computerised technologies and programming has created the possibility of more interactive and adaptable cCBT that may fit the needs of young people though use of gamification and 'serious games'. (Hollis et al., 2017) Typically, it has been presumed that children and young people

(CYP) will prefer DHIs considering their ubiquitous digital activity. Yet, evidence remains inconsistent as to whether: 1) DHIs for CYP are clinically and cost-effective; 2) CYP prefer DHIs to traditional services; 3) DHIs widen access to treatment: 4) traditional evaluation and adopted methods are the most appropriate. (Hollis et al., 2017)

The assessment of effectiveness of DHIs has been based on evidence from RCTs, with the majority conducted on CBT focused in domains of depression and anxiety in adolescents and young adults, with significantly less research focused on other clinical areas and therapeutic interventions. Generally speaking, there is limited support for the role of computerized cognitive behaviour therapy (cCBT) in improving symptoms of depression and anxiety in CYP. Further, there is evidence from 'head to head' trials that therapist-guided (remote) cCBT is as effective as face to FtF CBT. (Sethi, 2013) Trials have typically focused on older adolescents with mild and moderate symptomatology. Thus, it remains unclear as to whether DHIs are useful for CYP who present with more severe symptomatology typically found presenting to mental health services. (Hollis et al., 2017) Evidence indicates that trials with active comparators demonstrate reduced benefit of DHIs than those with non-active controls. There is some evidence that human support, either in the form of a therapist's guidance or researcher contact, may be favourable in terms of adherence and effectiveness. DHIs for Attention deficit hyperactivity disorder (ADHD), Autism Spectrum Disorder (ASD), eating disorders, psychosis and post-traumatic stress disorder (PTSD) demonstrate limited benefits. Also, there is a notable lack of evidence concerning the cost-effectiveness of DHIs in CYP. To summarize, the heterogeneity of DHIs and limited quality of many studies make it difficult to draw definitive conclusions about the effectiveness of DHIs and the role they should play in mental health services for CYP. (Hollis et al., 2017) Past research highlights a plethora of valid research questions and methodological issues that need to be considered for the field to move forward.

DHIs for Adults With Mental Health Problems

There are increasing numbers of DHIs available for use in adults with severe mental issues. Published literature unveils strong evidence for the feasibility of using smartphones to augment the care of people with schizophrenia (Firth & Torous, 2015). In fact, a systematic review of five studies focused on using smartphone apps for treating symptoms of schizophrenia demonstrated app retention was 92%, and approximately 3.95 patient-app interactions took place each day. (Firth & Torous, 2015) Self-reported patient experience survey results revealed high adherence, positive user experience, and broad-ranging clinical benefits. High rates of engagement and satisfaction with an array of apps indicates the nascent potential of this technology. Yet, overall evidence regarding the efficacy of such interventions remains limited. (Firth & Torous, 2015) Further, a meta-analysis of 18 randomized controlled trials (RCTs) covering 22 mobile apps demonstrated that using apps to relieve symptoms and self-manage depression significantly reduced patients' depressive symptoms compared to control conditions ($g=0.38$, $P<0.001$). (Firth et al., 2017) Authors noted that smartphone-based therapies yielded the most benefits for individuals with mild to moderate, rather than major, depression. (Firth et al., 2017) Findings from systematic review indicate that overall short-term usability and feasibility of technology are high in the SMI population, implying the potential utility of digital technology for incorporation into treatment of SMI. (Batra et al., 2017) Authors note that real-world, naturalistic studies using larger samples will further facilitate the integration of digital technology into everyday mental health care, meanwhile evaluating its long-term effectiveness.

DHIs for Seniors With Mental Health Problems

Evidence suggests that older adults (65+) have the potential to use tailored smartphone interventions to self-manage their illness. A group of researchers from Dartmouth developed a smartphone-based intervention using an adaptive systems engineering framework and principles of user-centered design. (Fortuna et al., 2018) The findings noted that a peer-delivered and technology-supported intervention designed to improve medical and psychiatric self-management is feasible, acceptable, and is potentially associated with improvements in psychiatric self-management, self-efficacy for managing chronic health conditions, hope, quality of life, medical self-management skills, and empowerment with older adults with serious mental illness (Fortuna et al., 2018). They found that even patients with limited technical abilities could use this app successfully (Fortuna et al., 2018). Evidence indicates that DHIs are associated with several advantages compared with traditional psychosocial interventions, such as: potential for individually tailored, just-in-time delivery along with wide dissemination and high population impact (Fortuna et al., 2018; Whiteman, Lohman, Gill, Bruce, & Bartels, 2017). But the process of adapting an existing psychosocial intervention to a DHIs mandates an adaptation for a high-risk group with limited health and technology literacy (Whiteman et al., 2017) and should be evaluated with studies containing larger and more representative population samples.

REFERENCES

Abdullah, S., Matthews, M., Frank, E., Doherty, G., Gay, G., & Choudhury, T. (2016). Automatic detection of social rhythms in bipolar disorder. *Journal of the American Medical Informatics Association*, *23*(3), 538–543. doi:10.1093/jamia/ocv200 PMID:26977102

Andersson, G., Cuijpers, P., Carlbring, P., Riper, H., & Hedman, E. (2014). Guided Internet-based vs. face-to-face cognitive behavior therapy for psychiatric and somatic disorders: A systematic review and meta-analysis. *World Psychiatry; Official Journal of the World Psychiatric Association (WPA)*, *13*(3), 288–295. doi:10.1002/wps.20151 PMID:25273302

Andersson, G., & Titov, N. (2014). Advantages and limitations of Internet-based interventions for common mental disorders. *World Psychiatry; Official Journal of the World Psychiatric Association (WPA)*, *13*(1), 4–11. doi:10.1002/wps.20083 PMID:24497236

Batra, S., Baker, R. A., Wang, T., Forma, F., DiBiasi, F., & Peters-Strickland, T. (2017). Digital health technology for use in patients with serious mental illness: A systematic review of the literature. *Medical Devices (Auckland, N.Z.)*, *10*, 237–251. doi:10.2147/MDER.S144158 PMID:29042823

Ben-Zeev, D., Schueller, S. M., Begale, M., Duffecy, J., Kane, J. M., & Mohr, D. C. (2015). Strategies for mHealth research: Lessons from 3 mobile intervention studies. *Administration and Policy in Mental Health*, *42*(2), 157–167. doi:10.100710488-014-0556-2 PMID:24824311

Biagianti, B., Hidalgo-Mazzei, D., & Meyer, N. (2017). Developing digital interventions for people living with serious mental illness: Perspectives from three mHealth studies. *Evidence-Based Mental Health*, *20*(4), 98–101. doi:10.1136/eb-2017-102765 PMID:29025862

Blackwell, S. E., Browning, M., Mathews, A., Pictet, A., Welch, J., Davies, J., ... Holmes, E. A. (2015). Positive Imagery-Based Cognitive Bias Modification as a Web-Based Treatment Tool for Depressed Adults: A Randomized Controlled Trial. *Clinical Psychological Science*, *3*(1), 91–111. doi:10.1177/2167702614560746 PMID:25984421

Borner, K., Contractor, N., Falk-Krzesinski, H. J., Fiore, S. M., Hall, K. L., Keyton, J., ... Uzzi, B. (2010). A multi-level systems perspective for the science of team science. *Science Translational Medicine*, *2*(49), 49cm24. doi:10.1126citranslmed.3001399 PMID:20844283

Chan, S., Torous, J., Hinton, L., & Yellowlees, P. (2015). Towards a Framework for Evaluating Mobile Mental Health Apps. *Telemedicine Journal and e-Health*, *21*(12), 1038–1041. doi:10.1089/tmj.2015.0002 PMID:26171663

Chandrashekar, P. (2018). Do mental health mobile apps work: Evidence and recommendations for designing high-efficacy mental health mobile apps. *mHealth*, *4*, 6. doi:10.21037/mhealth.2018.03.02 PMID:29682510

Craske, M. G., Rose, R. D., Lang, A., Welch, S. S., Campbell-Sills, L., Sullivan, G., ... Roy-Byrne, P. P. (2009). Computer-assisted delivery of cognitive behavioral therapy for anxiety disorders in primary-care settings. *Depression and Anxiety*, *26*(3), 235–242. doi:10.1002/da.20542 PMID:19212970

Donker, T., Bennett, K., Bennett, A., Mackinnon, A., van Straten, A., Cuijpers, P., ... Griffiths, K. M. (2013). Internet-delivered interpersonal psychotherapy versus internet-delivered cognitive behavioral therapy for adults with depressive symptoms: Randomized controlled noninferiority trial. *Journal of Medical Internet Research*, *15*(5), e82. doi:10.2196/jmir.2307 PMID:23669884

Donker, T., Petrie, K., Proudfoot, J., Clarke, J., Birch, M. R., & Christensen, H. (2013). Smartphones for smarter delivery of mental health programs: A systematic review. *Journal of Medical Internet Research*, *15*(11), e247. doi:10.2196/jmir.2791 PMID:24240579

Fairburn, C. G., & Patel, V. (2017). The impact of digital technology on psychological treatments and their dissemination. *Behaviour Research and Therapy*, *88*, 19–25. doi:10.1016/j.brat.2016.08.012 PMID:28110672

Firth, J., & Torous, J. (2015). Smartphone Apps for Schizophrenia: A Systematic Review. *JMIR mHealth and uHealth*, *3*(4), e102. doi:10.2196/mhealth.4930 PMID:26546039

Firth, J., Torous, J., Nicholas, J., Carney, R., Pratap, A., Rosenbaum, S., & Sarris, J. (2017). The efficacy of smartphone-based mental health interventions for depressive symptoms: A meta-analysis of randomized controlled trials. *World Psychiatry; Official Journal of the World Psychiatric Association (WPA)*, *16*(3), 287–298. doi:10.1002/wps.20472 PMID:28941113

Fortuna, K. L., DiMilia, P. R., Lohman, M. C., Bruce, M. L., Zubritsky, C. D., Halaby, M. R., ... Bartels, S. J. (2018). Feasibility, Acceptability, and Preliminary Effectiveness of a Peer-Delivered and Technology Supported Self-Management Intervention for Older Adults with Serious Mental Illness. *The Psychiatric Quarterly*, *89*(2), 293–305. doi:10.100711126-017-9534-7 PMID:28948424

Free, C., Knight, R., Robertson, S., Whittaker, R., Edwards, P., Zhou, W., ... Roberts, I. (2011). Smoking cessation support delivered via mobile phone text messaging (txt2stop): A single-blind, randomised trial. *Lancet*, *378*(9785), 49–55. doi:10.1016/S0140-6736(11)60701-0 PMID:21722952

Freeman, D., Bradley, J., Antley, A., Bourke, E., DeWeever, N., Evans, N., ... Clark, D. M. (2016). Virtual reality in the treatment of persecutory delusions: Randomised controlled experimental study testing how to reduce delusional conviction. *The British Journal of Psychiatry*, *209*(1), 62–67. doi:10.1192/bjp.bp.115.176438 PMID:27151071

Hollis, C., Falconer, C. J., Martin, J. L., Whittington, C., Stockton, S., Glazebrook, C., & Davies, E. B. (2017). Annual Research Review: Digital health interventions for children and young people with mental health problems - a systematic and meta-review. *Journal of Child Psychology and Psychiatry, and Allied Disciplines*, *58*(4), 474–503. doi:10.1111/jcpp.12663 PMID:27943285

Hunting,, G. S. N., Sahakyan, Y., Fan, I., Moneypenny, C.R., Stanimirovic, A., North, T., … Rac, V.E. (2015). A multi-level qualitative analysis of Telehomecare in Ontario: Challenges and opportunities. *BMC Health Services Research*, *15*(544). PMID:26645639

James, E. L., Bonsall, M. B., Hoppitt, L., Tunbridge, E. M., Geddes, J. R., Milton, A. L., & Holmes, E. A. (2015). Computer Game Play Reduces Intrusive Memories of Experimental Trauma via Reconsolidation-Update Mechanisms. *Psychological Science*, *26*(8), 1201–1215. doi:10.1177/0956797615583071 PMID:26133572

Killikelly, C., He, Z., Reeder, C., & Wykes, T. (2017). Improving Adherence to Web-Based and Mobile Technologies for People With Psychosis: Systematic Review of New Potential Predictors of Adherence. *JMIR mHealth and uHealth*, *5*(7), e94. doi:10.2196/mhealth.7088 PMID:28729235

Kleiboer, A., Donker, T., Seekles, W., van Straten, A., Riper, H., & Cuijpers, P. (2015). A randomized controlled trial on the role of support in Internet-based problem solving therapy for depression and anxiety. *Behaviour Research and Therapy*, *72*, 63–71. doi:10.1016/j.brat.2015.06.013 PMID:26188373

Lewis, T. L., & Wyatt, J. C. (2014). mHealth and mobile medical Apps: A framework to assess risk and promote safer use. *Journal of Medical Internet Research*, *16*(9), e210. doi:10.2196/jmir.3133 PMID:25223398

Ly, K. H., Truschel, A., Jarl, L., Magnusson, S., Windahl, T., Johansson, R., ... Andersson, G. (2014). Behavioural activation versus mindfulness-based guided self-help treatment administered through a smartphone application: A randomised controlled trial. *BMJ Open*, *4*(1), e003440. doi:10.1136/bmjopen-2013-003440 PMID:24413342

McLean, G., Band, R., Saunderson, K., Hanlon, P., Murray, E., Little, P., ... Mair, F. S. (2016). Digital interventions to promote self-management in adults with hypertension systematic review and meta-analysis. *Journal of Hypertension*, *34*(4), 600–612. doi:10.1097/HJH.0000000000000859 PMID:26845284

Merry, S. N., Stasiak, K., Shepherd, M., Frampton, C., Fleming, T., & Lucassen, M. F. (2012). The effectiveness of SPARX, a computerised self help intervention for adolescents seeking help for depression: Randomised controlled non-inferiority trial. *BMJ (Clinical Research Ed.)*, *344*, e2598. doi:10.1136/bmj.e2598 PMID:22517917

Michie, S., Yardley, L., West, R., Patrick, K., & Greaves, F. (2017). Developing and Evaluating Digital Interventions to Promote Behavior Change in Health and Health Care: Recommendations Resulting From an International Workshop. *Journal of Medical Internet Research, 19*(6), e232. doi:10.2196/jmir.7126 PMID:28663162

Murray, E., Hekler, E. B., Andersson, G., Collins, L. M., Doherty, A., Hollis, C., ... Wyatt, J. C. (2016). Evaluating Digital Health Interventions: Key Questions and Approaches. *American Journal of Preventive Medicine, 51*(5), 843–851. doi:10.1016/j.amepre.2016.06.008 PMID:27745684

Naslund, J. A., Aschbrenner, K. A., & Bartels, S. J. (2016). Wearable Devices and Smartphones for Activity Tracking Among People with Serious Mental Illness. *Mental Health and Physical Activity, 10*, 10–17. doi:10.1016/j.mhpa.2016.02.001 PMID:27134654

Pal, K., Eastwood, S. V., Michie, S., Farmer, A., Barnard, M. L., Peacock, R., ... Murray, E. (2014). Computer-based interventions to improve self-management in adults with type 2 diabetes: A systematic review and meta-analysis. *Diabetes Care, 37*(6), 1759–1766. doi:10.2337/dc13-1386 PMID:24855158

Pots, W. T., Fledderus, M., Meulenbeek, P. A., ten Klooster, P. M., Schreurs, K. M., & Bohlmeijer, E. T. (2016). Acceptance and commitment therapy as a web-based intervention for depressive symptoms: Randomised controlled trial. *The British Journal of Psychiatry, 208*(1), 69–77. doi:10.1192/bjp.bp.114.146068 PMID:26250745

Riek, L. D. (2016). Robotics technology in mental health care. In *Artificial intelligence in behavioral and mental health care. London*. London: D.D. Luxton, Academic Press. doi:10.1016/B978-0-12-420248-1.00008-8

Rotondi, A. J., Eack, S. M., Hanusa, B. H., Spring, M. B., & Haas, G. L. (2015). Critical design elements of e-health applications for users with severe mental illness: Singular focus, simple architecture, prominent contents, explicit navigation, and inclusive hyperlinks. *Schizophrenia Bulletin, 41*(2), 440–448. doi:10.1093chbulbt194 PMID:24375458

Sethi, S. (2013). Treating Youth Depression and Anxiety: A Randomised Controlled Trial Examining the Efficacy of Computerised versus Face-to-face Cognitive Behaviour Therapy. *Australian Psychologist*, *48*(4), 249–257. doi:10.1111/ap.12006

Spijkerman, M. P., Pots, W. T., & Bohlmeijer, E. T. (2016). Effectiveness of online mindfulness-based interventions in improving mental health: A review and meta-analysis of randomised controlled trials. *Clinical Psychology Review*, *45*, 102–114. doi:10.1016/j.cpr.2016.03.009 PMID:27111302

Stott, R., Wild, J., Grey, N., Liness, S., Warnock-Parkes, E., Commins, S., ... Clark, D. M. (2013). Internet-delivered cognitive therapy for social anxiety disorder: A development pilot series. *Behavioural and Cognitive Psychotherapy*, *41*(4), 383–397. doi:10.1017/S1352465813000404 PMID:23676553

Titov, N., Dear, B. F., Schwencke, G., Andrews, G., Johnston, L., Craske, M. G., & McEvoy, P. (2011). Transdiagnostic internet treatment for anxiety and depression: A randomised controlled trial. *Behaviour Research and Therapy*, *49*(8), 441–452. doi:10.1016/j.brat.2011.03.007 PMID:21679925

Torous, J., Kiang, M. V., Lorme, J., & Onnela, J. P. (2016). New Tools for New Research in Psychiatry: A Scalable and Customizable Platform to Empower Data Driven Smartphone Research. *JMIR Ment Health*, *3*(2), e16. doi:10.2196/mental.5165 PMID:27150677

Torous, J., & Roberts, L. W. (2017). Needed Innovation in Digital Health and Smartphone Applications for Mental Health: Transparency and Trust. *JAMA Psychiatry*, *74*(5), 437–438. doi:10.1001/jamapsychiatry.2017.0262 PMID:28384700

Torous, J. B., Chan, S. R., Yellowlees, P. M., & Boland, R. (2016). To Use or Not? Evaluating ASPECTS of Smartphone Apps and Mobile Technology for Clinical Care in Psychiatry. *The Journal of Clinical Psychiatry*, *77*(6), e734–e738. doi:10.4088/JCP.15com10619 PMID:27136691

Valmaggia, L. R., Latif, L., Kempton, M. J., & Rus-Calafell, M. (2016). Virtual reality in the psychological treatment for mental health problems: An systematic review of recent evidence. *Psychiatry Research*, *236*, 189–195. doi:10.1016/j.psychres.2016.01.015 PMID:26795129

van Beugen, S., Ferwerda, M., Hoeve, D., Rovers, M. M., Spillekom-van Koulil, S., van Middendorp, H., & Evers, A. W. (2014). Internet-based cognitive behavioral therapy for patients with chronic somatic conditions: A meta-analytic review. *Journal of Medical Internet Research*, *16*(3), e88. doi:10.2196/jmir.2777 PMID:24675372

van Spijker, B. A., van Straten, A., & Kerkhof, A. J. (2014). Effectiveness of online self-help for suicidal thoughts: Results of a randomised controlled trial. *PLoS One*, *9*(2), e90118. doi:10.1371/journal.pone.0090118 PMID:24587233

Vandelanotte, C., Spathonis, K. M., Eakin, E. G., & Owen, N. (2007). Website-delivered physical activity interventions a review of the literature. *American Journal of Preventive Medicine*, *33*(1), 54–64. doi:10.1016/j.amepre.2007.02.041 PMID:17572313

Whiteman, K. L., Lohman, M. C., Gill, L. E., Bruce, M. L., & Bartels, S. J. (2017). Adapting a Psychosocial Intervention for Smartphone Delivery to Middle-Aged and Older Adults with Serious Mental Illness. *The American Journal of Geriatric Psychiatry*, *25*(8), 819–828. doi:10.1016/j.jagp.2016.12.007 PMID:28169129

Wild, J., Warnock-Parkes, E., Grey, N., Stott, R., Wiedemann, M., Canvin, L., ... Ehlers, A. (2016). Internet-delivered cognitive therapy for PTSD: A development pilot series. *European Journal of Psychotraumatology*, *7*(1), 31019. doi:10.3402/ejpt.v7.31019 PMID:27837579

Zhuo, X., Zhang, P., Kahn, H. S., Bardenheier, B. H., Li, R., & Gregg, E. W. (2015). Change in medical spending attributable to diabetes: National data from 1987 to 2011. *Diabetes Care*, *38*(4), 581–587. doi:10.2337/dc14-1687 PMID:25592194

Chapter 10
The Increase of How Mass Media Coverage Manipulates Our Minds

David Brian Ross
Nova Southeastern University, USA

Richard Louis
Broward College, USA

Melissa T. Sasso
Nova Southeastern University, USA

ABSTRACT

This chapter explores the insight of how the mind is negatively impacted by the news media. The purpose of this chapter is to introduce readers to how the human brain processes good and adverse effects of the news. The chapter begins with the overview that delves into the various aspects such as our brain and how it processes emotions, the theoretical frameworks of mass society, Marxism, functionalism, social constructionism, the historical context of the media in various countries, journalists and pundits, how the media divides communities, and how the media reports world events causing individuals to suffer from adverse psychological effects. This chapter then ends with a conclusion that consists of suggested future research.

DOI: 10.4018/978-1-5225-7513-9.ch010

OVERVIEW

In today's technological, virtual, and global world, people have access to 24/7 media news coverage. This news coverage has changed over the decades from reporting news to newscast personnel giving their opinions and commentaries based on their political views and personal agendas (i.e., appearing to know or not), to include the advertising from sponsors (Hopmann & Stromback, 2010). This different focus of the media news programming has become more of a business with pundits and so-called strategists who evoke stress on the viewers. Constant exposure to negative news coverage influences viewers' mental health, to include stress (Gregoire, 2015; Hamilton, 2014; Yeager, 2013). Gregoire (2015) stated, "The news can be violent, depressing, and emotionally-charged" (para. 1). As a result, this book chapter is based on media and the psychological effects (e.g., stress/ PTSD) it has on individuals. The chapter will begin with a theoretical framework, which will comprise of various theories and theorists, such as (a) Mass society theory, (b) Marxist media theory, (c) Functionalist theory, (d) Social constructionism, and (e) other aligning theories. The chapter will then unfold to a synthesis, which will discuss the types of media and the effects it has on individuals. Furthermore, it will illustrate the content of international news presented by media, such as war and natural disasters, politics, religion, and other issues for debate. Points are discussed in detail in regards to how it results in viewers suffering from stress, to the point of suffering from Post-Traumatic Stress Disorder.

The Negative Mind

The many forms of mass media have enhanced our lives toward how we view the world. Parents, ever since the beginning of radio and television restrained their children from listening and watching media due to the need for censorship. Viewing perceptions have changed since television edits had censored the pelvic movement of Elvis Presley on the Ed Sullivan show in 1956; this is compared to the many music videos and reality television shows of today. Due to the popularity and the public intrigue, the show reached over 80% of the television audience, while Elvis' contract started at $5,000 per engagement and increased to $300,000 (Gibson, n.d.).

Exposure to catastrophic events, regardless who their viewers are, exhibit a startled response, which is linked to a negative affect to any sudden or threatening stimuli, posttraumatic emotional/psychological and physical complications (Busso, McLaughlin, & Sheridan, 2014; Courtois & Gold, 2009). The emergence of many stress symptoms is brought about the continual exposure to media coverage of terrorism, war, natural disasters, and murders. Saylor, Cowart, Lipovsky, Jackson, and Finch (2003), and Lau, Lau, Kim, and Tsui (2006) defined that no matter how traumatic an event is, it will cause stress amongst all individuals no matter the type of disaster to include terrorist attacks throughout the world. Although the media informs viewers on what is occurring and how to stay safe, they also at the same time create mass anxiety. For example, in the United States, with all the school shootings, the media will demonstrate graphic images while attempting to set their agenda on gun control and mental health. Based on many graphic accounts, especially individuals who are vulnerable and unable to recognize and/or assimilate can inflict traumatic symptoms (Courtois & Gold, 2009).

People can assess different information from mass media whether they decide if it is enjoyable or it is volatile; people view media throughout their life to meet their satisfaction level as they change through life. Media psychology focuses on how human behavior is connected to the media and by understanding social cognitive theories. By definition, media psychology is the study of violence in mass media as well as how it is associated with violence and real-life aggression over a person's life. Hampton, Lou, and Shin (2016) feel that media is linked with high levels of psychological stress, which can lead to negative health outcomes. Hampton et al. and Goodwin, Palgi, Lavenda, Hamama-raz, and Ben-Ezra (2015) indicated that media is associated with the changes to the individuals' environment, however, once it is continuously with direct exposure via the media, higher levels of stress are present. Many external sources of stress stem from numerous traumatic events and chronic and ambient stressors. When individuals are in contact with all these stressors, anxiety and depression arises.

Both the sympathetic-adrenal medullary axis as well as the hypothalamic pituitary adrenal axis are activated when the brain becomes aware that a threat is to occur. This, in turn, leads to the excretion of the stress hormones (i.e., catecholamines, glucocorticoids). As Marin et al. (2012) indicated, glucocorticoids "is particularly interesting since it is a steroid that rapidly crosses the blood-brain-barrier and that binds to receptors in different brain regions, notably the hippocampus, the amygdala and the prefrontal cortex" (p. 1). It is also critical to note that there is a great association between stress hormones as well as dissimilar memory processes. When a person has an increase in catecholamines, it can cause a considerable amount of stress.

Whereas too little creates distraction, disorganization, or being indifferent. Furthermore, stress hormones have been illustrated to advance memory strengthening. The pre-frontal cortex, which is responsible for the high function of cognition and how people monitor behavior; also, can heighten one's arousal state, causing people to be more emotional rather than thinking rationally, especially when confronted with stressful situations. People are not rationale when watching the news as the media could manipulate and cause a person to be placed in a stressful state of mind.

THEORETICAL FRAMEWORK

The current media that is linked with the nineteenth and twentieth centuries are known as the (a) press, (b) radio, (c) television, and the (d) cinema and record industry and traditionally have been placed with each other under the term "mass media" (Bennett, 1982). There are a plethora of theories that have emerged based on mass media in which the following will reveal what the writers felt to be most critical to touch on.

Mass society theory. Bennett (1982) indicated that there are various theorists that are associated with the mass society theory and who contributed to this theory. Some of these theorists are Matthew Arnold, T. S. Eliot, Friedrich Nietzsche, and Ortega y Gasset, as well as political theorists John Stuart Mill and Alexis de Tocqueville, in addition to Vilfredo Pareto and Gaetano Mosca, who are the representatives of the Italian school of Sociology. Bennett revealed that the mass society theory should be looked at not as a whole, but as a theory with themes that are converged, such as, "the decline of the organic community, the rise of mass culture, the social atomization of mass man" (p. 32). When looked at as a whole, these themes have expressed an arrangement of negative as well as pessimistic reactions to the associated processes of, "industrialization, urbanization, the development of political democracy, the beginnings of popular education and the emergence of contemporary forms of mass communication" (Bennett, 1982, p. 32).

The mass society theory is based on the ideals that society is structured in the middle and on a massive scale. It is further based on the notion that the public becomes destroyed and that the media is centralized with a "one-way transmission" and that people rely on media to identify themselves. Lastly, this theory holds on the fact that media is utilized as a means to control and manipulate their audience (Bennett, 1982; McQuail, 2010).

Marxist media theory. Karl Marx was only familiar with the press prior to it being a real mass medium. However, there is still pertinence in terms of the tradition of Marxist analysis of the media in capitalist society. The idea of power is the main theme when explicating mass media in Marx's views (McQuail, 2010). Although there are variations, there has been a continuous emphasis on the notion that mass media are methods of controlling by as well as for a ruling class. As stated in Marx's German Ideology, "The class that has the means of material production has control at the same time over the means of mental production so that, thereby, generally speaking, the ideas of those who lack the means of mental production are subject to it" (as cited in McQuail, 2010, p. 96).

The Marxist media theory hypothesizes a direct association betwixt economic ownership in addition to the distribution of messages that confirm the legitimacy and worth of class society (McQuail, 2010). Within the twentieth century, there were those who created revised versions of the Marxist media theory, which emphasized on the ideological effects of media in regards to, "the interests of a ruling class, in reproducing the essentially exploitative relationships and manipulation, and in legitimating the dominance of capitalism and the subordination of the working class" (McQuail, 2010, p. 96). It has been noted that the political economy theory falls next in line to the Marxist media theory. The political economic theory focuses mainly on the association between the economic structure as well as the dynamics of media industries and the ideas of the content within media (McQuail, 2010).

Functionalist theory. Merton (as cited in McQuail, 2010) stated that the functionalist theory explicates social practices and institutions in regards to what society and individuals require. Society is seen as a continuing system of associated functioning parts in which each component makes a crucial contribution to progression and order. That stated; media could be viewed as one of these systems. This theory portrays media as independent and self-correcting. This theory is seen as having a conservative bias to the point where the media is viewed as keeping society where it is, rather than as a means of creating any drastic change to society. Within the early versions of functionalism, it had been rejected in sociology. However, it is still utilized as a means to approach media in novel methods and plays a role in answering research questions that pertain to media (McQuail, 2010). Laswell (as cited in McQuail, 2010) indicated that the primary functions of communication in society were watching over the environment, the interaction of the aspects of the society in how it reacts to its environment, as well as the transference of the cultural heritage. Wright (as cited in McQuail, 2010) added entertainment as the fourth primary media function. Lastly, a fifth function, which was mobilization, was added to the list of media functions (McQuail, 2010).

Social constructionism. The term social constructionism, in essence, was coined when Berger and Luckman's book, The Social Construction of Reality, was published in 1967 (McQuail, 2010). Social constructionism is based on the notion that society is a construct and not a fixed reality. Furthermore, this theory indicates that media offers the required materials for reality construction and the media provide the meanings. However, they can be either negotiated or declined (McQuail, 2010). The social constructionism theory also illustrates that the media will carefully reproduce specific meanings and that media cannot offer an objective explanation of social reality (McQuail, 2010).

Historical Context of the Media

Worldwide statistics illustrate that people access news from four areas: television, radio, print, and online, which includes many opportunities for social media. Statista (2018) in particular investigated 12 different countries to show the usage of these four areas to access information. In 2016, for television viewing the average usage of these 12 countries was 73.7%, radio was 32.2%, print was 40.4%, and online was 79.1%. Prior to radio, television, and the Internet, the public was able to obtain their news from print. The following information regarding regulation, advertising, and commercial broadcasting from various countries illustrates the inception of existence.

Due to the launch of broadcasting, many countries had to create regulations for broadcasting. In the late 1930s, the Federal Communications Commission was formed to regulate broadcasting in the United States. In addition to this change in how broadcasting began, was a need for regulations in other countries such as Canada. During the pioneer stage of broadcasting, radio, and television followed the emergence of public ownership and regulations between the years of 1928 and 1936. Graham Spry, a co-founder of the Canadian Radio League in 1930 felt there was a need for public control of the airwaves, as radio was listened to by those who had access to this type of media. Similarly, to Canada's pioneer days, England from 1920 to 1922 had the birth of British broadcasting, which led to England's present-day British Broadcasting Corporation. The British Broadcasting Corporation was formed in 1932 as the BBC Empire Service. The BBC's public service format is based on the Reithian motto of "to inform, to educate and to entertain" (Open Society Institute, 2005, p. 736).

In the case of Germany, broadcasting was reestablished after the end of World War II by the allied occupational forces. However, prior to World War II, the press in Germany opposed democratic institutions as the Nazi regime "abused all media, and the whole cultural sector, for propaganda and manipulation of the public" (Open Society Institute, 2005, p. 735). During the 1920s and into the 1930s, known as the Weimar Republic, is when this type of behavior occurred, therefore the need for regulations for this media not to become an anti-democratic power. As years approached the end of World War II, the American Federal Communications Commission, the model of free-market and commercial broadcasting; and England's British Broadcasting Corporation system designed for public service had influence in the changes for the Federal Republic of Germany's liberated free market system and the need for independence and pluralism. This type of service is to serve the public without bias for politics, the economy, or other interest groups. Hugh Carleton Greene, the BBC's senior manager, became the leader to oversee this new broadcasting organizational structure for Germany's North-Western regions. Therefore, with Greene's input and expertise, the BBC became the role model for Nordwestdeutscher Rundfunk, the new German broadcaster (Open Society Institute, 2005).

The Japan Broadcasting Corporation, which is known as the Nippon Hoso Kyokai (NHK) is publicly owned since 1924. Although the NHK was modeled after the BBC system, it was a semi-governmental institution. This radio broadcasting system assisted the Japanese government transfer military propaganda over the airwaves prior to and during World War II (Valaskivi, 2007). After the war in 1950, commercial companies began to broadcast throughout Japan. Radio broadcasting continued to enter the AM and FM radio station community into the 21st century (Fujitake, 2005; Valaskivi, 2007). According to Valaskivi (2007), in 1953 via the public broadcaster and Nippon Television Network Corporation, regular television broadcasting was underway.

Most of the European broadcasting market started years later as France began advertising on television in 1968. The 1960s were known as the decade of State television as the French government controlled its networks. Through the years, the French market is now a semi public-private system; however, "in reality, it is dominated by one single private company" (Open Society Institute, 2005, p. 642). The French broadcasting has three layers to the system: (a) the government designs broadcasting policies, drafts laws, and issues decrees to implement the laws; (b) the Parliament passes laws and controls funding, and (c) the High Council for Broadcasting (CSA) grants licenses, appoints heads of public broadcasters, and supervises the programming.

Hungary in the early 1990s consisted of only two national television channels; however, presently a majority of the population have the ability to view over 40 various Hungarian language channels. Although at the national level, public service television and commercial television is viewed in Hungary, this country was rather late in regards to passing broadcasting regulation (Open Society Institute, 2005). Due to political broadcasting laws and government voting, Czechoslovakia and Poland surpassed Hungary by four to five years respectively. The purpose of the 1996 Radio and Television Act was to terminate the political differences and power of control of media and societal values. “These disputes and the subsequent media policy measures were often referred to as Hungary’s media war” (Open Society Institute, 2005, p. 793). As a result of the Radio and Television Act, the National Radio and Television Board (ORTT) generated broadcasting rules for licensing, supervision, funding, as well as protecting media freedom.

The Radio Audizioni Italiane (RAI) is the Italian broadcasting system, which is known to have governmental and political controversial involvement; the government solely controls this. Similar to France, Italy began airing commercial television in the 1970s, which had no regulations as it transformed the media scene in addition to the advertising market and lastly, the political stakes. Like the majority of the countries discussed that have had strong political influence during the transition for regulation, (e.g., Germany, Japan), the mid-1990s deemed to play a critical role in Italy for voters to elect Prime Minister Silvio Berlusconi.

Within the country of Latvia, television is the most predominant source of information for individuals who reside in this country. Research revealed that television viewing is almost 100%, whereas due to the lack of recovery from eliminating the Soviet frequencies in the 1990s, listening to the radio to attain information is not as popular. Furthermore, media such as newspapers were also spread has fallen, due to the effect of economic reforms on buying power. It is evident that broadcasting in Latvia has been subjected to basic changes since 1990, however, the expansion of public broadcasting as well as broadcasting regulation in general has been restricted due to the constant outdated attitude of broadcasting being utilized for the political elite to reach out to the public, instead of using it as a means for democratic debate or even to integrate various groups within society (Open Society Institute, 2005).

Like Hungary, Latvia also has minimal television channels as there are a total of four national terrestrial television channels, of which two are public (LTV1 and LTV7) as well as two private (LNT and TV3). The migration of cable television, which comprises the main form of information for those who speak Russian, occurred due to the termination of broadcasting of Russia's State channel ORT in Latvia. That said, cable television takes on a somewhat critical spot within the broadcasting sector. The broadcasting district in Latvia is regulated by the National Radio and Television Council (NRTP). The NRTP regulates the public as well as the private broadcasters, in addition to disperses commercial broadcast licenses (Open Society Institute, 2005).

After the collapse of the Soviet Union, Russia underwent a plethora of changes in regards to the mass media system. In fact, laws were adopted to prevent the censorship that occurred through the Soviet Union Era (Strovsky, 2006). However, there are still scholars that believe that similarities are still evident when comparing the old Soviet system to the new Soviet system. Due to Russia's war on terrorism and the devastating apartment bombings in August 1999 that killed over 1,000 individuals, gave authorities an abundance of excuses to restrict what is reported. An abundance of bills was debated on in regards to limiting the reports by mass media that pertain to incidents (Strovsky, 2006). However, when analyzing the Russian media history, it has been illustrated that journalistic censorship and self-censorship have always been around, as in comparison to other European countries, Russia has always kept its authoritarian tradition, which was infiltrated among all aspects of their lives. Prior to 1804, there were regulations on the press by a series of individual laws. However, a special statute combined all the media laws, and 22 years later a new document was born, entitled and nicknamed the cast iron statute (Strovsky, 2006).

After 1917, Russia was under a stricter authoritarian rule, which was reinforced by the ideology that accepted the Soviet society and was made a portion of the state institutions (Simons & Strovsky, 2006; von Seth, 2011). The press's main function was to publicize party policies as well as to educate and raise the masses. The journalistic depictions were meant to be interpreted and in agreement with the Socialists view, where the outcome that the truth in reporting had nothing to do with the objectiveness (von Seth, 2011).

The implementation of the new media law in 1990 made massive changes for journalism as censorship was eradicated, journalists were independent of the publishers, and the concept of privately owning media outlets was allowed. However, once the Soviet Union was destroyed, the press lost its strength as the main mode of attaining news, and therefore the circulation of daily press dropped tremendously (von Seth, 2011). In the post-Soviet state, media freedom was diminished due to other media forms taking over, such as (a) TV 6, (b) NTV, and (c) national daily papers. These were taken over by both corporations and the state during the early 2000s. However, as of the 2000s, authorities indicated that the media is irresponsible and are inappropriately utilizing their freedom of expression. The post-Soviet experience demonstrates that the media did not take an independent position in regards to political actors. This was illustrated during the 1996 presidential election campaign when all leading broadcast media backed Yeltsin's candidacy.

Journalistic Perspectives and Punditry

In 1924, the White House Correspondents Association, in the United States, holds a dinner to celebrate journalism and raise funds for scholarships of future journalists. Journalists by definition are those who collect, assess, create, write, and present news and information. Pundits are defined as individuals who are summoned and paid to give their personal opinions, which are based on their agenda. Pundits, who talk as though they are experts in their field or actually in any field, appear as though they have the only insight of information that they relay to their audience. Did the true journalists of the 1950s and 1960s report the news or were talking heads by reading the teleprompter. As compared to today's pundits who never read a teleprompter because they babble on and on about their agenda, not facts. Hopmann and Stromback (2010) stated that due to the influence of political actors, journalists perceive themselves pressured and discover ways to guard their independence by "being impartial or objective in the news reporting" (para. 2). In addition, Hopmann and Stromback used a phrase of journalists to fight back against political actors to (a) adopt an interpretive journalistic style, (b) focus on the why rather than the what with regards to politics, (c) frame the political landscape away from issues and place more emphasis on the strategic game format, and (d) use pundits to provide their commentary.

Referring back to the White House Correspondent's dinner, there were individuals (e.g., pundits, comedians), as in every year, who were asked to comment on the current Presidential Office of individuals, to include the President of the United States. Keep in mind that this is a fundraiser for future journalists and the celebration of journalists' First Amendment Rights. In the past two years, the focus of these monologues has become very partisan with venomous speech. Izaguirre (2015) mentioned that this type of speech had been imposed upon the media viewing audience by pundits and television talk show hosts. When society is impacted with this venomous speech of unease and pundits continue with their obstruction and negativity will "win the day" by creating this type of behavior (Izaguirre, 2015, p. 163). Is the public obtaining the accurate facts and stories regarding world issues that they need to be aware? When the public turns to newscasts and/or social media, they want full transparency, yet the media and these rising political pundits set their narratives via the views of amateur punditry. Considering the widespread presence within mainstream media of pundits, whose job it is to pronounce the political process, the concept of amateur punditry is encouraged. These amateur pundits utilize a great deal of time discussing parties, leaders, and media coverage of the election, with no referencing to issues (Jansen & Koop, 2005).

When listening to the constant news cycles, the public needs to look at who has the interests and motives in putting out what is selling the stories. In addition, the viewers should always look at who has this interest in what is leaked to the media and what the media wants the public to hear. There is no more relaying accurate news; instead, it is more of relaying the pundits preferred choice of spin regarding the world issues. It is a shame and disservice to the public who desires the real stories to make an educated and informed decision on world issues, political parties, and other issues of strong debate; however, the media manipulates it. Letukas (2012) mentioned the pundits who are on cable news, "have the ability to have quick, provocative interpretations and quotable material that could be reproduced off screen and manipulated into a sound bite" (pp. 58-59).

Schulten (2015) illustrated that the idea of media literacy is nothing new; however, this cannot be said of news literacy, which is a novel field that is expanding. Schulten further explicated that the newest form of communication since the invention of the Gutenberg's printing press, has made it far more difficult to decide what is the truth. Thanks to the digital revolution, a plethora of information as well as misinformation is accessible to the public through various channels at any time of the day. According to Barclay (2015), a pundit is an individual who appears to be an expert in their field and will be found commenting or writing about current issues. Barclay indicated that political pundits could be found everywhere, from television to the radio, to newspapers and even writing blogs on the Internet. Barclay further revealed that pundits are consistently needed as some will quit, others will be fired, and ultimately some will pass away. As such, media outlets are desperate to quickly discover other pundits, of which some so happen to be inadequately trained in their field (Barclay, 2015). It is astonishing how pundits, who continue to be fascinated by their narrow understandings of world issues, dictate to politicians regarding how to conduct business based on their so-called strategies at both the national and international levels. However, one would ask what makes them the experts in all the world issues and where did they receive formal training concerning these issues? When media outlets so happen to make these hasty decisions, pundits who have no clue as to what they are saying will be employed and even speak on national television or write in national newspapers and thus display a deficiency in their supposed knowledge on such topics that they are presumed experts (Barclay, 2015). Schulten (2015) added that commentators, bloggers, as well as pundits had been found battling against traditional journalists for public attention. Therefore, an abundance of ignorant opinions is being utilized and covered up as news. As a result, deciphering between legitimate journalism and propaganda has become far more difficult (Schulten, 2015). The trend of negative convergence by state-run propaganda and censorship, "in which the space for meaningful political expression online shrinks and moves in the direction of less free traditional media, has profoundly troubling implications" (Walker & Orttung, 2014, p. 79). Due to this overflow of information, it is critical that the public is capable of judging what is and is not reliable information when scrolling through their social media (Schulten, 2015).

Not only could information from pundits be valid or reliable for the public concern, but even the journalists' perspectives are skewed. For many years in the United States, there had been three major news outlets, which reported the same stories at the local, national, and international levels. With the increase of the 24/7 cable news outlets and just about every world news incident, news anchors repeat the same story-of-the-day repeatedly until it is deep-seated in the viewers' minds, which is intended to manipulate the minds of individuals who have difficulty making a decision. According to Claster (2010), prior research was conducted that revealed that audiences from television news are feeling broken in regards to their sentiments toward mainstream media. This prior research further demonstrates that people will discern a bias or lack of objectivity when they discern the show as being slanted in opposition to their own beliefs, despite their political outlook. Claster further indicated an additional study that discovered that people would view news media based on the sources they deem to be precise as well as objective. At the moment, people can choose which media they utilize and can research information that strengthens what they already believe and have knowledge on. Parenti (as cited in Claster, 2010) indicated that power is far more potent when it is hidden. That said, objectivity claims become a critical technique to attain faithful viewers. As pundits declare to be objective as well as neutral, they also attempt to convince the viewers that the topic is neutralized; however, actually twist the story.

In addition, since the 1980s, opinionated broadcasting programs (e.g., radio, television) have been developed, as producers are aware there are specific audiences who want to hear the engaged debate and rapid-fire arguments regarding politics and other social issues. According to Letukas (2012), since news can be viewed in such a constant state, the opinionated programs have targeted primetime with the increase of pundits who, by preaching their pre-existing ideologies, have framed a substantial role in setting the public agenda in America. Letukas (2012) additionally indicated that Gaye Tuchman and Todd Gitlin, who are sociologists, were the first to administer the idea of framing in regards to the method that news media, as well as other claim makers, introduce information. Tuchman (as cited in Letukas, 2012) indicated that framing is born when editors determine what story will be published and framing evolves when journalists depict particular parts of the story to the public. Journalists, as well as other claims-makers, supply the context through which pertinent information can be spoken about as well as debated. By doing it in this fashion, various forms of issues can be interpreted by the media as well as the public in various ways, and that communication theory has to be sensitive to these dissimilarities (Letukas, 2012).

Lee (2004, 2010) stated that in the profession of journalism, the truth is essential. Researchers continued to point out the critical role of a journalist, which is, to tell the truth, more than most professions and then give a balanced story, otherwise, it can become misleading (Lee, 2004; Lewandowsky, Ecker, Seifert, Schwarz, & Cook, 2012). However, there are inconsistent opinions about how journalists choose to deceive and manipulate the viewers' minds. Journalists knowingly resort to deception because it makes getting a story easier and more objective" (Lee, 2010, p. 68) and that it could be the only means to obtain essential information. Although journalists should tell the truth, media scholars consider that some deception and manipulation is warranted (Lee, 2004). "The news business is following an unconscious rule that offhand, casual deception is okay, but elaborate and carefully planned deceptions are wicked" (Meyer, 1987, p. 81). Elliot and Culver (1992) defined journalistic deception as "it is sometimes just as morally problematic for journalists to withhold true information as it is to give false information" (p. 77). There are still great role model journalists who want the public to hear the truth of world issues and will report on journalists who have described untruths in their stories. Many of these untruths, which could lose the credibility with the audiences, are listed as false claims, journalistic fraud, altered photos, favoritism of a specific political party, deception, smearing a person's character, negligence, plagiarism, quote tampering, staging, and other fabrication of the news as long as it meets their agenda (Elliot, 1989; Elliot & Culver, 1992; Lee 2004, 2010).

Division of Communities

Race and ethnicity. Mass media whether it is through television, radio, newspapers, and now through social media and streaming services distribute some form of ideology. The ideology is created through the method of framing, which is the way that information is organized and presented (Powell, 2011; Scheufele, 1999). As the viewing public, we understand and process the information through the frames created for us (Powell, 2011; Scheufele, 1999). The frames are constructed via angles or story focus that makes sense to news writers and the influence of public opinion (Takahashi, 2010). Courtois and Gold (2009) spoke about many events from terrorism to widespread disasters, which "have been increasingly framed through the lens of trauma by both professionals and the news media" (p. 3). Powell (2011) indicated that primarily the frames constructed in the United States are of a Caucasian Christian male perspective, as they are the primary framers of media ideology. The mass media utilizes framing as a critical process to tell stories. The framing process can also be a significant factor in our relationships, which can be driven by the paradigms of culture, gender, as well as vocation.

Mastro (2015) emphasized that race and ethnic relations continue to be a significant and controversial issue in the 21st century. The Internet has also had an impact regarding tense race relations via social media on college campuses (Chan, 2017). The factors that contribute to race relations are extensive and complex, although many conceptualizations and characterizations are framed in the mass media, including news and entertainment offerings (Mastro, 2015). Media portrayals are incredibly important as our primary viewpoint of other races and cultures are shaped by the media. Our perspective is formed in this fashion due to our society still living in a segregated manner. Mastro indicated that the average Caucasian American lives in a neighborhood and attends a school that is 75% Caucasian. African Americans and Hispanics live in neighborhoods and go to schools, which make up their own racial or ethnic groups. The numbers are similar to Caucasian, as 70% of African

Americans and 80% of Hispanics live in neighborhoods and attend schools that are predominantly non-Caucasian (Mastro, 2015). Through the mix of news and entertainment media, the quality of race and ethnic representations have not been favorable. Mastro emphasized that although there has been an improvement of African Americans on primetime television, they are still commonly depicted as violent and menacing criminals in print and television news. "Many media outlets reinforce the public's racial misconceptions about crime by presenting African Americans and Latinos differently than Whites . . . Television news programs and newspapers over-represent racial minorities as crime suspects and Whites as crime victims" (Prince, 2014, para. 2). The social norms of our society frown on overt racial expressions and hostilities; however, the rise in hate groups since 2012 seem to dispute those social norms (Mastro, 2015). Mass media does very little to offer comprehensive explanations of race and ethnic portrayals; rather groups are simply linked to desirable as well as undesirable characterizations. This type of linkage only enflames societal racial tensions where more deliberate accurate delivering and framing of the news could discourage bias and promote optimal intergroup relations (Mastro, 2015).

Banjo (2013) emphasized Mastro's findings that our understanding of the social world is not only dictated by what we are shown, but also through the exclusion of selected race and ethnic groups. African Americans have historically been ignored and misrepresented by the media. The misrepresentation has taken place to the extent that it significantly reinforces the stereotypes and attitudes towards African Americans by other race and ethnic groups (Banjo, 2013). Ramasubramanian (2011) agreed that African Americans in mass media had a long history of demeaning and violent stereotypes portrayed of them specifically through news media, although entertainment programming has also presented portrayals through limited use of these stereotypes. The stereotypes presented by the media can significantly shape real-world beliefs, causal interpretations, and emotions between race and ethnic groups (Prince, 2014; Ramasubramanian, 2011).

The media's history of framing in such a fashion that dictates the actions of the masses can go back as far as the Tulsa (Oklahoma) Riot of 1921. The framing not only emphasized the paradigm in which was seen through racial frames but could also have signaled the commencement of the negative relationships between law enforcement officials and African Americans. On May 31, 1921, in Tulsa, Oklahoma was the scene of the most (at the time) devastating single episode of racial conflict in the post-slavery United States. The riot was precipitated by the arrest of an African American man who was accused of an assault against a Caucasian female. The May 31st edition of the Tulsa Tribune framed the story in such a fashion to inflame passions of Caucasian citizens. The riot erupted when Caucasian citizens, who were also deputized by law enforcement officials, attempted to break into the jail where the African American man was held in custody for the purposes of lynching him. Upon reaching the jail, the Caucasian citizens were confronted by African American citizens who seek to protect the accused from being lynched. At that time, several violent episodes erupted and resulted in the riot-taking place between both groups in Tulsa's Greenwood section, which was designated for African Americans (Messer & Bell, 2010). The riot resulted in extensive damage to Greenwood, which resulted in 35 city blocks being looted or damaged to the result of 36 reported deaths and $1.8 million in damages (Messer & Bell, 2010). The number of fatalities had long been disputed given that several citizens were not given proper burials.

The Tulsa Tribune's framing of the pre and post-riot incidents continued to frame the African American man as a criminal and those who came to protect him as agitators. The Caucasian citizens were portrayed as citizens seeking justice, although they were not law enforcement (though later deputized) and the African American man was already in the custody of law enforcement. The law enforcement officials were viewed as incompetent and inept not only for lack of instituting order in a smoldering situation but also for deputizing citizens who had an objective of vengeance and terrorism based on the framed narrative in the Tulsa Tribune (Messer & Bell, 2010). The framing still affected the efforts for reparations sought by survivors nearly 75 years later. Messer and Bell (2010) believed that the time gap between the riot and the reparations movement as well as the media framing of the riot in 1921 had prevented African American survivors from receiving justice.

Black lives matter and minority relations with law enforcement. Black Lives Matter is an activist movement in the United States resulting from the July 2013 acquittal of George Zimmerman in the killing of Trayvon Martin. The phrase "Black lives matter" first appeared in social media and received increased attention in the subsequent deaths of Michael Brown, Tamir Rice, and Freddie Gray (Ince, Rojas, & Davis, 2017). The decentralization of the movement, invited audiences to frame the movement Black lives matter into a myriad of issues affecting African Americans through the utilization of social media and the hashtag (#, which categorizes issues, under one umbrella within social media), #blacklivesmatter (Ince, Rojas, & Davis, 2017). The decentralization of the movement allowed for the framing of the movement via social media and mass media platforms. The reach of many populations seems to spread even faster through social media and mass media attention. The framing of the movement and the issues it brought attention to, only seemed to further entrench individuals in their narratives depending primarily on the race and ethnic group one belonged to.

Black Lives Matter has brought attention through social media and mass media the relationship between minority communities and law enforcement. The frequent presentation of random violence in mass media has increased the importance and awareness of crime in people's lives, which increases their assessment of risk and level of fear (Callanan, 2012). This presentation of violence disproportionally portrays Black suspects in a mug shot or handcuffed, which creates resentment on the view and value of African Americans by Black Lives Matter supporters while re-examining public trust and confidence in law enforcement by all (Callanan & Rosenberger, 2011). One's experience significantly influences the public trust and confidence in law enforcement. Overall, there is a high value and opinion of police in democratic societies, although African Americans have a lower opinion of law enforcement than Caucasians (Callanan & Rosenberger, 2011). Callanan and Rosenberger (2011) attributed the prevailing African American opinion of law enforcement due to the historical as well as contemporary, aggressive police tactics, which has led to a long history of mistrust and low opinion of law enforcement.

The framing of relations between minorities and law enforcement as well as the viewpoint of Caucasians on minority relations and law enforcement is very real to each group. Framing once again, goes to how a story is told which can be reinforced by one's experiences. The police shootings of unarmed men continue to be of an increased concern coupled with 24-hour news coverage of African American men losing their lives along with the framing of riots and scenes of destruction in various cities in the United States that continue to sow seeds of racial tension and anger in urban neighborhoods (Crichlow & Fulcher, 2017). The framing of these narratives brings viewership to mass media outlets, which brings ratings and then brings revenue. The mass media are owned and supported by corporations with influence to fulfill agendas by managing news content that is broadcasted (Crichlow & Fulcher, 2017). African Americans and Hispanics are often portrayed as violent criminals could lead to more punitive criminal justice approaches starting with law enforcement interactions, these interactions and approaches are often dictated by media depictions after an incident that stirs racial passions and forms public opinion (Crichlow & Fulcher, 2017).

The mass media serves as many individuals' main source of criminal justice information. The method in which information is framed has a significant influence towards views on crime and criminal justice. Commercial pressures and advertising dollars drive the need for higher viewership, which pushes for the priority to present the most sensational stories. This push drives the concern from healing relationships and eradicating racial injustice to promoting fear and increased support for repressive criminal justice policies (Crichlow & Fulcher, 2017). Weitzer (2015) also chronicled that public confidence in the police erodes after the mass media heavily publicizes a controversial incident. In the days and weeks following the 1991 beating of Los Angeles motorist, Rodney King, police confidence was only 31% among Hispanics, and only 14% among African Americans (Weitzer, 2015). The confidence meter in police does increase over time once an incident has passed but can decrease again after the next highly media publicized incident.

Welch, Price, and Yankey (2004) emphasized that part of mass media's sensationalism of crime is to create a new label of menace with African Americans and Hispanics as the face of that label. In 1989, the Central Park Jogger rape case had the New York City press emerge with the term "wilding" (Welch, Price, & Yankey, 2004). The lines of factual news reporting and entertainment were blurred into a new form called info-tainment. Info-tainment gave birth to the term "wilding" which was a new menacing phrase in a pre-social media period designed to sensationalize the story of the Central Park jogger case (Welch, Price, & Yankey, 2004). As part of this info-tainment strategy, the New York City media as a practice withheld names of accused assailants who were minors. However, in this case, the minors' names, addresses, and photos were published with the phrase of "wilding" being associated with them. In the years following the case, the term "wilding" was used as a racially biased buzzword to describe African American and Hispanic lawbreakers as well as those accused in the minority community. In 2002, 13 years after the trial and after all the individuals served their sentences, DNA evidence proved their innocence by excluding them from having any connection to the crime, and their convictions were vacated. Due to the mass media framing, and info-tainment of the case, there was still a significant population who refused to accept objective scientific evidence disputing their media-constructed beliefs about the case.

Gender and the media. As it pertains to gender and the media, women are often under-represented across the range of media (Collins, 2011). When women are often represented in media, they are often portrayed negatively. Women are often sexualized through the presentation of provocative clothing or traditionally feminine (stereotyped) roles such as a homemaker, wife, or parent (Collins, 2011). It is agreed that increasing the representation of women is valuable; the manner in which they are portrayed should be examined to avoid an increase in stereotypical depictions (Collins, 2011). Gender roles (stereotyping) in advertising have persisted for years particularly when it comes to women and thus have shaped our paradigms when it comes to societal roles (Eisend, 2010). Stereotyping is a set of concepts in a social category, which is not necessarily an adverse judgment since stereotypes can provide a useful orientation to everyday living (Eisend, 2010). However, stereotypes do lead to oversimplified conceptions and misapplied knowledge, which becomes problematic as it can lead to judgments and expectations that restrict life opportunities (Eisend, 2010). As it pertains to gender stereotyping, it can limit life opportunities for women regarding standards of beauty and restrictions on career income aspirations (Eisend, 2010). An example of these restrictions would be the participation of women in sports through Title IX (which provided equitable funding in collegiate athletics without consideration of gender). The experiences of girls and women in sports have positively increased in the United States since the advent of Title IX; however, the mass media depiction still presents sports as the sanctuary of men (Hardin & Greer, 2009). Female athletes are vastly underrepresented in media coverage due to the most popular spectator sports in the United States are still considered to be masculine (Hardin & Greer, 2009). Gender stereotyping via media messages through given names (of girls and boys), and labeling the color pink for girls and the color blue for boys, plays into the world of sports that although women to participate as much (even more in some sports) as men in athletics. The view of sports as made centered has not changed through the framing mechanisms of the mass media (Hardin & Greer, 2009).

World Events

Natural disasters. Numerous disasters have brought on critical psychological impacts to the general population (Lau, Lau, Kim, & Tsui, 2004). Current research has illustrated how media plays a significant role in increasing one's anxiety and stress levels in which people respond to natural disasters (Goodwin, Palgi, Lavenda, Hamama-Raz, & Ben-Ezra, 2014; Weems, Scott, Banks, & Graham, 2012). In fact, the term media amplification has been utilized to demonstrate post-traumatic stress responses, as media exposure has been linked with far more significant stress than if one were to be directly exposed to the traumatic event (Goodwin, Palgi, Lavenda, Hamama-Raz, & Ben-Ezra, 2014).

It is also critical to note that these impacts also affect children. The American Academy of Pediatrics recommends that pediatricians shed light on parents about the damaging effects of indirect natural disaster exposure to children (Hagan & American Academy of Pediatrics, 2005). A study conducted by Weems, Scott, Banks, and Graham (2012) evaluated the link between the amount of TV disaster coverage viewed by children with PTSD symptoms that followed a disaster, even after the researchers controlled for pre-disaster PTSD symptoms. This study further examined if viewing media coverage is associated with preexisting PTSD symptoms. The study comprised of two sets of samples of which one sample consisted of 141 children from fourth to eighth grade, the second sample consisted of 191 children whose age ranged from 9 through 16 years (Weems et al., 2012).

An additional study conducted by Yeung, Yu, Xu, Zhang, Lau, Zhang, Choi, Mak, and Lui (2016) analyzed the longitudinal effect of media exposure associated to the Sichuan Earthquake on probable PTSD amid children and adolescents in Kunming, China. This study further delved into identifying causes, which were assessed at baseline that deemed to be predictive of probable PTSD at a six-month follow-up. The study comprised of 3,577 students, who were attained from six primary schools and six secondary schools in Kumming. Yunnan, which is 444 miles away from the earthquake that had occurred (Yeung et al., 2016). Unlike Weems et al. and Yeung et al. study that utilized youths as their sample, a study conducted by Lau et al. (2004) which comprised of 292 men and 312 women, determined the predominance of signs of posttraumatic stress symptoms as well as other related responses in regards to a 2004 tsunami that occurred in Hong Kong on December 26, 2004. Lau et al. (2004) population comprised of men and women aged 18 through 60.

To attain the results, Weems et al. (2012) utilized direct impact exposure to Hurricane Katrina, TV coverage exposure from hurricane Gustav, as well as an assessment to measure PTSD symptoms, which was a modified version of the University of California at Los Angeles Posttraumatic Stress Disorder Reaction Index. Unlike Weems et al. (2012) study, Lau et al. (2004) utilized a survey that was administered via the phone. Furthermore, sociodemographic characteristics, as well as the connection with the affected areas, were measured. The assessment tools used were the locally validated life orientation test scale utilized to measure optimism, as well as the Chinese version of the impact of event scale, which measured signs of post-traumatic stress. To measure Post Traumatic Stress Symptoms, and attain Yeung et al. (2016) results, one of the many tools utilized included the Children's Revised Impact of Event Scale.

Results for Weems et al. (2012) study indicated that the association between being exposed to TV viewing of disasters and PTSD symptoms in children is not only due to preexisting symptoms. The data attained for this study further revealed that the children with pre-existing elevated symptoms would maintain their symptoms even after viewing more media coverage of natural disasters. Lastly, it is for those children who have already preexisting hardships, that the adverse effect of viewing a vast amount of media coverage of a disaster is most significant. Just like Weems et al. (2012) study, Yeung et al. (2016) investigation revealed that 38% and 53% of those who took part in the study stated that they were repeatedly exposed to both distant and close up pictures of dead bodies in addition to other disturbing images. A total of 80% of the participants were exposed to different forms of unrest content in media coverage. Results revealed that a range of 34.3% to 72.5% of participants felt much or very much disturbed by the 11 forms of earthquake-related unrest news contents. Results further indicated that 54.6% of the participants felt emotionally disturbed, 58.6% felt horrified, and 60.0% were apprehensive because of the earthquake. Lastly, results revealed the prevalence of probable PTSD at 16.9% at the baseline and 11.1% at six months. As time progressed, participants illustrated substantial changes in regards to their levels of risk of probable PTSD. Those who had a lower risk of probable PTSD, 8.8% developed probable PTSD at the six months follow up. A total of 22.4% of those who have a high risk of probable PTSD at baseline illustrated persistent probable PTSD at six months.

Similarly, Lau et al. (2004) results demonstrated that the viewing of visual images as well as the contents of the messages created a plethora of psychological disturbances. This was illustrated due to the excessive amounts of information provided by the media. Therefore, high levels of stress were found among the participants, and 79%, as well as 73.4% of the participants, felt terrified or concerned of the tsunami, and 40.6% felt emotionally disturbed. Elements of media coverage, such as (a) frequency of coverage, (b) visual images, in addition to (c) distressful contents heavily predicted stressful responses related to the tsunami. It was further indicated that coverage on (a) children, (b) dead bodies, and (c) death tolls had stronger correlations with post-traumatic stress symptoms (Lau et al., 2004).

Terrorism. As stated in Johnson, Ross, Matteson, Henry, Link, Axler, Lopez, and, Grace (2015), "Acts of terrorism are designed to create psychological instability and fear" (p. 4). A significant amount of research indicated that being exposed to terrorist attacks could have a substantial effect on one's mental health, for adults and even children. Such an impact includes the beginning of post-traumatic stress disorder symptoms. According to a survey administered in 2012, the September 11th attack deemed to be the most impactful occurrence that television viewers have ever witnessed over the past 50 years (Silver, Holman, Andersen, Poulin, McIntosh, and Gil-Rivas, 2013). The September 11th attack also proved to have an effect on children in the United Kingdom, as studies illustrated that, children in London who viewed the attacks on television suffered from posttraumatic stress symptoms as well as functional impairment throughout the six months after September 11th (Silver et al., 2013). Evidence illustrated that over 20% of individuals who resided in New York City, who lived near the World Trade Center during the September 11th attacks illustrated all required symptoms to be diagnosed for PTSD two months after the incident occurred (Busso, McLaughlin, & Sheridan, 2014). Time after the September 11th attack occurred, traumatic symptoms across the board were evident and present to individuals who were indirectly exposed to the attacks (Monfort & Afzali, 2017). These symptoms were linked with media exposure three to five days as well as nine to 23 days after the September 11th attack and two to four weeks following the Boston Marathon bombings in 2013 (Monfort & Afzali, 2017). Chronic stress symptoms were also related to media exposure one to two months as well as three years following the September 11th attack. It has further been illustrated that significant levels of media exposure to terrorist attacks can be somewhat damaging for those who are already at risk for developing PTSD (Busso et al., 2014). A total of 36 studies examined the relation between psychopathological outcome and media viewing, of which mainly dealt with the September 11th attacks. A majority of these 36 studies investigated individuals who viewed television related to terrorism and established an association between numerous psychological outcomes and viewing television that related to disasters (Monfort & Afzali, 2017).

A study conducted by Duarte, Wu, Cheung, Mandell, Fan, Wicks, Musa, and Hoven (2011) examined the utilization of three forms of media: (a) TV, (b) the web, and (c) the combination of radio as well as print media six months after 9/11 by utilizing a representative sample of public school children who reside in New York City within various levels of World Trade Center exposure. The study comprised of 8,236 students in New York City public schools who were 9-21 years of age in Grades 4-12. The gender/ ethnic/ racial distribution mirrored that of what one would find at a New York City public school population. Like Duarte et al.'s study, a study conducted by Saylor, Cowart, Lipovsky, Jackson, and Finch (2003) examined the experiences, both as the events unfolded as well as the days and weeks that followed, of elementary school children who were exposed to media during the World Trade Center Terrorist attack, who was in a geographical location that was not directly impacted by the catastrophic event. Furthermore, the study examined the association between distinct exposure experiences as well as post-traumatic stress symptoms in children who were only exposed to the traumatic event via media coverage. The sample size for Saylor et al.'s study was 179 students from four schools, which comprised of 49% boys and 51% girls whose age ranged from 5 to 11 years old, of which 75% are Caucasian, 16% are African American, and 9% are Other. A further three-year study conducted by Silver et al. (2013) observed the physical and mental health outcomes of American participants who were exposed to the September 11th attacks via the media. As this was a three-year longitudinal study, there were three sets of participants, of which the first set comprised of 2,033 participants, the second set included of 1,571 participants, and the third set consisted of 1,771 participants.

To attain the data for Duarte et al. (2011) study, the students were given a paper, and pencil self-reported questionnaire to be completed. Although Duarte et al.'s study comprised of one survey, Saylor et al. (2003) utilized three measurement tools, which were (a) Pediatric Emotional Distress Scale, and (b) The Parent Report of Post Traumatic Symptoms, and the Children's Report of Post Traumatic Symptoms. For Silver et al.'s (2013) study, data was attained through Internet-based surveys, utilizing a sample taken from a national probability panel of the U.S population who were gathered using stratified random digit dial telephone sampling and managed by Knowledge Networks, a company that offers Internet access.

Results for Duarte et al. (2011) study illustrated that six months after the World Trade Center attack, 62% of the students indicated that they viewed an abundance of TV in regards to the attack, which was then followed by radio and print at 31%, and finally the Web at 7%. Students who were in Grades 9 through 12 indicated more TV viewing with 67% versus students in Grades 4 through 8. Of those students, students who identified themselves as White illustrated the highest rate of watching World Trade Center coverage on TV, followed by Hispanic students with 64%, and finally African American students with the lowest utilization at 55% (Duarte et al., 2011). Whereas Saylor et al. (2003) study indicated that 64% of the participants received the information about the world trade center attack through their parents, however, approximately half of the third through fifth graders viewed television coverage in their schools, with 32% of the participants having this as their first exposure from this form of media. In regards to the hours and days following the terrorist attack, a minimum of 85% of the participants was exposed to some media of the World Trade Center attack and its impact. There were 68% of students who viewed negative media (footage of attack, footage of individuals escaping, crying, and yelling) and 69% of students who viewed positive media (pictures of celebrities helping attack victims, observed President Bush address nation, saw pictures of heroes aiding or rescuing victims) (Saylor et al., 2003). Whereas Silver et al.'s (2013) results revealed that 63% of the participants indicated that they viewed the September 11th attacks as it took place live on television and 33% stated that they did not view any live exposure. In regards to the week after September 11th, 0.7% of the participants reported they did not view any September 11th associated television news coverage, with 13% seeing less than one hour per day, 42% stated one to three hours per day, and finally 44% reported watching four or more hours per day. A total of 11.85% of participants indicated high levels of September 11th associated acute stress symptoms. Viewing four or more hours of September 11th associated television predicted a 51% increased possibility of reporting high September 11th associated acute stress after it was controlled for prior September 11th mental health, demographics, as well as lifetime trauma. That stated, results indicated that early September 11th associated television viewing was linked with posttraumatic stress symptoms both two and three years after September 11th. This was based on one to three hours of viewing television per day at two years, one to three hours per day at three years and four or more hours per day at two years, and four or more hours per day at three years past the September 11th. Results revealed that viewing one or more hours per day of early post-September 11th television coverage, predicted an incline in posttraumatic stress over three years post-September 11th. Moreover, results indicated that media exposure as well as acute stress greatly predicted September 11th related posttraumatic stress, when cumulative acute stress was tested as a mediator.

An interesting result within Duarte et al. (2011) study, illustrated that students who indicated exhaustive utilization of TV, as well as the combined category six months following the World Trade Center attack, were far more likely in comparison to the other students who did not utilize this form of media exhaustively to have been directly exposed to the World Trade Center attack, whereas the utilization of the Web did not illustrate any effect. In comparison, Saylor et al.'s (2003) study demonstrated that there was no difference in PTSD symptoms among the various forms of media. Lastly, overall probable PTSD was linked more-so with the utilization of a considerable amount of media for both TV and radio as well as print, however not with the usage of the Web (Duarte et al., 2011). An additional interesting result indicated in Saylor et al.'s (2003) study revealed that the amount of positive media images were substantially related to PTSD symptoms, however as the amount of positive images increased, so did the amount of PTSD symptoms. Nevertheless, anxiety was significantly related to negative media images, but it was not associated with positive media images.

Wars. Research conducted utilizing children as participants for studies on the Oklahoma City bombing as well as the 1990 Gulf War illustrated that there was an association between television exposure and trauma-related symptoms (Silver et al., 2013). As previously mentioned, a study conducted by Silver et al. (2013) observed how the media played a role in Americans physical and mental state, and stress responses after being exposed to the September 11th attack as well as the Iraq War that took place after September 11th through the media, more specifically, TV media. Whereas, a study conducted by Kira, Hammad, Lewandowski, Templin, Ramaswamy, Ozkan, and Mohanesh (2007) tried to determine the cause of elevated levels of poor health and mental health in Iraqi refugees. The participants who comprised Kira et al. study were 274 males whose age ranged from 12 to 79 years old. The participants were required to complete a survey that consisted of numerous scales, of which one included media exposure to the war in Iraq.

In regards to the data attained for the study conducted by Silver et al. and the results that pertained to the Iraq War, when it came to media exposure and the Iraq War, 6.4% of war survey participants revealed that they never saw media images of war, whereas 19% indicated that they rarely saw pictures, and 55% acknowledged seeing them sometimes, with 20% reporting that they saw Iraq war images often. Following the beginning of the Iraq War, 3.0% of the participants revealed that they viewed no war-related television, 21.7% stated that they observed less than 1 hour per day, 55.6% indicated seeing 1 to 3 hours per day, and 19.7% indicated that they watched 4 or more hours per day (Silver et al., 2013).

In terms of the Iraq War-related acute stress within Silver et al. (2013) study, 7.3% of the participants reported high acute stress when the Iraq War commenced. Results further indicated viewing 4 or more hours of war associated television and the frequency of seeing war-related images both were linked with war-related acute stress symptoms. Moreover, more recurrent exposure to war associated media images predicted a 40% increased possibility of high war-related acute stress. The two particular images that were significantly linked with war-related acute stress symptoms were images of allied prisoners of war as well as dead Iraqi children (Silver et al., 2013).

Lastly, Silver et al. (2013) study determined that war-related media exposure predicted September 11th associated post-traumatic stress symptoms two to three years after September 11th. Results further illustrated that viewing one or more hours per day of early post-September 11th television coverage, viewing four or more hours per day of war-related television coverage, as well as repeated viewing of Iraq war images all predicted an influx in post-traumatic stress over three years following September 11th. When Silver et al. tested cumulative acute stress as a mediator, evidence illustrated that media exposure as well as acute stress greatly predicted September 11th related posttraumatic stress. Therefore, results propose that media image exposure is "independently and indirectly" linked with posttraumatic stress. Similar to Silver et al. results, Kira et al. (2007) study revealed that more than 14% of the participants indicated that they met the full criteria for PTSD, with adolescents having a higher chance of being diagnosed (19.6%) than adults. Various factors resulted in the participants acquiring PTSD, which included; (a) the downward social, economic, and occupational mobility and (b) lack of acculturation. However, the most significant factors that caused poor health and mental health were (a) cumulative trauma, (b) collective identity trauma/ discrimination, and (c) exposure to media news of the war in Iraq. It was further illustrated that when participants were exposed to the news on war in comparison to other past traumas, there was equal or stronger on health as well as PTSD.

CONCLUSION OF WHAT WE LEARNED

Based on the research provided within this chapter, it is evident that media is associated with or causes PTSD disorder among other adverse psychological effects to humankind. "Media coverage of disturbing news events via television, radio, and print sources may be a greater source of stress then has been assumed" (McNaughton-Cassill, 2001, p. 193).

Mass media can control individuals' minds, whether good or bad. Due to the good effect-bad effect, it is up to the individuals to seek through all the agendas and propaganda by news outlets and by countries to develop their ideas without being manipulated by the media. It is evident in the research and public opinion that the mass media creates stories to generate a viewing audience. Even within countries, there are news outlets that support different political parties and are selective in how they report world events. It is in the best interest of marketers to align themselves with news outlets who have a broader viewing audience, as there are more people to view that product. Even news outlets that have book authors, pundits, and strategists on their broadcasts sometimes pay to be on that particular show to promote their agenda; to sway the viewing audience.

Based on research, the media intend to obtain the larger audience no matter how horrific the visualization of war, terrorism, natural disasters as well as the divisions of race, gender, and culture worldwide. They utilize strategic verbiage to attract viewers' attention on events that the average person would most likely not want to see. However, due to the continuous borage of negative news, it seems as though it is the norm for viewers to be subjected to this. The method the media draws people in, makes them want to view more. For example, everyone wants to see an accident that they are not in. The media provides instant gratification by sensationalizing terrible events. For instance, beheadings and lighting people on fire in cages, as seen, performed by terrorists.

It would be best for media to commence showing positive news, in a non-biased approach. The media should be more positive to disrupt the negativity and shed a positive light on viewers. For example the show Vice, which is a documentary series of groundbreaking news from all over the world. This is not like the typical news, as they are attempting to create harmony amongst groups. Some of their shows were based on topics such as Afghan women's rights, and the Cold War. There should be more shows like this, rather than what is currently being aired, which promotes division and hatred. As we have all seen in the past, what occurs after we witness a tragic school shooting being aired on the news? A subsequent school shooting will transpire. Media focuses far too much on giving attention to individuals who engage in devastations, and not on individuals who engage in positive behaviors.

Based on research within all areas, the media is well aware of how the brain works and based on all countries regulations, whether by advertising or propaganda, it places fear in people. Advertisers are also mindful of how the mind works, which is why they pay so much per spot during commercial airtime. It has been revealed that just alone in the last couple of years, cable news has had an increase of viewers, which is an increase in marketing sales. Also, when authors have a time slot on cable or local news, those authors are paying the media outlet for that time. Most of those books are political and controversial.

Future research is to conduct several mixed methods studies on several news outlets to discuss their business models on advertising and their agenda regarding their manipulation of minds. Research should also reach to government legislatures regarding their regulations as well as psychiatrists and psychologists experiences with media psychology. Media psychology has become a new area of study beginning from the 1980s. Rutledge (2008) stated during this timeframe, "technological advances have revolutionized the media environment, generating opportunities and raising concerns" (para. 1). Rutledge (2008) and Luskin (2012) continued to explain that media psychology is not only for psychologists, but also in other fields as education, researchers, healthcare, business, entertainment, and lay individuals; all individuals who have an interest in how the mind and media correlate. To look more into media psychology, it should be defined more by investigating standards of the field by practitioners to include collaboration while informing the public. Luskin commented that media psychology has evolved since its inception and has many components to include online education, consulting, media interviews, and the money-making elements of consumer products, marketing, advertising, product placement, and game theory. Game theory is interesting in the manipulation of minds as it compares the relationships between contributors in a particular model and forecasts their optimal decisions.

REFERENCES

Banjo, O. O. (2013). For us only? Examining the effect of viewing context on Black audiences' perceived influence of Black entertainment. *Race and Social Problems*, *5*(4), 309–322. doi:10.100712552-013-9106-x

Barclay, L. (2005). *What will we do when the pundits are all gone?* Retrieved from https://search-proquest-com.ezproxylocal.library.nova.edu/central /docview/438893939/23CE7DA458FE417BPQ/1?accountid=6579

Bennett, T. (1982). *Culture, society and the media* (1st ed.). Methuen & Co Ltd.

Busso, D. S., McLaughlin, K. A., & Sheridan, M. A. (2014). Media exposure and sympathetic nervous system reactivity predict PTSD symptoms after the Boston Marathon bombings. *Depression and Anxiety*, *31*(7), 551–558. doi:10.1002/da.22282 PMID:24995832

Callanan, V. J. (2012). Media consumption, perceptions of crime, risk and fear of crime: Examining race/ethnic differences. *Sociological Perspectives*, *55*(1), 93–115. doi:10.1525op.2012.55.1.93

Callanan, V. J., & Rosenberger, J. S. (2011). Media and public perceptions of the police: Examining the impact of race and personal experience. *Policing and Society*, *21*(2), 167–189. doi:10.1080/10439463.2010.540655

Chan, J. (2017). Racial identity in online spaces: Social media's impact on students of color. *Journal of Student Affairs Research and Practice*, *54*(2), 163–174. doi:10.1080/19496591.2017.1284672

Claster, S. M. (2012). *Pundit wars: An investigation into the pragmatics of news talk programs* (Doctoral dissertation). Available from ProQuest Dissertations and Theses database. (UMI No. 3484262)

Collins, R. L. (2011). Content analysis of gender roles in media: Where are we now and where should we go? *Sex Roles*, *64*(3-4), 290–298. doi:10.100711199-010-9929-5

Courtois, C. A., & Gold, S. N. (2009). The need for inclusion of psychological trauma in the professional curriculum: A call to action. *Psychological Trauma: Theory, Research, Practice, and Policy*, *1*(1), 3–23. doi:10.1037/a0015224

Crichlow, V. J., & Fulcher, C. (2017). Black men down: An assessment of experts' quotes on deadly encounters with the police. *Race and Social Problems*, *9*(3), 171–180. doi:10.100712552-017-9197-x

Duarte, C. S., Wu, P., Cheung, A., Mandell, D. J., Fan, B., Wicks, J., ... Hoven, C. W. (2011). Media use by children and adolescents from New York City 6 months after the WTC attack. *Journal of Traumatic Stress*, *24*(5), 553–556. doi:10.1002/jts.20687 PMID:21882251

Eisend, M. (2010). A meta-analysis of gender roles in advertising. *Journal of the Academy of Marketing Science*, *38*(4), 418–440. doi:10.100711747-009-0181-x

Elliot, D. (1989). Journalistic deception. In P. Y. Windt, P. C. Appleby, M. P. Battin, L. P. Francis, & B. M. Landesman (Eds.), *Ethical issues in the professions* (pp. 144–146). Englewood Cliffs, NJ: Prentice Hall.

Elliot, D., & Culver, C. (1992). Defining and analyzing journalistic deception. *Journal of Mass Media Ethics*, *7*(2), 69–84. doi:10.120715327728jmme0702_1

Fujitake, A. (2005). *Nihon no masumedia* (2nd ed.). Tokyo, Japan: Nihon Hoso Shuppan Kyokai.

Gibson, C. (n.d.). *Elvis on the Ed Sullivan show: The real story*. Retrieved from www.elvispresleymusic.com.au/pictures/1956-september-9-ed-sullivan-show.html

Goodwin, R., Palgi, Y., Lavenda, O., Hamama-Raz, Y., & Ben-Ezra, M. (2015). Association between media use, acute stress disorder and psychological distress. *Psychotherapy and Psychosomatics*, *84*, 253-254. doi:10.1159/000377706

Gregoire, C. (2015). *What constant exposure to negative news is doing to our mental health*. Retrieved from https://www.huffingtonpot.com/2015/02/19/violent-media -anxiety_n_6671732.html

Hagan, J. F. Jr. (2005). Psychosocial implications of disaster or terrorism on children: A guide for the pediatrician. *Pediatrics*, *116*(3), 787–795. doi:10.1542/peds.2005-1498 PMID:16140724

Hamilton, J. (2014). *Bingeing on bad news can fuel daily stress*. Retrieved from https://www.npr.org/sections/health-shots/2014/07/10/323355132/binging-on

Hampton, K. N., Lu, W., & Shin, I. (2016). Digital media and stress: The cost of caring 2.0. *Information Communication and Society*, *19*(9), 1267–1286. doi:10.1080/1369118X.2016.1186714

Hardin, M., & Greer, J. D. (2009). The influence of gender-role socialization, media use and sports participation on perceptions of gender-appropriate sports. *Journal of Sport Behavior*, *32*, 207–225.

Historica Canada. (n.d.). *Radio and television broadcasting*. Retrieved April 14, 2018 from, http://www.thecanadianencyclopedia.ca/en/article/radio-and-television-broadcasting/

Hopmann, D. N., & Stromback, J. (2010). *The rise of the media punditocracy? Journalists and media pundits in Danish election news 1994-2007*. Retrieved from journals.sagepub.com/doi/abs/10.1177/0163443710379666

Ince, J., Rojas, F., & Davis, C. A. (2017). The social media response to Black lives matter: How twitter users interact with Black lives matter through hashtag use. *Ethnic and Racial Studies*, *40*(11), 1814–1830. doi:10.1080/01419870.2017.1334931

Izaguirre, J. G. III. (2015). Prophets, gurus, and pundits: Rhetorical styles and public engagement. *The Quarterly Journal of Speech*, *101*(4), 673–677. doi:10.1080/00335630.2015.1128052

Jansen, H. J., & Kopp, R. (2005). Pundits, ideologues, and ranters: The British Columbia Election online. *Canadian Journal of Communication*, *30*(4). doi:10.22230/cjc.2005v30n4a1483

Johnson, R., Ross, D. B., Matteson, R., Henry, S., Link, M., Axler, D., . . . Grace, E. (2015). *A Forensic psychological assessment of terrorists: An anti-terrorism approach for radicalized westerners*. Fischler College of Education. Retrieved from http://nsuworks.nova.edu/fse_facarticles/244

Kira, I., Hammad, A., Lewandowski, L., Templin, T., Ramaswamy, V., Ozkan, B., & Mohanesh, J. (2007). The physical and mental status of Iraqi Refugees and its etiology. *Ethnicity & Disease*, *17*, 79–82. Retrieved from https://www.ethndis .org/priorsuparchives/ethn-17-02s3-79.pdf PMID:17985465

Lau, J. T., Lau, M., Kim, J. H., & Tsui, H. Y. (2006). Impacts of media coverage on the community stress level in Hong Kong after the tsunami on 26 December 2004. *Journal of Epidemiology and Community Health, 60*(8), 675–682. doi:10.1136/jech.2005.041897 PMID:16840756

Lee, S. T. (2004). Lying to tell the truth: Journalists and the social context of deception. *Mass Communication & Society, 7*(1), 97–120. doi:10.120715327825mcs0701_7

Lee, S. T. (2010). Truth telling as a journalistic imperative. In M. S. McGlone & M. L. Knapp (Eds.), *The interplay of truth and deception: New agendas in communication* (pp. 66–88). New York, NY: Routledge.

Letukas, L. (2012). *The ascent of punditry: Media and the news construction of cable news* (Doctoral dissertation). Available from ProQuest Dissertations and Theses database. (UMI No. 3526446)

Lewandowsky, S., Ecker, U. K. H., Seifert, C. M., Schwarz, N., & Cook, J. (2012). Misinformation and its correction: Continued influence and successful debiasing. *Psychological Science in the Public Interest, 13*(3), 106–131. doi:10.1177 /1529100612451018

Luskin, B. J. (2012). Defining and describing media psychology. *Psychology Today*. Retrieved from https://www.psychologytoday.com/us/blog/the-media-psychology-effect/201211/defining-and-describing-media-psychology

Mastro, D. (2015). Why the media's role in issues of race and ethnicity should be in the spotlight. *The Journal of Social Issues, 71*(1), 1–16. doi:10.1111/josi.12093

McQuail, D. (2010). *McQuail's Mass Communication Theory* (6th ed.). Thousand Oaks, CA: Sage.

Messer, C. M., & Bell, P. A. (2010). Mass media and governmental framing of riots. *Journal of Black Studies, 40*(5), 851–870. doi:10.1177/0021934708318607

Meyer, P. (1987). *Ethical journalism*. Lanham, MD: University Press of America.

Monfort, E., & Afzali, M. H. (2017). Traumatic stress symptoms after the November 13th 2015 terrorist attacks among young adults: The relation to media and emotion regulation. *Comprehensive Psychiatry*, *75*, 68–74. doi:10.1016/j.comppsych.2017.02.015 PMID:28324678

Open Society Institute. (2005). *Television across Europe: Regulation, policy and independence* (Volume 2). Retrieved from https://www. opensocietyfoundations .org/sites/default/files/voltwo_20051011_0.pdf

Powell, K. A. (2011). Framing Islam: An analysis of U.S. media coverage of terrorism since 9/11. *Communication Studies*, *62*(1), 90–112. doi:10.108 0/10510974.2011.533599

Prince, R. (2014). *How media have shaped our perception of race and crime. Journal-isms*. Gizmodo Media Group. Retrieved from https:// journalisms.theroot.com /how-media-have-shaped-our-perception-of-race-and-crime-1790885677

Prior, M. (2013). Media and political polarization. *Annual Review of Political Science*, *16*(1), 101–127. doi:10.1146/annurev-polisci-100711-135242

Ramasubramanian, S. (2011). The impact of stereotypical versus counterstereotypical media exemplars on racial attitudes, causal attributions, and support for affirmative action. *Communication Research*, *38*(4), 497–516. doi:10.1177/0093650210384854

Rutledge, P. (2008). The evolving definition of media psychology. *The Media Psychology Review*, *7*(2). Retrieved from mprcenetr.org/review/evolving-definition-media-psychology/?print=print

Saylor, C. F., Cowart, B. L., Lipovsky, J. A., Jackson, C., & Finch, A. Jr. (2003). Media exposure to September 11: Elementary school students' experiences and posttraumatic symptoms. *The American Behavioral Scientist*, *46*(12), 1622–1641. doi:10.1177/0002764203254619

Scheufele, D. A. (1991). Framing as a theory of media effects. *Journal of Communication*, *49*(1), 103–122. doi:10.1111/j.1460-2466.1999.tb02784.x

Schulten, K. (2015). Skills and strategies: Fake news vs. real news: Determining the reliability of sources. *The New York Times*. Retrieved from https://learning.blogs.nytimes.com/2015/10/02/skills-and-strategies-fake-news-vs-real-news-determining-the-reliability-of-sources/

Silver, R. C., Holman, E. A., Andersen, J. P., Poulin, M., McIntosh, D. N., & Gil-Rivas, V. (2013). Mental-and physical-health effects of acute exposure to media images of the September 11, 2001, attacks and the Iraq War. *Psychological Science*, *24*(9), 1623–1634. doi:10.1177/0956797612460406 PMID:23907546

Simons, G., & Strovsky, D. (2006). Censorship in contemporary Russian journalism in the age of the war against terrorism. *European Journal of Communication*, *21*(2), 189–211. doi:10.1177/0267323105064045

Statista. (2018). *News industry - statistics & facts*. Retrieved April 20, 2018 from, https://www.statista.com/topics/1640/news/

Takahashi, B. (2010). Framing and sources: A study of mass media coverage of climate change in Peru during V ALCUE. *Public Understanding of Science (Bristol, England)*, *20*(4), 543–557. doi:10.1177/0963662509356502 PMID:21936267

Valaskivi, K. (2007). *Mapping media and communication research*. Department of Communication: University of Helsinki. Retrieved from www.helsinki.fi/crc /Julkaisut/ReportJapan.pdf

von Seth, R. (2011). The language of the press in Soviet and post-Soviet Russia: Creation of the citizen role through newspaper discourse. *Journalism*, *13*(1), 53–70. doi:10.1177/1464884911400844

Walker, C., & Orttung, R. W. (2014). Breaking the news: The role of state-run media. *Journal of Democracy*, *25*(1), 71–85. doi:10.1353/jod.2014.0015

Weems, C. F., Scott, B. G., & Banks, D. M. (2012). Is TV traumatic for all youths? The role of preexisting posttraumatic-stress symptoms in the link between disaster coverage and stress. *Psychological Science, 23*(11), 1293-1297. doi:10.1177 /0956797612446952

Weitzer, R. (2015). American policing under fire: Misconduct and reform. *Social Science and Public Policy*, *52*, 475–480.

Welch, M., Price, E., & Yankey, N. (2004). Youth violence and race in the media: The emergence of "wilding" as an invention of the press. *Race, Gender, & Class*, *11*, 36–48.

Yeager, A. (2013). Watching media coverage of disasters linked to stress. *Science News*. Retrieved from https://www.sciencenews.org/blog/science-ticker/watching-media-coverage-disasters-linked-stress

Yeung, N. C. A., Yu, N. X., Xu, Z., Zhang, Q., Lau, J. T. F., Zhang, J., ... Lui, W. W. S. (2016). Media exposure related to the 2008 Sichuan earthquake predicted probable PTSD among Chinese adolescents in Kunming, China: A longitudinal study. *Psychological Trauma: Theory, Research, Practice, and Policy*, *10*(2), 253–262. doi:10.1037/tra0000121 PMID:27428553

Compilation of References

Abdullah, S., Matthews, M., Frank, E., Doherty, G., Gay, G., & Choudhury, T. (2016). Automatic detection of social rhythms in bipolar disorder. *Journal of the American Medical Informatics Association*, *23*(3), 538–543. doi:10.1093/jamia/ocv200 PMID:26977102

Abe, J., Zane, N., & Chun, K. (1994). Differential responses to trauma: Migration-related discriminants of post-traumatic stress disorder among Southeast Asian refugees. *Journal of Community Psychology*, *22*(2), 121–135. doi:10.1002/1520-6629(199404)22:2<121::AID-JCOP2290220208>3.0.CO;2-D

Ahmad, A. (2008). Posttraumatic stress among children in Kurdistan. *Acta Paediatrica (Oslo, Norway)*, *97*(7), 884–888. doi:10.1111/j.1651-2227.2008.00873.x PMID:18532935

Ahmad, A. (2014). Crisis intervention program for children and adolescents (CIPCA) to prevent posttraumatic psychopathology, preliminary report. *Duhok Medical Journal*, *8*(2), 1–11.

Ahmad, A., Sofi, M., Sundelin-Wahlsten, V., & Von Knorring, A.-L. (2000). Posttraumatic stress disorder in children after the military operation "Anfal" in Iraqi Kurdistan. *European Child & Adolescent Psychiatry*, *9*(4), 235–243. doi:10.1007007870070026 PMID:11202098

Ainamani, H. E., Elbert, T., Olema, D. K., & Hecker, T. (2017). PTSD symptom severity relates to cognitive and psycho-social dysfunctioning–a study with Congolese refugees in Uganda. *European Journal of Psychotraumatology*, *8*(1), 1283086. doi:10.1080/20008198.2017.1283086 PMID:28326164

Albert, P. R., Vahid-Ansari, F., & Luckhart, C. (2014). Serotonin-prefrontal cortical circuitry in anxiety and depression phenotypes: Pivotal role of pre- and post-synaptic 5-HT1A receptor expression. *Frontiers in Behavioral Neuroscience*, *8*, 199. doi:10.3389/fnbeh.2014.00199 PMID:24936175

Allais, M. (1953). Le comportement de l'homme rationnel devant le risque: Critique des postulats et axiomes de l'ecole Americaine. *Econometrica*, *21*(4), 503–546. doi:10.2307/1907921

American Academy of Otolaryngology — Head and Neck Surgery portal. (2018). *Cochlear Implants*. Retrieved from http://www.entnet.org/content/cochlearimplants

American Association of Orthodontics. (2012). *Glossary of Orthodontists*. AAO.

Andersen, P. (2007). *The Hippocampus Book*. London, UK: Oxford University Press.

Andersson, G., Cuijpers, P., Carlbring, P., Riper, H., & Hedman, E. (2014). Guided Internet-based vs. face-to-face cognitive behavior therapy for psychiatric and somatic disorders: A systematic review and meta-analysis. *World Psychiatry; Official Journal of the World Psychiatric Association (WPA)*, *13*(3), 288–295. doi:10.1002/wps.20151 PMID:25273302

Andersson, G., & Titov, N. (2014). Advantages and limitations of Internet-based interventions for common mental disorders. *World Psychiatry; Official Journal of the World Psychiatric Association (WPA)*, *13*(1), 4–11. doi:10.1002/wps.20083 PMID:24497236

Angle, E. H. (1913). *Okklusions Anomalien der Zahne*. Veri.H.

Angoa-Perez, M., Kane, M. J., Briggs, D. I., Herrera-Mundo, N., Sykes, C. E., Francescutti, D. M., & Kuhn, D. M. (2014). Mice genetically depleted of brain serotonin do not display a depression-like behavioral phenotype. *ACS Chemical Neuroscience*, *5*(10), 908–919. doi:10.1021/cn500096g PMID:25089765

Antidepressant Medications for Children and Adolescents: Information for Parents and Caregivers. (n.d.). Retrieved 1 April 2018 from https://www.nimh.nih.gov/health/topics/child-and-adolescent-mental-health/antidepressant-medic ations-for-children-and-adolescents-information-for-parents-and-caregivers.shtml

Arean, P. A., Hallgren, K. A., Jordan, J. T., Gazzaley, A., Atkins, D. C., Heagerty, P. J., & Anguera, J. A. (2016). The use and effectiveness of mobile apps for depression: Results from a fully remote clinical trial. *Journal of Medical Internet Research, 18*(12), e330. doi:10.2196/jmir.6482 PMID:27998876

Ari, A. B., Peri, T., Margalit, D., Galili-Weisstub, E., Udassin, R., & Benarroch, F. (2017). Surgical procedures and pediatric medical traumatic stress (PMTS) syndrome: Assessment and future directions. *Journal of Pediatric Surgery*. PMID:29129330

Attanayake, V., McKay, R., Joffres, M., Singh, S., Burkle, F. Jr, & Mills, E. (2009). Prevalence of mental disorders among children exposed to war: A systematic review of 7,920 children. *Medicine, Conflict, and Survival, 25*(1), 4–19. doi:10.1080/13623690802568913 PMID:19413154

Attkisson, C., Cook, J., Karno, M., Lehman, A., McGlashan, T. H., Meltzer, H. Y., ... Hohmann, A. A. (1992). Clinical services research. *Schizophrenia Bulletin, 18*(4), 561–626. doi:10.1093chbul/18.4.561 PMID:1439613

Baker, D. H., Quittner, A. L., Fink, N. E., Eisenberg, L. S., Tobey, E. A., & Niparko, J. K. (2009). Predicting behavior problems in deaf and hearing children: The influences of language, attention, and parent-child communication. *Development and Psychopathology, 21*(2), 373–392. doi:10.1017/S0954579409000212 PMID:19338689

Bakker, D., Kazantzis, N., Rickwood, D., & Rickard, N. (2016). Mental health smartphone apps: Review and evidence-based recommendations for future developments. *JMIR Mental Health, 3*(1). Retrieved 30 March 2018 from https://www.ncbi.nlm.nih.gov/pmc/articles/PMC4795320/

Banjo, O. O. (2013). For us only? Examining the effect of viewing context on Black audiences' perceived influence of Black entertainment. *Race and Social Problems*, *5*(4), 309–322. doi:10.100712552-013-9106-x

Barclay, L. (2005). *What will we do when the pundits are all gone?* Retrieved from https://search-proquest-com.ezproxylocal.library.nova.edu/central/doc view/438893939/23CE7DA458FE417BPQ/1?accountid=6579

Barrera, M., Calderón, L., & Bell, V. (2013). The cognitive impact of sexual abuse and PTSD in children: A neuropsychological study. *Journal of Child Sexual Abuse*, *22*(6), 625–638. doi:10.1080/10538712.2013.811141 PMID:23924174

Batra, S., Baker, R. A., Wang, T., Forma, F., DiBiasi, F., & Peters-Strickland, T. (2017). Digital health technology for use in patients with serious mental illness: A systematic review of the literature. *Medical Devices (Auckland, N.Z.)*, *10*, 237–251. doi:10.2147/MDER.S144158 PMID:29042823

Bean, T. M., Eurelings-Bontekoe, E., & Spinhoven, P. (2007). Course and predictors of mental health of unaccompanied refugee minors in the Netherlands: One year follow-up. *Social Science & Medicine*, *64*(6), 1204–1215. doi:10.1016/j.socscimed.2006.11.010 PMID:17188787

Beckham, J. C., Vrana, S. R., Barefoot, J. C., Feldman, M. E., Fairbank, J., & Moore, S. D. (2002). Magnitude and duration of cardiovascular responses to anger in Vietnam veterans with and without posttraumatic stress disorder. *Journal of Consulting and Clinical Psychology*, *70*(1), 228–234. doi:10.1037/0022-006X.70.1.228 PMID:11860049

Beer, J., Pisoni, D. B., & Kronenberger, W. (2009). Executive function in children with cochlear implants: The role of organizational integrative processes. *Volta Voices*, *16*, 18–23. PMID:23687425

Beers, S. R., & De Bellis, M. D. (2002). Neuropsychological function in children with maltreatment-related posttraumatic stress disorder. *The American Journal of Psychiatry*, *159*(3), 483–486. doi:10.1176/appi.ajp.159.3.483 PMID:11870018

Beitchman, J. H., Wilson, B., Atkinson, L., Young, A., & Adalf, E. (2001). Fourteen year follow up of speech impaired and control children: Psychiatric outcome. *Journal of the American Academy of Child and Adolescent Psychiatry, 40*(1), 75–82. doi:10.1097/00004583-200101000-00019 PMID:11195567

Bench, J., Kowal, A., & Bamford, J. (1979). The BKB (Bamford-Kowal-Bench) sentence lists for partially-hearing children. *British Journal of Audiology, 13*(3), 108–112. doi:10.3109/03005367909078884 PMID:486816

Bennett, T. (1982). *Culture, society and the media* (1st ed.). Methuen & Co Ltd.

Ben-Zeev, D., Schueller, S. M., Begale, M., Duffecy, J., Kane, J. M., & Mohr, D. C. (2015). Strategies for mHealth research: Lessons from 3 mobile intervention studies. *Administration and Policy in Mental Health, 42*(2), 157–167. doi:10.100710488-014-0556-2 PMID:24824311

Berlim, M. T., McGirr, A., Van den Eynde, F., Fleck, M. P., & Giacobbe, P. (2014). Effectiveness and acceptability of deep brain stimulation (DBS) of the subgenual cingulate cortex for treatment-resistant depression: A systematic review and exploratory meta-analysis. *Journal of Affective Disorders, 159*, 31–38. doi:10.1016/j.jad.2014.02.016 PMID:24679386

Bersani, F. S., Minichino, A., Fojanesi, M., Gallo, M., Maglio, G., Valeriani, G., ... Fitzgerald, P. B. (2014). Cingulate Cortex in Schizophrenia: Its relation with negative symptoms and psychotic onset. A review study. *European Review for Medical and Pharmacological Sciences, 18*(22), 3354–3367. PMID:25491609

Besser, M. J., Ganor, Y., & Levite, M. (2005). Dopamine by itself activates either D2, D3 or D1/D5 dopaminergic receptors in normal human T-cells and triggers the selective secretion of either IL-10, TNFalpha or both. *Journal of Neuroimmunology, 169*(1-2), 161–171. doi:10.1016/j.jneuroim.2005.07.013 PMID:16150496

Bess, F. H. (2000). The role of generic health-related quality of life measures in establishing audiological rehabilitation outcomes. *Ear and Hearing, 21*(Supplement), 74S–79S. doi:10.1097/00003446-200008001-00009 PMID:10981596

Betancourt, T. S., Abdi, S., Ito, B. S., Lilienthal, G. M., Agalab, N., & Ellis, H. (2015). We left one war and came to another: Resource loss, acculturative stress, and caregiver–child relationships in Somali refugee families. *Cultural Diversity & Ethnic Minority Psychology, 21*(1), 114–125. doi:10.1037/a0037538 PMID:25090142

Betancourt, T. S., Speelman, L., Onyango, G., & Bolton, P. (2009). A qualitative study of mental health problems among children displaced by war in northern Uganda. *Transcultural Psychiatry, 46*(2), 238–256. doi:10.1177/1363461509105815 PMID:19541749

Bhatia, S. K., & Bhatia, S. C. (2007). Childhood and adolescent depression. *American Family Physician, 75*(1), 73–80. Retrieved from http://citeseerx.ist.psu.edu/viewdoc/download?doi=10.1.1.629.8098&rep=rep1&type=pdf PMID:17225707

Biagianti, B., Hidalgo-Mazzei, D., & Meyer, N. (2017). Developing digital interventions for people living with serious mental illness: Perspectives from three mHealth studies. *Evidence-Based Mental Health, 20*(4), 98–101. doi:10.1136/eb-2017-102765 PMID:29025862

Bishara ES Textbook of Orthodontics. (2001). WB Saunders Company.

Blackwell, S. E., Browning, M., Mathews, A., Pictet, A., Welch, J., Davies, J., ... Holmes, E. A. (2015). Positive Imagery-Based Cognitive Bias Modification as a Web-Based Treatment Tool for Depressed Adults: A Randomized Controlled Trial. *Clinical Psychological Science, 3*(1), 91–111. doi:10.1177/2167702614560746 PMID:25984421

Blanchard, E., & Hickling, E. (1997). *After the crash: assessment and treatment of motor vehicle accident survivors*. Washington, DC: APA.

Blanchfield, B. B., Feldman, J. J., Dunbar, J. L., & Gardner, E. N. (2001). The severely to profoundly hearing-impaired population in the United States: Prevalence estimates and demographics. *Journal of the American Academy of Audiology, 12*, 183–189. PMID:11332518

Bohs, E. S., Ladd, G. W., & Herald, S. L. (2006). Peer exclusion and victimization: Processes that mediate the relation between peer group rejection and children's classroom engagement and achievement? *Journal of Educational Psychology, 98*(1), 1–13. doi:10.1037/0022-0663.98.1.1

Bolton, D., O'Ryan, D., Udwin, O., Boyle, S., & Yule, W. (2000). The long-term psychological effects of a disaster experienced in adolescence: II: General psychopathology. *Journal of Child Psychology and Psychiatry, and Allied Disciplines*, *41*(4), 513–523. doi:10.1111/1469-7610.00636 PMID:10836681

Borner, K., Contractor, N., Falk-Krzesinski, H. J., Fiore, S. M., Hall, K. L., Keyton, J., ... Uzzi, B. (2010). A multi-level systems perspective for the science of team science. *Science Translational Medicine*, *2*(49), 49cm24. doi:10.1126citranslmed.3001399 PMID:20844283

Bowe, F. G., McMahon, B. T., Chang, T., & Louvi, J. (2005). Workplace discrimination, deafness and learning impairment the national, EEEC ADA research project. *Work (Reading, Mass.)*, *25*, 19–25. PMID:16006672

Bradley, A. J., & Lenox-Smith, A. J. (2013). Does adding noradrenaline reuptake inhibition to selective serotonin reuptake inhibition improve efficacy in patients with depression? A systematic review of meta-analyses and large randomised pragmatic trials. *Journal of Psychopharmacology (Oxford, England)*, *27*(8), 740–758. doi:10.1177/0269881113494937 PMID:23832963

Branche, C., Oyebite, K., Hyder, A., Ozanne-Smith, J., Bartolomeos, K., & Rivara, F. (2008). *World report on child injury prevention*. World Health Organization.

Bremner, J. D. (2016). Posttraumatic stress disorder from neurobiology to treatment. Wiley Blackwell.

Breslau, N. (2012). *Epidemiology of posttraumatic stress disorder in adults*. In *The Oxford Handbook of Traumatic Stress Disorders* (pp. 84–97). New York: Oxford University Press. doi:10.1093/oxfordhb/9780195399066.013.0007

Bressan, R. A., & Crippa, J. A. (2005). The role of dopamine in reward and pleasure behaviour--review of data from preclinical research. *Acta Psychiatrica Scandinavica. Supplementum*, *111*(427), 14–21. doi:10.1111/j.1600-0447.2005.00540.x PMID:15877719

Broberg, A. G., Dyregrov, A., & Lilled, L. (2005). The Göteborg discotheque fire: Posttraumatic stress, and school adjustment as reported by the primary victims 18 months later. *Journal of Child Psychology and Psychiatry, and Allied Disciplines*, *46*(12), 1279–1286. doi:10.1111/j.1469-7610.2005.01439.x PMID:16313428

Bronstein, I., & Montgomery, P. (2011). Psychological distress in refugee children: A systematic review. *Clinical Child and Family Psychology Review*, *14*(1), 44–56. doi:10.100710567-010-0081-0 PMID:21181268

Bullinger, M., Anderson, R., Cella, D., & Aaronson, N. (1993). Developing and evaluating cross- cultural instruments from minimum requirements to optimal models. *Quality of Life Research: An International Journal of Quality of Life Aspects of Treatment, Care and Rehabilitation*, *2*(6), 451–459. doi:10.1007/BF00422219 PMID:8161979

Burkhauser, R. V., & Heutenville, A. J. (2010). Employment among working-age people with disabilities: What current data can tell us. In R. Parker & E. M. Szymanski (Eds.), *Work and disability: Contexts, issues, and strategies for enhancing employment outcomes for people with disabilities* (3rd ed.; pp. 49–86). Austin, TX: Pro-Ed.

Busso, D. S., McLaughlin, K. A., & Sheridan, M. A. (2014). Media exposure and sympathetic nervous system reactivity predict PTSD symptoms after the Boston Marathon bombings. *Depression and Anxiety*, *31*(7), 551–558. doi:10.1002/da.22282 PMID:24995832

Byrne, D., & Noble, W. (1998). Optimising sound localisation with hearing aids. *Trends in Amplification*, *3*(2), 51–73. doi:10.1177/108471389800300202 PMID:25425879

Callanan, V. J. (2012). Media consumption, perceptions of crime, risk and fear of crime: Examining race/ethnic differences. *Sociological Perspectives*, *55*(1), 93–115. doi:10.1525op.2012.55.1.93

Callanan, V. J., & Rosenberger, J. S. (2011). Media and public perceptions of the police: Examining the impact of race and personal experience. *Policing and Society*, *21*(2), 167–189. doi:10.1080/10439463.2010.540655

Cannon, R. C., Wheal, H. V., & Turner, D. A. (1999). Dendrites of classes of hippocampal neurons differ in structural complexity and branching patterns. *The Journal of Comparative Neurology*, *413*(4), 619–633. doi:10.1002/(SICI)1096-9861(19991101)413:4<619::AID-CNE10>3.0.CO;2-B PMID:10495447

Cannon, W. B. (1987). The James-Lange theory of emotions: A critical examination and an alternative theory. By Walter B. Cannon, 1927. *The American Journal of Psychology*, *100*(3-4), 567–586. doi:10.2307/1422695 PMID:3322057

Carr, H. J., & Higginson, I. J. (2001). Are quality of life measures patient centered? *BMJ (Clinical Research Ed.)*.

Catani, C., Schauer, E., Elbert, T., Missmahl, I., Bette, J. P., & Neuner, F. (2009). War trauma, child labor, and family violence: Life adversities and PTSD in a sample of school children in Kabul. *Journal of Traumatic Stress: Official Publication ofThe International Societyfor Traumatic Stress Studies*, *22*(3), 163–171. doi:10.1002/jts.20415 PMID:19462436

Caves, C. M., Fuchs, C. A., & Schack, R. (2002). Quantum probabilities as Bayesian probabilities. *Physical Review A.*, *65*(2), 022305. doi:10.1103/PhysRevA.65.022305

Ceri, V., Özlü-Erkilic, Z., Özer, Ü., Yalcin, M., Popow, C., & Akkaya-Kalayci, T. (2016). Psychiatric symptoms and disorders among Yazidi children and adolescents immediately after forced migration following ISIS attacks. *Neuropsychiatrie, 30*(3), 145-50.

Ceri, V., & Ahmad, A. (2018). Exploring Psychological Vaccination for Potentially Traumatized Children. *Journal of Psychology and Clinical Psychiatry*, *9*(1), 143–147. doi:10.15406/jpcpy.2018.09.00512

Çeri, V., Beşer, C., Fiş, N. P., & Arman, A. (2018). Findings From A Specialized Child Psychiatry Unit For Care of Refugee Children in Istanbul. *J Clin Psy*, *21*(2), 113–121. doi:10.5505/kpd.2018.57070

Ceri, V., Özlü-Erkilic, Z., Özer, Ü., Kadak, T., Winkler, D., Dogangün, B., & … . (2017). Mental health problems of second generation children and adolescents with migration background. *International Journal of Psychiatry in Clinical Practice*, 1–6. PMID:28498088

Chandrashekar, P. (2018). Do mental health mobile apps work: Evidence and recommendations for designing high-efficacy mental health mobile apps. *mHealth*, *4*, 6. doi:10.21037/mhealth.2018.03.02 PMID:29682510

Chan, J. (2017). Racial identity in online spaces: Social media's impact on students of color. *Journal of Student Affairs Research and Practice*, *54*(2), 163–174. doi:10.1080/19496591.2017.1284672

Chan, S., Torous, J., Hinton, L., & Yellowlees, P. (2015). Towards a Framework for Evaluating Mobile Mental Health Apps. *Telemedicine Journal and e-Health*, *21*(12), 1038–1041. doi:10.1089/tmj.2015.0002 PMID:26171663

Chemtob, C. M., Nomura, Y., & Abramovitz, R. A. (2008). Impact of conjoined exposure to the World Trade Center attacks and to other traumatic events on the behavioral problems of preschool children. *Archives of Pediatrics & Adolescent Medicine*, *162*(2), 126–133. doi:10.1001/archpediatrics.2007.36 PMID:18250236

Chwalisz, K., & Vaux, A. (2000). Psychology, Social support and adjustment to disability. In Handbook of rehabilitation psychology. American Psychological Association.

Cipriani, A., Furukawa, T. A., Salanti, G., Chaimani, A., Atkinson, L. Z., Ogawa, Y., . . . Geddes, J. R. (2018). Comparative efficacy and acceptability of 21 antidepressant drugs for the acute treatment of adults with major depressive disorder: A systematic review and network meta-analysis. *The Lancet*. Retrieved 1 April 2018 from http://www.thelancet.com/pdfs/journals/lancet/PIIS0140-6736(17)32802-7.pdf

Cipriani, A. (2003). Review: Selective serotonin reuptake inhibitors as effective as tricyclic antidepressants for major depression, and may have fewer adverse effects. *Evidence-Based Mental Health*, *6*(4), 117. doi:10.1136/ebmh.6.4.117 PMID:14585790

Clarke-Stewart, K. A., Allhusen, V. D., McDowell, D. J., Thelen, L., & Call, J. D. (2003). Identifying psychological problems in young children: How do mothers compare with child psychologists? *Journal of Applied Developmental Psychology*, *23*(6), 589–624. doi:10.1016/S0193-3973(03)00006-6

Claster, S. M. (2012). *Pundit wars: An investigation into the pragmatics of news talk programs* (Doctoral dissertation). Available from ProQuest Dissertations and Theses database. (UMI No. 3484262)

Cohen, J. A. (2010). Practice parameter for the assessment and treatment of children and adolescents with posttraumatic stress disorder. *Journal of the American Academy of Child and Adolescent Psychiatry*, *49*(4), 414–430. PMID:20410735

Cohen, J. A., Deblinger, E., Mannarino, A. P., & Steer, R. A. (2004). A multisite, randomized controlled trial for children with sexual abuse–related PTSD symptoms. *Journal of the American Academy of Child and Adolescent Psychiatry*, *43*(4), 393–402. doi:10.1097/00004583-200404000-00005 PMID:15187799

Collins, R. L. (2011). Content analysis of gender roles in media: Where are we now and where should we go? *Sex Roles*, *64*(3-4), 290–298. doi:10.100711199-010-9929-5

Courtois, C. A., & Gold, S. N. (2009). The need for inclusion of psychological trauma in the professional curriculum: A call to action. *Psychological Trauma: Theory, Research, Practice, and Policy*, *1*(1), 3–23. doi:10.1037/a0015224

Cox, C. M., Kenardy, J. A., & Hendrikz, J. K. (2008). A meta-analysis of risk factors that predict psychopathology following accidental trauma. *Journal for Specialists in Pediatric Nursing*, *13*(2), 98–110. doi:10.1111/j.1744-6155.2008.00141.x PMID:18366377

Craft, L. L., & Perna, F. M. (2004). The benefits of exercise for the clinically depressed. *Primary Care Companion to the Journal of Clinical Psychiatry*, *6*(3), 104–111. doi:10.4088/PCC.v06n0301 PMID:15361924

Craske, M. G., Rose, R. D., Lang, A., Welch, S. S., Campbell-Sills, L., Sullivan, G., ... Roy-Byrne, P. P. (2009). Computer-assisted delivery of cognitive behavioral therapy for anxiety disorders in primary-care settings. *Depression and Anxiety*, *26*(3), 235–242. doi:10.1002/da.20542 PMID:19212970

Crichlow, V. J., & Fulcher, C. (2017). Black men down: An assessment of experts' quotes on deadly encounters with the police. *Race and Social Problems*, *9*(3), 171–180. doi:10.100712552-017-9197-x

Çuhadaroğlu Çetin, F., Coşkun, A., & İşeri, E. (2008). *Çocuk ve ergen psikiyatrisi temel kitabı. 1*. Ankara: Baskı Hekimler Yayın Birliği.

Dai, W., Chen, L., Lai, Z., Li, Y., Wang, J., & Liu, A. (2016). The incidence of post-traumatic stress disorder among survivors after earthquakes: A systematic review and meta-analysis. *BMC Psychiatry*, *16*(1), 188. doi:10.118612888-016-0891-9 PMID:27267874

Dascaloglannakis, J. (2000). *Glossary of Orthodontics Terms*. Ouintessence Publishing Co, Inc.

Davis, A. (1997). Epidemiology of hearing impairment. In A. G. Kerr & D. Stephens (Eds.), *Scott Brownis Otolaryngology* (6th ed.; Vol. 4, pp. 18–19). Oxford, UK: Butterworth Heiremann.

De Beilis, M. D., & Putnam, F. W. (1994). The psychobiology of childhood maltreatment. *Child and Adolescent Psychiatric Clinics of North America*, *3*(4), 663–678. doi:10.1016/S1056-4993(18)30463-2

De Bellis, M. D., Hooper, S. R., Spratt, E. G., & Woolley, D. P. (2009). Neuropsychological findings in childhood neglect and their relationships to pediatric PTSD. *Journal of the International Neuropsychological Society*, *15*(6), 868–878. doi:10.1017/S1355617709990464 PMID:19703321

De Bellis, M. D., Keshavan, M. S., Clark, D. B., Casey, B., Giedd, J. N., Boring, A. M., ... Ryan, N. D. (1999). Developmental traumatology part II: Brain development. *Biological Psychiatry*, *45*(10), 1271–1284. doi:10.1016/S0006-3223(99)00045-1 PMID:10349033

De Bellis, M. D., Woolley, D. P., & Hooper, S. R. (2013). Neuropsychological findings in pediatric maltreatment: Relationship of PTSD, dissociative symptoms, and abuse/neglect indices to neurocognitive outcomes. *Child Maltreatment*, *18*(3), 171–183. doi:10.1177/1077559513497420 PMID:23886642

De Jong, J. T., Komproe, I. H., Van Ommeren, M., El Masri, M., Araya, M., & Khaled, N. (2001). Lifetime events and posttraumatic stress disorder in 4 postconflict settings. *Journal of the American Medical Association*, *286*(5), 555–562. doi:10.1001/jama.286.5.555 PMID:11476657

Deblinger, E., Stauffer, L. B., & Steer, R. A. (2001). Comparative efficacies of supportive and cognitive behavioral group therapies for young children who have been sexually abused and their nonoffending mothers. *Child Maltreatment*, *6*(4), 332–343. doi:10.1177/1077559501006004006 PMID:11675816

Demyttenaere, K., & Jaspers, L. (2008). Review: Bupropion and SSRI-induced side effects. *Journal of Psychopharmacology (Oxford, England)*, *22*(7), 792–804. doi:10.1177/0269881107083798 PMID:18308785

Depression, T. (n.d.). *The Pros and Cons of Medication*. Retrieved 1 April 2018 from https://www.psycom.net/depression.central.teens.medication.html

DePrince, A. P., Weinzierl, K. M., & Combs, M. D. (2009). Executive function performance and trauma exposure in a community sample of children. *Child Abuse & Neglect*, *33*(6), 353–361. doi:10.1016/j.chiabu.2008.08.002 PMID:19477515

Dhillon, S., Yang, L. P., & Curran, M. P. (2008). Bupropion: A review of its use in the management of major depressive disorder. *Drugs*, *68*(5), 653–689. doi:10.2165/00003495-200868050-00011 PMID:18370448

Donker, T., Bennett, K., Bennett, A., Mackinnon, A., van Straten, A., Cuijpers, P., ... Griffiths, K. M. (2013). Internet-delivered interpersonal psychotherapy versus internet-delivered cognitive behavioral therapy for adults with depressive symptoms: Randomized controlled noninferiority trial. *Journal of Medical Internet Research*, *15*(5), e82. doi:10.2196/jmir.2307 PMID:23669884

Donker, T., Petrie, K., Proudfoot, J., Clarke, J., Birch, M., & Christensen, H. (2013). Smartphones for smarter delivery of mental health programs: A systematic review. *Journal of Medical Internet Research*, *15*(11), e247. doi:10.2196/jmir.2791 PMID:24240579

Donnelly, C. L., & Amaya-Jackson, L. (2002). Post-traumatic stress disorder in children and adolescents. *Paediatric Drugs*, *4*(3), 159–170. doi:10.2165/00128072-200204030-00003 PMID:11909008

Donnelly, C., Amaya-Jackson, L., & March, J. (1999). Psychopharmacology of pediatric posttraumatic stress disorder. *Journal of Child and Adolescent Psychopharmacology*, *9*(3), 203–220. doi:10.1089/cap.1999.9.203 PMID:10521013

Dopheide, J. A. (2006). Recognizing and treating depression in children and adolescents. *American Journal of Health-System Pharmacy*, *63*(3), 233–243. doi:10.2146/ajhp050264 PMID:16434782

Dows, W. R., & Harrison, L. (1998). Childhood maltreatment and the risk of substance problems in later life. *Health & Social Care in the Community*, *6*(1), 35–46. doi:10.1046/j.1365-2524.1998.00097.x PMID:11560575

Drevets, W. C., Thase, M. E., Moses-Kolko, E. L., Price, J., Frank, E., Kupfer, D. J., & Mathis, C. (2007). Serotonin-1A receptor imaging in recurrent depression: Replication and literature review. *Nuclear Medicine and Biology*, *34*(7), 865–877. doi:10.1016/j.nucmedbio.2007.06.008 PMID:17921037

DSM-5®. (2013). *Diagnostic and Statistical Manual of Mental Disorders (DSM-5®)*. American Psychiatric Publication.

Du Feu, M., & Fergusson, K. (2003). Sensory impairment and mental health. *Advances in Psychiatric Treatment*, *9*(02), 95–103. doi:10.1192/apt.9.2.95

Duarte, C. S., Wu, P., Cheung, A., Mandell, D. J., Fan, B., Wicks, J., ... Hoven, C. W. (2011). Media use by children and adolescents from New York City 6 months after the WTC attack. *Journal of Traumatic Stress*, *24*(5), 553–556. doi:10.1002/jts.20687 PMID:21882251

Dubicka, B., & Brent, D. (2017). Editorial: Pharmacotherapy and adolescent depression - an important treatment option. *Child and Adolescent Mental Health*, *22*(2), 59–60. doi:10.1111/camh.12223

Dubner, A., & Motta, R. (1999). Sexually and physically abused foster care children and posttraumatic stress disorder. *Journal of Consulting and Clinical Psychology*, *67*(3), 367–373. doi:10.1037/0022-006X.67.3.367 PMID:10369057

Dyregrov, A., & Yule, W. (2006). A review of PTSD in children. *Child and Adolescent Mental Health*, *11*(4), 176–184. doi:10.1111/j.1475-3588.2005.00384.x

Dyson, F. (2004). Infinite in All Directions: Gifford Lectures Given at Aberdeen, Scotland April--November 1985. New York: Perennial.

Eide, A. H., & Roysamb, E. (2002). The relationship between level of disability, psychological problems, social activity and social networks. *Rehabilitation Psychology*, *47*(2), 165–183. doi:10.1037/0090-5550.47.2.165

Eisend, M. (2010). A meta-analysis of gender roles in advertising. *Journal of the Academy of Marketing Science*, *38*(4), 418–440. doi:10.100711747-009-0181-x

Elliot, D. (1989). Journalistic deception. In P. Y. Windt, P. C. Appleby, M. P. Battin, L. P. Francis, & B. M. Landesman (Eds.), *Ethical issues in the professions* (pp. 144–146). Englewood Cliffs, NJ: Prentice Hall.

Elliot, D., & Culver, C. (1992). Defining and analyzing journalistic deception. *Journal of Mass Media Ethics*, *7*(2), 69–84. doi:10.120715327728jmme0702_1

Ellsberg, D. (1961). Risk, ambiguity, and the Savage axioms. *The Quarterly Journal of Economics*, *75*(4), 643–669. doi:10.2307/1884324

Elwan, A. (1999). *Poverty and Disability: A Survey of the Literature*. Washington, DC: World Bank.

Fairbrother, G., Stuber, J., Galea, S., Fleischman, A. R., & Pfefferbaum, B. (2003). Posttraumatic stress reactions in New York City children after the September 11, 2001, terrorist attacks. *Ambulatory Pediatrics*, *3*(6), 304–311. doi:10.1367/1539-4409(2003)003<0304:PSRINY>2.0.CO;2 PMID:14616045

Fairburn, C. G., & Patel, V. (2017). The impact of digital technology on psychological treatments and their dissemination. *Behaviour Research and Therapy*, *88*, 19–25. doi:10.1016/j.brat.2016.08.012 PMID:28110672

Fareri, D. S., & Tottenham, N. (2016). Effects of early life stress on amygdala and striatal development. *Developmental Cognitive Neuroscience*, *19*, 233–247. doi:10.1016/j.dcn.2016.04.005 PMID:27174149

Fazel, M., & Betancourt, T. S. (2017). *Preventive mental health interventions for refugee children and adolescents in high-income settings*. The Lancet Child & Adolescent Health.

Fazel, M., Wheeler, J., & Danesh, J. (2005). Prevalence of serious mental disorder in 7000 refugees resettled in western countries: A systematic review. *Lancet*, *365*(9467), 1309–1314. doi:10.1016/S0140-6736(05)61027-6 PMID:15823380

Feldman, R., & Vengrober, A. (2011). Posttraumatic stress disorder in infants and young children exposed to war-related trauma. *Journal of the American Academy of Child and Adolescent Psychiatry*, *50*(7), 645–658. doi:10.1016/j.jaac.2011.03.001 PMID:21703492

Finkelhor, D. (1994). The international epidemiology of child sexual abuse. *Child Abuse & Neglect, 18*(5), 409–417. doi:10.1016/0145-2134(94)90026-4 PMID:8032971

Finkelhor, D., Hotaling, G., Lewis, I. A., & Smith, C. (1990). Sexual abuse in a national survey of adult men and women: Prevalence, characteristics, and risk factors. *Child Abuse & Neglect, 14*(1), 19–28. doi:10.1016/0145-2134(90)90077-7 PMID:2310970

Firth, J., & Torous, J. (2015). Smartphone Apps for Schizophrenia: A Systematic Review. *JMIR mHealth and uHealth, 3*(4), e102. doi:10.2196/mhealth.4930 PMID:26546039

Firth, J., Torous, J., Nicholas, J., Carney, R., Pratap, A., Rosenbaum, S., & Sarris, J. (2017). The efficacy of smartphone-based mental health interventions for depressive symptoms: A meta-analysis of randomized controlled trials. *World Psychiatry; Official Journal of the World Psychiatric Association (WPA), 16*(3), 287–298. doi:10.1002/wps.20472 PMID:28941113

Fletcher, K. E. (1996). Childhood posttraumatic stress disorder. *Child Psychopathology*, 242-76.

Fletcher, A., Gore, S., Jones, D., Fitzpatrick, R., Spiegelhalter, D., & Cox, D. (1992). Quality of life measures in health care: Design, analysis and interpretation. *BMJ (Clinical Research Ed.), 305*(6862), 1145–1148. doi:10.1136/bmj.305.6862.1145 PMID:1463954

Ford, T., Goodman, R., & Meltzer, H. (2003). The British child and adolescent mental health survey 1999: The prevalence of DSM-IV disorders. *Journal of the American Academy of Child and Adolescent Psychiatry, 42*(10), 1203–1211. doi:10.1097/00004583-200310000-00011 PMID:14560170

Forman-Hoffman, V., Bose, J., Batts, K., Glasheen, C., Hirsch, E., & Karg, R. (2012). *Correlates of lifetime exposure to one or more potentially traumatic events and subsequent posttraumatic stress among adults in the United States: results from the Mental Health Surveillance Study, 2008-2012*. Academic Press.

Fortuna, K. L., DiMilia, P. R., Lohman, M. C., Bruce, M. L., Zubritsky, C. D., Halaby, M. R., ... Bartels, S. J. (2018). Feasibility, Acceptability, and Preliminary Effectiveness of a Peer-Delivered and Technology Supported Self-Management Intervention for Older Adults with Serious Mental Illness. *The Psychiatric Quarterly*, *89*(2), 293–305. doi:10.100711126-017-9534-7 PMID:28948424

Foster, S., & Macleod, J. (2003). Deaf people at work: Assessment of communication among deaf and hearing persons in work settings. *International Journal of Audiology*, *42*(sup1), S128–S139. doi:10.3109/14992020309074634 PMID:12918620

Free, C., Knight, R., Robertson, S., Whittaker, R., Edwards, P., Zhou, W., ... Roberts, I. (2011). Smoking cessation support delivered via mobile phone text messaging (txt2stop): A single-blind, randomised trial. *Lancet*, *378*(9785), 49–55. doi:10.1016/S0140-6736(11)60701-0 PMID:21722952

Freeman, D., Bradley, J., Antley, A., Bourke, E., DeWeever, N., Evans, N., ... Clark, D. M. (2016). Virtual reality in the treatment of persecutory delusions: Randomised controlled experimental study testing how to reduce delusional conviction. *The British Journal of Psychiatry*, *209*(1), 62–67. doi:10.1192/bjp.bp.115.176438 PMID:27151071

Freeman, R. D., Malkin, S. F., & Hastings, J. O. (1975). Psychosocial problems of deaf children and their families: A comparative study. *American Annals of the Deaf*, *120*, 391–405. PMID:1163401

Fujitake, A. (2005). *Nihon no masumedia* (2nd ed.). Tokyo, Japan: Nihon Hoso Shuppan Kyokai.

Galea, S., Nandi, A., & Vlahov, D. (2005). The epidemiology of post-traumatic stress disorder after disasters. *Epidemiologic Reviews*, *27*(1), 78–91. doi:10.1093/epirev/mxi003 PMID:15958429

Gekker, M., Coutinho, E., Berger, W., Luz, M., Araújo, A., Pagotto, L., ... Mendlowicz, M. V. (2018). Early scars are forever: Childhood abuse in patients with adult-onset PTSD is associated with increased prevalence and severity of psychiatric comorbidity. *Psychiatry Research*, *267*, 1–6. doi:10.1016/j.psychres.2018.05.042 PMID:29879599

Gibson, C. (n.d.). *Elvis on the Ed Sullivan show: The real story*. Retrieved from www.elvispresleymusic.com.au/pictures/1956-september-9-ed-sullivan-show.html

Gillham, J. E., Reivich, K. J., Jaycox, L. H., & Seligman, M. E. (1995). Prevention of depressive symptoms in schoolchildren: Two-year follow-up. *Psychological Science*, *6*(6), 343–351. doi:10.1111/j.1467-9280.1995.tb00524.x

Gillies, D., Maiocchi, L., Bhandari, A. P., Taylor, F., Gray, C., & O'Brien, L. (2016). Psychological therapies for children and adolescents exposed to trauma. *The Cochrane Library*. PMID:27726123

Gil, T., Calev, A., Greenberg, D., Kugelmass, S., & Lerer, B. (1990). Cognitive functioning in post-traumatic stress disorder. *Journal of Traumatic Stress*, *3*(1), 29–45. doi:10.1002/jts.2490030104

Glassman, K. (2017). *13 Foods That Fight Stress*. Retrieved 2 April 2018 from https://www.prevention.com/mind-body/emotional-health/13-healthy-foods-that-reduce-stress-an d-depression/slide/4

Goldin, S., Hägglöf, B., Levin, L., & Persson, L. Å. (2008). Mental health of Bosnian refugee children: A comparison of clinician appraisal with parent, child and teacher reports. *Nordic Journal of Psychiatry*, *62*(3), 204–216. doi:10.1080/08039480801983604 PMID:18622884

Gold, M. R., Siegel, J. E., Russell, L. B., & Weinstein, M. C. (1996). *Cost effectiveness in Health and Medicine*. New York: Oxford University Press.

Goodwin, R., Palgi, Y., Lavenda, O., Hamama-Raz, Y., & Ben-Ezra, M. (2015). Association between media use, acute stress disorder and psychological distress. *Psychotherapy and Psychosomatics, 84*, 253-254. doi:10.1159/000377706

Graber, T. M. (1972). *Unfavorable sequelae of malocclusion*. Philadelphia: Orthodontics -Principles and Practice.

Green, B. L., Korol, M., Grace, M. C., Vary, M. G., Leonard, A. C., Gleser, G. C., & Smitson-Cohen, S. (1991). Children and disaster: Age, gender, and parental effects on PTSD symptoms. *Journal of the American Academy of Child and Adolescent Psychiatry*, *30*(6), 945–951. doi:10.1097/00004583-199111000-00012 PMID:1757444

Gregoire, C. (2015). *What constant exposure to negative news is doing to our mental health*. Retrieved from https://www.huffingtonpot.com/2015/02/19/violent-media -anxiety_n_6671732.html

Grenberg, M. T., & Krusche, C. A. (1993). *Promoting social and emotional development in deaf children*. Seattle, WA: The PATHS Project U of Washington Press.

Haas, B. K. (1999). Clarification and integration of similar quality of life concepts. *Image--the Journal of Nursing Scholarship*, *31*(9), 215–220. doi:10.1111/j.1547-5069.1999.tb00483.x PMID:10528449

Hagan, J. F. Jr. (2005). Psychosocial implications of disaster or terrorism on children: A guide for the pediatrician. *Pediatrics*, *116*(3), 787–795. doi:10.1542/peds.2005-1498 PMID:16140724

Hallberg, L. R., & Carlsson, S. G. (1993). A qualitative study of situations turning a hearing disability into a handicap. *Disability, Handicap & Society*, *8*(1), 71–85. doi:10.1080/02674649366780051

Haller, J. (2018). The role of central and medial amygdala in normal and abnormal aggression: A review of classical approaches. *Neuroscience and Biobehavioral Reviews*, *85*, 34–43. doi:10.1016/j.neubiorev.2017.09.017 PMID:28918358

Hamilton, J. (2014). *Bingeing on bad news can fuel daily stress*. Retrieved from https://www.npr.org/sections/health-shots/2014/07/10/323355132/binging-on

Hampton, K. N., Lu, W., & Shin, I. (2016). Digital media and stress: The cost of caring 2.0. *Information Communication and Society*, *19*(9), 1267–1286. doi:10.1080/1369118X.2016.1186714

Hardin, M., & Greer, J. D. (2009). The influence of gender-role socialization, media use and sports participation on perceptions of gender-appropriate sports. *Journal of Sport Behavior*, *32*, 207–225.

Harris, L. K., & Vanzandt, C. E. (1997). Counseling needs of students who are deaf and hard of hearing. *The School Counselor*, *44*, 271.

Hart, B., & Risley, T. R. (1995). *Meaningful differences in the everyday experience of young American children. Paul H.* Baltimore, MD: Brookes Publishing Co.

Haskins, B. G. (2004). Serving Deaf Adult Psychiatric Impairments. *Psychiatric Services (Washington, D.C.)*, *55*(4), 439–441. doi:10.1176/appi.ps.55.4.439 PMID:15067159

Hayes, J. P., Hayes, S. M., & Mikedis, A. M. (2012). Quantitative meta-analysis of neural activity in posttraumatic stress disorder. *Biology of Mood & Anxiety Disorders*, *2*(1), 9. doi:10.1186/2045-5380-2-9 PMID:22738125

Hayman, L. A., Fuller, G. N., Cavazos, J. E., Pfleger, M. J., Meyers, C. A., & Jackson, E. F. (1998). The hippocampus: Normal anatomy and pathology. *AJR. American Journal of Roentgenology*, *171*(4), 1139–1146. doi:10.2214/ajr.171.4.9763010 PMID:9763010

Health at a Glance. (2013). *OECD indicators*. Retrieved 30 March 2018 from https://www.oecd.org/els/health-systems/Health-at-a-Glance-2013.pdf

Heptinstall, E., Sethna, V., & Taylor, E. (2004). PTSD and depression in refugee children. *European Child & Adolescent Psychiatry*, *13*(6), 373–380. doi:10.100700787-004-0422-y PMID:15619050

Herbst, K. G., & Humphrey, C. (1980). Hearing impairment and mental state in the elderly living at home. *British Medical Journal*, *281*(6245), 903–905. doi:10.1136/bmj.281.6245.903 PMID:7427503

Herringa, R. J. (2017). Trauma, PTSD, and the developing brain. *Current Psychiatry Reports*, *19*(10), 69. doi:10.100711920-017-0825-3 PMID:28823091

Higginson, I. (1994). Clinical teams, general practice, audit and outcomes. In *Outcomes into clinical practice*. London: BMJ Books.

Hindley, P., & VanGent, T. (2004). Psychiatric aspects of specific sensory impairments. In M. Rytter & E. Taylor (Eds.), *Child and Adolescent Psychiatry* (4th ed.; pp. 842–857). Blackwell.

Hinton, D. E., Rasmussen, A., Nou, L., Pollack, M. H., & Good, M.-J. (2009). Anger, PTSD, and the nuclear family: A study of Cambodian refugees. *Social Science & Medicine*, *69*(9), 1387–1394. doi:10.1016/j.socscimed.2009.08.018 PMID:19748169

Historica Canada. (n.d.). *Radio and television broadcasting*. Retrieved April 14, 2018 from, http://www.thecanadianencyclopedia.ca/en/article/radio-and-television-broadcasting/

Hock, E., Hart, M., Kang, M. J., & Lutz, W. J. (2004). Predicting children's reactions to terrorist attacks: The importance of self-reports and preexisting characteristics. *The American Journal of Orthopsychiatry*, *74*(3), 253–262. doi:10.1037/0002-9432.74.3.253 PMID:15291702

Hodes, M. (2008). Psychopathology in refugee and asylum seeking children. In Rutter's Child and Adolescent Psychiatry (5th ed.). Wiley.

Hodes, M., Jagdev, D., Chandra, N., & Cunniff, A. (2008). Risk and resilience for psychological distress amongst unaccompanied asylum seeking adolescents. *Journal of Child Psychology and Psychiatry, and Allied Disciplines*, *49*(7), 723–732. doi:10.1111/j.1469-7610.2008.01912.x PMID:18492037

Hodgkinson, P. E., & Stewart, M. (1991). Coping with catastrophe: A handbook of disaster management. Taylor & Frances/Routledge.

Hollis, C., Falconer, C. J., Martin, J. L., Whittington, C., Stockton, S., Glazebrook, C., & Davies, E. B. (2017). Annual Research Review: Digital health interventions for children and young people with mental health problems - a systematic and meta-review. *Journal of Child Psychology and Psychiatry, and Allied Disciplines*, *58*(4), 474–503. doi:10.1111/jcpp.12663 PMID:27943285

Hopmann, D. N., & Stromback, J. (2010). *The rise of the media punditocracy? Journalists and media pundits in Danish election news 1994-2007*. Retrieved from journals.sagepub.com/doi/abs/10.1177/0163443710379666

Hoskins, M., Pearce, J., Bethell, A., Dankova, L., Barbui, C., Tol, W. A., ... Bisson, J. I. (2015). Pharmacotherapy for post-traumatic stress disorder: Systematic review and meta-analysis. *The British Journal of Psychiatry*, *206*(2), 93–100. doi:10.1192/bjp.bp.114.148551 PMID:25644881

Howie, L., Pastor, P., & Lukacs, S. (2014). *Use of Medication Prescribed for Emotional or Behavioral Difficulties Among Children Aged 6–17 Years in the United States, 2011–2012*. Retrieved 8 March 2018 from https://www.cdc.gov/nchs/data/databriefs/db148.htm

Hsu, C.-C., Chong, M.-Y., Yang, P., & Yen, C.-F. (2002). Posttraumatic stress disorder among adolescent earthquake victims in Taiwan. *Journal of the American Academy of Child and Adolescent Psychiatry*, *41*(7), 875–881. doi:10.1097/00004583-200207000-00022 PMID:12108814

Huguet, A., Rao, S., Mcgrath, P. J., Wozney, L., Wheaton, M., Conrod, J., & Rozario, S. (2016). A systematic review of cognitive behavioral therapy and behavioral activation apps for depression. *PLoS One*, *11*(5), e0154248. doi:10.1371/journal.pone.0154248 PMID:27135410

Humphries, T., Kushalnagar, P., Mathur, G., Napoli, D. J., Padden, C., Rathmann, C., & Smith, S. R. (2012). Language acquisition for deaf children: Reducing the harms of zero tolerance to the use of alternative approaches. *Harm Reduction Journal*, *9*(16). PMID:22472091

Hunting,, G. S. N., Sahakyan, Y., Fan, I., Moneypenny, C.R., Stanimirovic, A., North, T., … Rac, V.E. (2015). A multi-level qualitative analysis of Telehomecare in Ontario: Challenges and opportunities. *BMC Health Services Research*, *15*(544). PMID:26645639

Hytoglou-Antoniadou. M. (2003). The Social Cerebrum. Thessaloniki, Greece: Publish City. (in Greek)

Ibrahim, H., & Hassan, C. Q. (2017). Post-traumatic stress disorder symptoms resulting from torture and other traumatic events among Syrian Kurdish refugees in Kurdistan Region, Iraq. *Frontiers in Psychology, 8*, 241.

Ince, J., Rojas, F., & Davis, C. A. (2017). The social media response to Black lives matter: How twitter users interact with Black lives matter through hashtag use. *Ethnic and Racial Studies*, *40*(11), 1814–1830. doi:10.1080/01419870.2017.1334931

Izaguirre, J. G. III. (2015). Prophets, gurus, and pundits: Rhetorical styles and public engagement. *The Quarterly Journal of Speech*, *101*(4), 673–677. doi:10.1080/00335630.2015.1128052

James, E. L., Bonsall, M. B., Hoppitt, L., Tunbridge, E. M., Geddes, J. R., Milton, A. L., & Holmes, E. A. (2015). Computer Game Play Reduces Intrusive Memories of Experimental Trauma via Reconsolidation-Update Mechanisms. *Psychological Science*, *26*(8), 1201–1215. doi:10.1177/0956797615583071 PMID:26133572

Jansen, H. J., & Kopp, R. (2005). Pundits, ideologues, and ranters: The British Columbia Election online. *Canadian Journal of Communication*, *30*(4). doi:10.22230/cjc.2005v30n4a1483

Jaycox, L. H., Reivich, K. J., Gillham, J., & Seligman, M. E. (1994). Prevention of depressive symptoms in school children. *Behaviour Research and Therapy*, *32*(8), 801–816. doi:10.1016/0005-7967(94)90160-0 PMID:7993324

Jerger, J., & Hayes, D. (1977). Diagnostic speech audiometry. *Archives of Otolaryngology (Chicago, Ill.)*, *103*(4), 216–222. doi:10.1001/archotol.1977.00780210072008 PMID:849199

John, P. B., Russell, S., & Russell, P. S. S. (2007). The prevalence of posttraumatic stress disorder among children and adolescents affected by tsunami disaster in Tamil Nadu. *Disaster Management & Response*, *5*(1), 3–7. doi:10.1016/j.dmr.2006.11.001 PMID:17306747

Johnson, R., Ross, D. B., Matteson, R., Henry, S., Link, M., Axler, D., . . . Grace, E. (2015). *A Forensic psychological assessment of terrorists: An anti-terrorism approach for radicalized westerners*. Fischler College of Education. Retrieved from http://nsuworks.nova.edu/fse_facarticles/244

Kandemir, H., Karataş, H., Çeri, V., Solmaz, F., Kandemir, S. B., & Solmaz, A. (2018). Prevalence of war-related adverse events, depression and anxiety among Syrian refugee children settled in Turkey. *European Child & Adolescent Psychiatry*, 1–5. PMID:29948231

Karakaya, I., & Çolak, B. (2007). Çocuk ve Ergenlerde Travma Sonrası Stres Bozukluğu ve Adli Tıbbi Değerlendirme. *The Bulletin of Legal Medicine*, *12*(2), 82–87. doi:10.17986/blm.2007122642

Kaufman, J., & Charney, D. (2001). Effects of early stress on brain structure and function: Implications for understanding the relationship between child maltreatment and depression. *Development and Psychopathology*, *13*(3), 451–471. doi:10.1017/S0954579401003030 PMID:11523843

Kent, K.A. (2003). Identity issues for hard of hearing adolescents ages 11, 13 and 15 in mainstream settings. *Journal of Deaf Studies and Deaf Education, 8*, 315-324.

Keppel-Benson, J. M., Ollendick, T. H., & Benson, M. J. (2002). Post-traumatic stress in children following motor vehicle accidents. *Journal of Child Psychology and Psychiatry, and Allied Disciplines*, *43*(2), 203–212. doi:10.1111/1469-7610.00013 PMID:11902599

Kessler, R. C., Sonnega, A., Bromet, E., Hughes, M., & Nelson, C. B. (1995). Posttraumatic stress disorder in the National Comorbidity Survey. *Archives of General Psychiatry*, *52*(12), 1048–1060. doi:10.1001/archpsyc.1995.03950240066012 PMID:7492257

Khrennikov, A. (2008). The Quantum-Like Brain on the Cognitive and Subcognitive Time Scales. *Journal of Consciousness Studies*, *15*(7).

Khrennikov, A. (2009). *Contextual Approach to Quantum Formalism (Fundamental Theories of Physics 160)*. Springer. doi:10.1007/978-1-4020-9593-1

Killikelly, C., He, Z., Reeder, C., & Wykes, T. (2017). Improving Adherence to Web-Based and Mobile Technologies for People With Psychosis: Systematic Review of New Potential Predictors of Adherence. *JMIR mHealth and uHealth*, *5*(7), e94. doi:10.2196/mhealth.7088 PMID:28729235

Kilpatrick, D. G., Ruggiero, K. J., Acierno, R., Saunders, B. E., Resnick, H. S., & Best, C. L. (2003). Violence and Risk of PTSD, Major Depression, Substance Abuse/Dependence, and Comorbidity: Results From the National Survey of Adolescents. *Journal of Consulting and Clinical Psychology*, *71*(4), 692–700. doi:10.1037/0022-006X.71.4.692 PMID:12924674

Kim, D. R., Snell, J. L., Ewing, G. C., & O'Reardon, J. (2015). Neuromodulation and antenatal depression: A review. *Neuropsychiatric Disease and Treatment*, *11*, 975–982. doi:10.2147/NDT.S80480 PMID:25897234

Kim, S. K., & Jeon, S. (2012). Simultaneous determination of serotonin and dopamine at the PEDOP/MWCNTs-Pd nanoparticle modified glassy carbon electrode. *Journal of Nanoscience and Nanotechnology*, *12*(3), 1903–1909. doi:10.1166/jnn.2012.5169 PMID:22754997

King, N. J., Tonge, B. J., Mullen, P., Myerson, N., Heyne, D., Rollings, S., ... Ollendick, T. H. (2000). Treating sexually abused children with posttraumatic stress symptoms: A randomized clinical trial. *Journal of the American Academy of Child and Adolescent Psychiatry*, *39*(11), 1347–1355. doi:10.1097/00004583-200011000-00008 PMID:11068889

Kinzie, J. D., Sack, W. H., Angell, R. H., Manson, S., & Rath, B. (1986). The psychiatric effects of massive trauma on Cambodian children: I. The children. *Journal of the American Academy of Child Psychiatry*, *25*(3), 370–376. doi:10.1016/S0002-7138(09)60259-4

Kira, I., Hammad, A., Lewandowski, L., Templin, T., Ramaswamy, V., Ozkan, B., & Mohanesh, J. (2007). The physical and mental status of Iraqi Refugees and its etiology. *Ethnicity & Disease*, *17*, 79–82. Retrieved from https://www.ethndis .org/priorsuparchives/ethn-17-02s3-79.pdf PMID:17985465

Kizilhan, J. I., & Noll-Hussong, M. (2018). Post-traumatic stress disorder among former Islamic State child soldiers in northern Iraq. *The British Journal of Psychiatry*, 1–5. PMID:29852882

Kleiboer, A., Donker, T., Seekles, W., van Straten, A., Riper, H., & Cuijpers, P. (2015). A randomized controlled trial on the role of support in Internet-based problem solving therapy for depression and anxiety. *Behaviour Research and Therapy*, *72*, 63–71. doi:10.1016/j.brat.2015.06.013 PMID:26188373

Knutson, J. F., Johnson, C. R., & Sullivan, P. M. (2004). Disciplinary choices of mothers of deaf children and mothers of normally hearing children. *Child Abuse & Neglect*, *28*(9), 925–937. doi:10.1016/j.chiabu.2004.04.005 PMID:15450759

Koçak, E. E., & Kılıç, C. (2017). Travma Sonrası Stres Bozukluğunda Bilişsel Bozukluklar. *Türk Psikiyatri Dergisi*, *28*(2), 124–131. PMID:29192945

Kochkin, S., Luxford, W., Northern, J., Mason, P., & Tharpe, A. M. (2007). Are a million dependents with hearing loss in America being left behind? *Hearing Review*. Retrieved from http://www.betterhearing.org/sites/default/files/hearingpedia-resources/M7_children_hearing_loss_left_behind.pdf

Koren, D., Arnon, I., & Klein, E. (1999). Acute stress response and posttraumatic stress disorder in traffic accident victims: A one-year prospective, follow-up study. *The American Journal of Psychiatry*, *156*(3), 367–373. PMID:10080550

Kovacs, M., & Devlin, B. (1998). Internalizing disorders in childhood. *Journal of Child Psychology and Psychiatry, and Allied Disciplines*, *39*(1), 47–63. doi:10.1017/S0021963097001765 PMID:9534086

Kraashen, S. (1973). Lateralization, language learning, and the critical period. Some new evidence. *Language Learning*, *26*(1), 63–71. doi:10.1111/j.1467-1770.1973.tb00097.x

Krabbe, P. F. M., Hinderink, J. B., & Vanden Broek, P. (2000). The effect of cochlear implant use in postlingually deaf results. *International Journal of Technology Assessment in Health Care*, *16*(03), 864–873. doi:10.1017/S0266462300102132 PMID:11028141

Kruse, D. (1997). *Employment and Disability: Characteristics of Employed and Non- Employed People with Disabilities*. Washington, DC: US Department of Labor.

Kyriafinis, G. (2005). *Cochlear implantation*. Thessaloniki, Greece: Publish City. (in Greek)

La forge, R.G., Spector, W.D., & Sternberg, J. (1992). The relationship of vision and hearing impairment to one-year mortality and functional decline. *J. Aging Health, 4*, 126-148.

La Greca, A. M., Silverman, W. K., Vernberg, E. M., & Prinstein, M. J. (1996). Symptoms of posttraumatic stress in children after Hurricane Andrew: A prospective study. *Journal of Consulting and Clinical Psychology*, *64*(4), 712–723. doi:10.1037/0022-006X.64.4.712 PMID:8803361

Lai, B. S., Kelley, M. L., Harrison, K. M., Thompson, J. E., & Self-Brown, S. (2015). Posttraumatic stress, anxiety, and depression symptoms among children after Hurricane Katrina: A latent profile analysis. *Journal of Child and Family Studies*, *24*(5), 1262–1270. doi:10.100710826-014-9934-3 PMID:25892902

Langeland, W., & Olff, M. (2008). Psychobiology of posttraumatic stress disorder in pediatric injury patients: A review of the literature. *Neuroscience and Biobehavioral Reviews*, *32*(1), 161–174. doi:10.1016/j.neubiorev.2007.07.002 PMID:17825911

Laroche, C., Garcia, L. J., & Barrette, J. (2000). Perceptions by persons with hearing impairment, audiologists and employers of the obstacles to work integration. *Journal of the Academy of Rehabilitative Audiology*, *33*, 63–90.

Laufer, A., & Solomon, Z. (2009). Gender differences in PTSD in Israeli youth exposed to terror attacks. *Journal of Interpersonal Violence*, *24*(6), 959–976. doi:10.1177/0886260508319367 PMID:18663245

Lau, J. T., Lau, M., Kim, J. H., & Tsui, H. Y. (2006). Impacts of media coverage on the community stress level in Hong Kong after the tsunami on 26 December 2004. *Journal of Epidemiology and Community Health*, *60*(8), 675–682. doi:10.1136/jech.2005.041897 PMID:16840756

Lee, C. H., Choi, C. H., Yoon, S.-Y., & Lee, J. K. (2015). Posttraumatic Stress Disorder Associated With Orthopaedic Trauma: A Study in Patients With Extremity Fractures. *Journal of Orthopaedic Trauma*, *29*(6), e198–e202. doi:10.1097/BOT.0000000000000255 PMID:25463428

Lee, D. J., Schnitzlein, C. W., Wolf, J. P., Vythilingam, M., Rasmusson, A. M., & Hoge, C. W. (2016). Psychotherapy versus pharmacotherapy for posttraumatic stress disorder: Systemic review and meta-analyses to determine first-line treatments. *Depression and Anxiety*, *33*(9), 792–806. doi:10.1002/da.22511 PMID:27126398

Lee, S. T. (2004). Lying to tell the truth: Journalists and the social context of deception. *Mass Communication & Society*, *7*(1), 97–120. doi:10.120715327825mcs0701_7

Lee, S. T. (2010). Truth telling as a journalistic imperative. In M. S. McGlone & M. L. Knapp (Eds.), *The interplay of truth and deception: New agendas in communication* (pp. 66–88). New York, NY: Routledge.

Lehman, A. F. (1988). A Quality of Life Interview for the Chronically Mentally Ill. *Evaluation and Program Planning*, *II*(1), 51–62. doi:10.1016/0149-7189(88)90033-X

Leigh, J., Dettman, S., Holland, J., Dowell, R., & Briggs, R. J. (2008). Long-term language, speech production and speech perception outcomes for children who received a cochlear implant at or before 12 months of age. Reflecting Connections: A Joint Conference Between New Zealand Speech-Language Therapists Association and Speech Pathology Australia, Auckland, New Zealand.

Lenneberg, E. (1967). *Biological Foundations of Language*. New York: Willey.

Leonard, B. E. (1997). The role of noradrenaline in depression: A review. *Journal of Psychopharmacology (Oxford, England)*, *11*(4Suppl), S39–S47. PMID:9438232

Letukas, L. (2012). *The ascent of punditry: Media and the news construction of cable news* (Doctoral dissertation). Available from ProQuest Dissertations and Theses database. (UMI No. 3526446)

Lewandowsky, S., Ecker, U. K. H., Seifert, C. M., Schwarz, N., & Cook, J. (2012). Misinformation and its correction: Continued influence and successful debiasing. *Psychological Science in the Public Interest, 13*(3), 106–131. doi:10.1177 /1529100612451018

Lewis, T. L., & Wyatt, J. C. (2014). mHealth and mobile medical Apps: A framework to assess risk and promote safer use. *Journal of Medical Internet Research*, *16*(9), e210. doi:10.2196/jmir.3133 PMID:25223398

Lovheim, H. (2012). A new three-dimensional model for emotions and monoamine neurotransmitters. *Medical Hypotheses*, *78*(2), 341–348. doi:10.1016/j.mehy.2011.11.016 PMID:22153577

Luria, A. R. (1961). *The role of speech in normal and abnormal behavior*. New York: Liveright.

Luskin, B. J. (2012). Defining and describing media psychology. *Psychology Today*. Retrieved from https://www.psychologytoday.com/us/blog/the-media-psychology-effect/201211/defining-and-describing-media-psychology

Ly, K. H., Truschel, A., Jarl, L., Magnusson, S., Windahl, T., Johansson, R., ... Andersson, G. (2014). Behavioural activation versus mindfulness-based guided self-help treatment administered through a smartphone application: A randomised controlled trial. *BMJ Open*, *4*(1), e003440. doi:10.1136/ bmjopen-2013-003440 PMID:24413342

Machina, M. J. (2009). Risk, ambiguity, and the dark-dependence axioms. *American Econonomical Review*, *99*(1), 385–392. doi:10.1257/aer.99.1.385

MacSweeney, M. (1998). Cognition and Deafness. In S. Gregory, P. Knight, W. MacCracken, S. Powers, & L. Watson (Eds.), *Issues in Deaf Education* (pp. 20–27). London: David Fulton Publishers.

Mangerud, W., Bjerkeset, O., Lydersen, S., & Indredavik, M. (2014). Physical activity in adolescents with psychiatric disorders and in the general population. *Child and Adolescent Psychiatry and Mental Health*, *8*(1), 2. doi:10.1186/1753-2000-8-2 PMID:24450542

March, J. S., Amaya-Jackson, L., Murray, M. C., & Schulte, A. (1998). Cognitive-behavioral psychotherapy for children and adolescents with posttraumatic stress disorder after a single-incident stressor. *Journal of the American Academy of Child and Adolescent Psychiatry*, *37*(6), 585–593. doi:10.1097/00004583-199806000-00008 PMID:9628078

Mastro, D. (2015). Why the media's role in issues of race and ethnicity should be in the spotlight. *The Journal of Social Issues*, *71*(1), 1–16. doi:10.1111/josi.12093

Mc Elwain, N. L., & Volling, B. L. (2005). Preschool children's interactions with friends and older siblings: Relationship specificity and joint contributions to problem behavior. *Journal of Family Psychology*, *19*(4), 486–496. doi:10.1037/0893-3200.19.4.486 PMID:16402863

McCarthy, M., MacKenzie, E. J., Edwin, D., Bosse, M. J., Castillo, R. C., & Starr, A. (2003). Psychological distress associated with severe lower limb injury. *JBJS*, *85-A*(9), 1689–1697. doi:10.2106/00004623-200309000-00006 PMID:12954826

Mc, L. E. E. R. S. V., Deblinger, E., Atkins, M. S., Foa, E. B., & Ralphe, D. L. (1988). Post-traumatic stress disorder in sexually abused children. *Journal of the American Academy of Child and Adolescent Psychiatry*, *27*(5), 650–654. doi:10.1097/00004583-198809000-00024 PMID:3182633

McLaughlin, K. A., Koenen, K. C., Hill, E. D., Petukhova, M., Sampson, N. A., & Zaslavsky, A. M. (2013). Trauma exposure and posttraumatic stress disorder in a national sample of adolescents. *Journal of the American Academy of Child & Adolescent Psychiatry, 52*(8), 815-30.

McLean, G., Band, R., Saunderson, K., Hanlon, P., Murray, E., Little, P., ... Mair, F. S. (2016). Digital interventions to promote self-management in adults with hypertension systematic review and meta-analysis. *Journal of Hypertension, 34*(4), 600–612. doi:10.1097/HJH.0000000000000859 PMID:26845284

McQuail, D. (2010). *McQuail's Mass Communication Theory* (6th ed.). Thousand Oaks, CA: Sage.

Meadow, K. P., & Trybus, R. J. (1979). Behavioral and emotional problems of deaf children: an overview In Hearing and Hearing Impairment. Grune and Stratton.

Meiser-Stedman, R. (2002). Towards a cognitive–behavioral model of PTSD in children and adolescents. *Clinical Child and Family Psychology Review, 5*(4), 217–232. doi:10.1023/A:1020982122107 PMID:12495267

Mercola, J. (2015). *10 Superfoods That Reduce Stress.* Retrieved 2 April 2018 from https://articles.mercola.com/sites/articles/archive/2015/04/27/10-stress-relieving-superfoods.aspx

Merry, S. N., Stasiak, K., Shepherd, M., Frampton, C., Fleming, T., & Lucassen, M. F. (2012). The effectiveness of SPARX, a computerised self help intervention for adolescents seeking help for depression: Randomised controlled non-inferiority trial. *BMJ (Clinical Research Ed.), 344*, e2598. doi:10.1136/bmj.e2598 PMID:22517917

Messer, C. M., & Bell, P. A. (2010). Mass media and governmental framing of riots. *Journal of Black Studies, 40*(5), 851–870. doi:10.1177/0021934708318607

Meyer, P. (1987). *Ethical journalism.* Lanham, MD: University Press of America.

Michie, S., Yardley, L., West, R., Patrick, K., & Greaves, F. (2017). Developing and Evaluating Digital Interventions to Promote Behavior Change in Health and Health Care: Recommendations Resulting From an International Workshop. *Journal of Medical Internet Research, 19*(6), e232. doi:10.2196/jmir.7126 PMID:28663162

Middelweerd, A., Mollee, J. S., Wal, C. N., Brug, J., & Velde, S. J. (2014). Apps to promote physical activity among adults: A review and content analysis. *The International Journal of Behavioral Nutrition and Physical Activity*, *11*(1), 97. doi:10.118612966-014-0097-9 PMID:25059981

Milgram, N. A., Toubiana, Y. H., Klingman, A., Raviv, A., & Goldstein, I. (1988). Situational exposure and personal loss in children's acute and chronic stress reactions to a school bus disaster. *Journal of Traumatic Stress*, *1*(3), 339–352. doi:10.1002/jts.2490010306

Mills, R., Kisely, S., Alati, R., Strathearn, L., & Najman, J. (2016). Self-reported and agency-notified child sexual abuse in a population-based birth cohort. *Journal of Psychiatric Research*, *74*, 87–93. doi:10.1016/j.jpsychires.2015.12.021 PMID:26774419

Mitchell, T., & Quittner, A. (1996). Multimethod study of attention and behavior problems in hearing impaired children. *Journal of Clinical Child Psychology*, *25*(1), 83–96. doi:10.120715374424jccp2501_10

Mohammadi, S., Haghir, H., Fazel, A. R., & Vafaei, A. (2013). Analysis of Amygdala Nucleus in the Rat Brain: A review study. *Electronic Physician*, *5*(2), 639–642. doi:10.14661/2013.639-642 PMID:26120396

Mollica, R., Culhane, A., & Hovelson, D. (2001). The special psychiatric problems of refugees. In M. Gelder, N. Andreasen, J. Lopez-Ibor, & J. Geddes (Eds.), New Oxford Textbook of Psychiatry (2nd ed.; pp. 1493–1500).Oxford University Press.

Molnar, B., Buka, S., & Kessler, R. (2001). Child sexual abuse and subsequent psychopathology: Results from the national comorbidity survey. *American Journal of Public Health*, *91*(5), 753–760. doi:10.2105/AJPH.91.5.753 PMID:11344883

Monfort, E., & Afzali, M. H. (2017). Traumatic stress symptoms after the November 13th 2015 terrorist attacks among young adults: The relation to media and emotion regulation. *Comprehensive Psychiatry*, *75*, 68–74. doi:10.1016/j.comppsych.2017.02.015 PMID:28324678

Morgan, L., Scourfield, J., Williams, D., Jasper, A., & Lewis, G. (2003). The Aberfan disaster: 33-year follow-up of survivors. *The British Journal of Psychiatry*, *182*(6), 532–536. doi:10.1192/bjp.182.6.532 PMID:12777345

Morgos, D., Worden, J. W., & Gupta, L. (2008). Psychosocial effects of war experiences among displaced children in southern Darfur. *Omega*, *56*(3), 229–253. doi:10.2190/OM.56.3.b PMID:18300649

Moss, M.L. (n.d.). The functionalal matrix. *U Vistas in Orthodontics*.

Murphy, M. B., Laurie-Rose, C., Brinkman, T. M., & McNamara, K. A. (2007). Sustained attention and social competence in typically developing preschool-aged children. *Early Child Development and Care*, *177*(2), 133–149. doi:10.1080/03004430500349559

Murray, E., Hekler, E. B., Andersson, G., Collins, L. M., Doherty, A., Hollis, C., ... Wyatt, J. C. (2016). Evaluating Digital Health Interventions: Key Questions and Approaches. *American Journal of Preventive Medicine*, *51*(5), 843–851. doi:10.1016/j.amepre.2016.06.008 PMID:27745684

Nader, K. O., Pynoos, R. S., Fairbanks, L. A., Al-Ajeel, M., & Al-Asfour, A. (1993). A preliminary study of PTSD and grief among the children of Kuwait following the Gulf crisis. *British Journal of Clinical Psychology*, *32*(4), 407–416. doi:10.1111/j.2044-8260.1993.tb01075.x PMID:8298537

Najarian, L. M., Majeed, M. H., & Gasparyan, K. (2017). Effect of relocation after a natural disaster in Armenia: 20-year follow-up. *Asian Journal of Psychiatry*, *29*, 8–12. doi:10.1016/j.ajp.2017.03.030 PMID:29061434

Nasıroğlu, S., Çeri, V., Erkorkmaz, Ü., & Semerci, B. (2018). Determinants of psychiatric disorders in children refugees in Turkey's Yazidi refugee camp. *Psychiatry and Clinical Psychopharmacology*, 1-9.

Nasıroğlu, S., & Ceri, V. (2016). Posttraumatic stress and depression in Yazidi refugees. *Neuropsychiatric Disease and Treatment*, *12*, 2941–2948. doi:10.2147/NDT.S119506 PMID:27881919

Naslund, J. A., Aschbrenner, K. A., & Bartels, S. J. (2016). Wearable Devices and Smartphones for Activity Tracking Among People with Serious Mental Illness. *Mental Health and Physical Activity*, *10*, 10–17. doi:10.1016/j.mhpa.2016.02.001 PMID:27134654

Nathan, L., Goulandris, N., & Snowling, M. J. (2000). The development of early literacy skills among children with speech difficulties: A test of the critical age hypothesis. *Journal of Speech, Language, and Hearing Research: JSLHR*, *43*, 380–394. PMID:10757691

Navalta, C. P., Polcari, A., Webster, D. M., Boghossian, A., & Teicher, M. H. (2006). Effects of childhood sexual abuse on neuropsychological and cognitive function in college women. *The Journal of Neuropsychiatry and Clinical Neurosciences*, *18*(1), 45–53. doi:10.1176/jnp.18.1.45 PMID:16525070

Neigh, G. N., Gillespie, C. F., & Nemeroff, C. B. (2009). The neurobiological toll of child abuse and neglect. *Trauma, Violence & Abuse*, *10*(4), 389–410. doi:10.1177/1524838009339758 PMID:19661133

Newman, E., Pfefferbaum, B., Kirlic, N., Tett, R., Nelson, S., & Liles, B. (2014). Meta-analytic review of psychological interventions for children survivors of natural and man-made disasters. *Current Psychiatry Reports*, *16*(9), 462. doi:10.100711920-014-0462-z PMID:25085234

Nicholson, D. A., & Geinisman, Y. (2009). Axospinous synaptic subtype-specific differences in structure, size, ionotropic receptor expression, and connectivity in apical dendritic regions of rat hippocampal CA1 pyramidal neurons. *The Journal of Comparative Neurology*, *512*(3), 399–418. doi:10.1002/cne.21896 PMID:19006199

Nooner, K. B., Linares, L. O., Batinjane, J., Kramer, R. A., Silva, R., & Cloitre, M. (2012). Factors related to posttraumatic stress disorder in adolescence. *Trauma, Violence & Abuse*, *13*(3), 153–166. doi:10.1177/1524838012447698 PMID:22665437

Nunes, T., Pretzlik, U., & Olson, J. (2001). Deaf children's social relationships in mainstream schools. *Deafness & Education International*, *3*(3), 123–136. doi:10.1179/146431501790560972

O'Doherty, D. C., Chitty, K. M., Saddiqui, S., Bennett, M. R., & Lagopoulos, J. (2015). A systematic review and meta-analysis of magnetic resonance imaging measurement of structural volumes in posttraumatic stress disorder. *Psychiatry Research: Neuroimaging*, *232*(1), 1–33. doi:10.1016/j.pscychresns.2015.01.002 PMID:25735885

Oerger, M. (1989). Quality of Life, Health Status, and Clinical Research. *Medical Care*, (Supplement), S148–S156. PMID:2646487

Olofsson, E., Bunketorp, O., & Andersson, A. L. (2009). Children and adolescents injured in traffic–associated psychological consequences: A literature review. *Acta Paediatrica (Oslo, Norway)*, *98*(1), 17–22. doi:10.1111/j.1651-2227.2008.00998.x PMID:18795910

Open Society Institute. (2005). *Television across Europe: Regulation, policy and independence* (Volume 2). Retrieved from https://www.opensocietyfoundations .org/sites/default/files/voltwo_20051011_0.pdf

Owens, R. (2013). *Language Disorders: A Functional Approach to Assessment and Intervention* (6th ed.). Pearson.

Özgen, F., & Aydın, H. (1999). Travma sonrası stres bozukluğu. *Klinik Psikiyatri.*, *1*, 34–41.

Padovan, C. M. (2013). Serotonin in anxiety and depression. *Journal of Psychopharmacology (Oxford, England)*, *27*(12), 1083. doi:10.1177/0269881113508831 PMID:24227796

Pal, K., Eastwood, S. V., Michie, S., Farmer, A., Barnard, M. L., Peacock, R., ... Murray, E. (2014). Computer-based interventions to improve self-management in adults with type 2 diabetes: A systematic review and meta-analysis. *Diabetes Care*, *37*(6), 1759–1766. doi:10.2337/dc13-1386 PMID:24855158

Pantic, I., Dacic, S., Brkic, P., Lavrnja, I., Jovanovic, T., Pantic, S., & Pekovic, S. (2015). Discriminatory ability of fractal and grey level co-occurrence matrix methods in structural analysis of hippocampus layers. *Journal of Theoretical Biology*, *370*, 151–156. doi:10.1016/j.jtbi.2015.01.035 PMID:25665716

Paolucci, E. O., Genuis, M. L., & Violato, C. (2001). A meta-analysis of the published research on the effects of child sexual abuse. *The Journal of Psychology*, *135*(1), 17–36. doi:10.1080/00223980109603677 PMID:11235837

Papageorgiou, V., Frangou-Garunovic, A., Iordanidou, R., Yule, W., Smith, P., & Vostanis, P. (2000). War trauma and psychopathology in Bosnian refugee children. *European Child & Adolescent Psychiatry*, *9*(2), 84–90. doi:10.1007007870050002 PMID:10926057

Parving, A., & Christensen, B. (1993). Training and employment in hearing-impaired subjects at 20-35 years of age. *Scandinavian Audiology*, 22133–22139. PMID:8321998

Patel, K., Allen, S., Haque, M. N., Angelescu, I., Baumeister, D., & Tracy, D. K. (2016). Bupropion: A systematic review and meta-analysis of effectiveness as an antidepressant. *Therapeutic Advances in Psychopharmacology*, *6*(2), 99–144. doi:10.1177/2045125316629071 PMID:27141292

Pauc, R., & Young, A. (2010). Little-known neurons of the medial wall: A literature review of pyramidal cells of the cingulate gyrus. *Journal of Chiropractic Medicine*, *9*(3), 115–120. doi:10.1016/j.jcm.2010.05.001 PMID:22027033

Pecina, M., Mickey, B. J., Love, T., Wang, H., Langenecker, S. A., Hodgkinson, C., ... Zubieta, J. K. (2013). DRD2 polymorphisms modulate reward and emotion processing, dopamine neurotransmission and openness to experience. *Cortex*, *49*(3), 877–890. doi:10.1016/j.cortex.2012.01.010 PMID:22424959

Peden, M. (2008). World report on child injury prevention appeals to "Keep Kids Safe". *Injury Prevention*, *14*(6), 413–414. doi:10.1136/ip.2008.020693 PMID:19074252

Pedersen, D. (2002). Political violence, ethnic conflict, and contemporary wars: Broad implications for health and social well-being. *Social Science & Medicine*, *55*(2), 175–190. doi:10.1016/S0277-9536(01)00261-1 PMID:12144134

Percy-Smith, L., Caye-Thomasen, P., Gudman, M., Jensen, J., & Thomsen, J. (2008). Self-esteem and social well-being of children with cochlear implant compared to normal hearing children. *International Journal of Pediatric Otorhinolaryngology*, *72*(7), 1113–1120. doi:10.1016/j.ijporl.2008.03.028 PMID:18501436

Pérez-Pereira, M., Tinajero, C., Rodríguez, M. S., Peralbo, M., & Sabucedo, J. M. (2012). Academic effects of the Prestige oil spill disaster. *The Spanish Journal of Psychology*, *15*(3), 1055–1068. doi:10.5209/rev_SJOP.2012.v15.n3.39396 PMID:23156914

Perry, B. D., Pollard, R. A., Blakley, T. L., Baker, W. L., & Vigilante, D. (1995). Childhood trauma, the neurobiology of adaptation, and "use-dependent" development of the brain: How "states" become "traits". *Infant Mental Health Journal, 16*(4), 271–291. doi:10.1002/1097-0355(199524)16:4<271::AID-IMHJ2280160404>3.0.CO;2-B

Pfefferbaum, B. (1997). Posttraumatic stress disorder in children: A review of the past 10 years. *Journal of the American Academy of Child and Adolescent Psychiatry, 36*(11), 1503–1511. PMID:9394934

Pfefferbaum, B., Noffsinger, M. A., Jacobs, A. K., & Varma, V. (2016). Children's cognitive functioning in disasters and terrorism. *Current Psychiatry Reports, 18*(5), 48. doi:10.100711920-016-0685-2 PMID:26997166

Pine, D. S., & Cohen, J. A. (2002). Trauma in children and adolescents: Risk and treatment of psychiatric sequelae. *Biological Psychiatry, 51*(7), 519–531. doi:10.1016/S0006-3223(01)01352-X PMID:11950454

Pollard, R. Q. (1994). Public mental health service and diagnostic trends regarding individuals who are deaf or hard-of-hearing. *Rehabilitation Psychology, 39*(3), 147–160. doi:10.1037/h0080318

Pothos, E. M., & Busemeyer, J. R. (2009). A quantum probability explanation for violations of 'rational'decision theory. *Proceedings of the Royal Society B: Biological Sciences, 276*(1665), 2171–2178.

Pots, W. T., Fledderus, M., Meulenbeek, P. A., ten Klooster, P. M., Schreurs, K. M., & Bohlmeijer, E. T. (2016). Acceptance and commitment therapy as a web-based intervention for depressive symptoms: Randomised controlled trial. *The British Journal of Psychiatry, 208*(1), 69–77. doi:10.1192/bjp.bp.114.146068 PMID:26250745

Powell, K. A. (2011). Framing Islam: An analysis of U.S. media coverage of terrorism since 9/11. *Communication Studies, 62*(1), 90–112. doi:10.1080/10510974.2011.533599

Pratt, L., Brody, D., & Qiuping, G. (2017). *NCHS Data Brief. U.S. Department of Health and Human Services. No. 283. Centers for Disease Control and Prevention National Center for Health Statistics Antidepressant Use Among Persons Aged 12 and Over: United States 2011–2014*. Retrieved 30 March 2018 from https://www.cdc.gov/nchs/data/databriefs/db283.pdf

Prince, R. (2014). *How media have shaped our perception of race and crime. Journal-isms*. Gizmodo Media Group. Retrieved from https://journalisms.theroot.com /how-media-have-shaped-our-perception-of-race-and-crime-1790885677

Prior, M. (2013). Media and political polarization. *Annual Review of Political Science*, *16*(1), 101–127. doi:10.1146/annurev-polisci-100711-135242

Prizant, B., & Meyer, E. (1993). Socioemotional aspects of language and social-communication disorders in young children. *American Journal of Speech-Language Pathology*, *2*(3), 56–71. doi:10.1044/1058-0360.0203.56

Proffit, W. R., & Fields, H. W. (2000). *Contemporary Orthodontics* (3rd ed.). St. Louis, MO: Mosby.

Putnam, F. W. (2003). Ten-Year Research Update Review: Child Sexual Abuse. *Journal of the American Academy of Child and Adolescent Psychiatry*, *42*(3), 269–278. doi:10.1097/00004583-200303000-00006 PMID:12595779

Pynoos, R. S., Frederick, C., Nader, K., Arroyo, W., Steinberg, A., Eth, S., & ... . (1987). Life threat and posttraumatic stress in school-age children. *Archives of General Psychiatry*, *44*(12), 1057–1063. doi:10.1001/archpsyc.1987.01800240031005 PMID:3689093

Qouta, S., Punamäki, R.-L., & El Sarraj, E. (2003). Prevalence and determinants of PTSD among Palestinian children exposed to military violence. *European Child & Adolescent Psychiatry*, *12*(6), 265–272. doi:10.100700787-003-0328-0 PMID:14689258

Quantum Approaches to Consciousness. (2011). In Stanford Encyclopedia of Philosophy. Stanford University Press.

Quittner, A. L., Barker, D. H., Snell, C., Cruz, I., McDonald, L., & Grimley, M. E. (2007). Improvements in visual attention after cochlear implantation. *Audiological Medicine*, *5*, 242–249. doi:10.1080/16513860701745401

Ramasubramanian, S. (2011). The impact of stereotypical versus counterstereotypical media exemplars on racial attitudes, causal attributions, and support for affirmative action. *Communication Research*, *38*(4), 497–516. doi:10.1177/0093650210384854

Realmuto, G. M., Masten, A., Carole, L. F., Hubbard, J., Groteluschen, A., & Chhun, B. (1992). Adolescent survivors of massive childhood trauma in Cambodia: Life events and current symptoms. *Journal of Traumatic Stress*, *5*(4), 589–599. doi:10.1002/jts.2490050408

Remmel, E., & Peters, K. (2009). Theory of mind and language in children with cochlear implants. *Journal of Deaf Studies and Deaf Education*, *14*(2), 218–237. doi:10.1093/deafed/enn036 PMID:18796736

Rescorla, L. (2002). Language and reading outcomes to age 9 I late-talking toddlers. *Journal of Speech, Language, and Hearing Research: JSLHR*, *45*(2), 360–371. doi:10.1044/1092-4388(2002/028) PMID:12003517

Rheker, J., Winkler, A., Doering, B. K., & Rief, W. (2016). Learning to experience side effects after antidepressant intake – Results from a randomized, controlled, double-blind study. *Psychopharmacology*, *234*(3), 329–338. doi:10.100700213-016-4466-8 PMID:27807605

Riek, L. D. (2016). Robotics technology in mental health care. In *Artificial intelligence in behavioral and mental health care. London*. London: D.D. Luxton, Academic Press. doi:10.1016/B978-0-12-420248-1.00008-8

Robbins, A.M., Svirsky, M., & Kirk, K.I. (1997). Children with implants can speak but can they communicate? *Otolaryngol. Head Neck Surg.*, *117*(ph I), 155-160.

Robinson, K., Gatchouse, S., & Browning, G. G. (1996). Measuring benefit from otorhinolaryngological surgery and therapy. *The Annals of Otology, Rhinology, and Laryngology*, *105*(6), 415–422. doi:10.1177/000348949610500601 PMID:8638891

Rogers, M. A., Kasai, K., Koji, M., Fukuda, R., Iwanami, A., Nakagome, K., ... Kato, N. (2004). Executive and prefrontal dysfunction in unipolar depression: A review of neuropsychological and imaging evidence. *Neuroscience Research*, *50*(1), 1–11. doi:10.1016/j.neures.2004.05.003 PMID:15288493

Romeo, R. D. (2017). The impact of stress on the structure of the adolescent brain: Implications for adolescent mental health. *Brain Research*, *1654*, 185–191. doi:10.1016/j.brainres.2016.03.021 PMID:27021951

Ronnenberg, J. (2003). *Working memory, neuroscience, and language: Evidence from deaf and hard-of-hearing individuals.* In M. Marschark & P. Spencer (Eds.), *Handbook of Deaf Studies, Language, and Education* (pp. 478–490). Oxford University Press.

Rosenberger, P. H., Ickovics, J. R., Epel, E., Nadler, E., Jokl, P., Fulkerson, J. P., ... Dhabhar, F. S. (2009). Surgical Stress-Induced Immune Cell Redistribution Profiles Predict Short-Term and Long-Term Postsurgical Recovery A Prospective Study. *The Journal of Bone and Joint Surgery. American Volume*, *91*(12), 2783–2794. doi:10.2106/JBJS.H.00989 PMID:19952239

Rose, S. C., Bisson, J., Churchill, R., & Wessely, S. (2002). Psychological debriefing for preventing post traumatic stress disorder (PTSD). *The Cochrane Library*. PMID:12076399

Ross, R. A., Foster, S. L., & Ionescu, D. F. (2017). The role of chronic stress in anxious depression. *Chronic Stress*. Retrieved 30 March 2018 from http://journals.sagepub.com/doi/pdf/10.1177/2470547016689472

Rotondi, A. J., Eack, S. M., Hanusa, B. H., Spring, M. B., & Haas, G. L. (2015). Critical design elements of e-health applications for users with severe mental illness: Singular focus, simple architecture, prominent contents, explicit navigation, and inclusive hyperlinks. *Schizophrenia Bulletin*, *41*(2), 440–448. doi:10.1093chbulbt194 PMID:24375458

Rowan, A. B., & Foy, D. W. (1993). Post-traumatic stress disorder in child sexual abuse survivors: A literature review. *Journal of Traumatic Stress*, *6*(1), 3–20. doi:10.1002/jts.2490060103

Royal Society for Public Health. (2017). Retrieved 30 March 2018 from https://www.rsph.org.uk/our-work/campaigns/status-of-mind.html

Ruben, R. J. (2000). Redefining the survival of the fittest. Communication disorders in the 21st century. *Laryngoscope*, *110*(2), 241–245. doi:10.1097/00005537-200002010-00010 PMID:10680923

Ruff, H. A., & Rothbart, M. K. (1996). *Attention in early development: Themes and Variations*. New York: Oxford University Press.

Rutledge, P. (2008). The evolving definition of media psychology. *The Media Psychology Review*, *7*(2). Retrieved from mprcenetr.org/review/evolving-definition-media-psychology/?print=print

Sack, W. H., Him, C., & Dickason, D. (1999). Twelve-year follow-up study of Khmer youths who suffered massive war trauma as children. *Journal of the American Academy of Child and Adolescent Psychiatry*, *38*(9), 1173–1179. doi:10.1097/00004583-199909000-00023 PMID:10504817

Samuelson, K. W., Krueger, C. E., Burnett, C., & Wilson, C. K. (2010). Neuropsychological functioning in children with posttraumatic stress disorder. *Child Neuropsychology*, *16*(2), 119–133. doi:10.1080/09297040903190782 PMID:19787496

Sanders, D. A. (1975). Hearing aid orientation and counseling. In M. C. Pollack (Ed.), *Amplification for the Hearing-Impaired.* New York: Grune and Stratton.

Sanders, D. A. (1982). *Aural Rehabilitation: A Management Model* (2nd ed.). Englewood Cliffs, NJ: Prentice-Hall.

Sanders, G. H., & Jutai, J. W. (2004). Hearing specific and generic measures of the psychosocial impact of hearing aids. S. *Am Acad Audiol.*, *15*(3), 238–248. doi:10.3766/jaaa.15.3.6

Savage, L. J. (1954). *The Foundations of Statistics*. John Wiley & Sons.

Savin, D., Sack, W. H., Clarke, G. N., Meas, N., & Richart, I. (1996). The Khmer Adolescent Project: III. A study of trauma from Thailand's Site II refugee camp. *Journal of the American Academy of Child and Adolescent Psychiatry*, *35*(3), 384–391. doi:10.1097/00004583-199603000-00021 PMID:8714328

Saylor, C. F., Cowart, B. L., Lipovsky, J. A., Jackson, C., & Finch, A. Jr. (2003). Media exposure to September 11: Elementary school students' experiences and posttraumatic symptoms. *The American Behavioral Scientist*, *46*(12), 1622–1641. doi:10.1177/0002764203254619

Schachter, D. (2013). *The source of toxicity in CTAB and CTAB/stabilized gold nanorods: Rutgers*. New Brunswick, NJ: The State University of New Jersey.

Scheufele, D. A. (1991). Framing as a theory of media effects. *Journal of Communication*, *49*(1), 103–122. doi:10.1111/j.1460-2466.1999.tb02784.x

Schick, B., de Villiers, P., de Villiers, J., & Hoffmeister, R. (2007). Language and Theory of Mind: A study of deaf children. *Child Development*, *78*(2), 376–396. doi:10.1111/j.1467-8624.2007.01004.x PMID:17381779

Schirk, B., Williams, K., & Kupermintz, H. (2006). Look who's being left behind? Educational interpreters and access to education for deaf and hard of hearing students. *Journal of Deaf Studies and Deaf Education*, *11*, 3–20. PMID:16192404

Schneiderman, N., Ironson, G., & Siegel, S. D. (2005). Stress and health: Psychological, behavioral, and biological determinants. *Annual Review of Clinical Psychology*, *1*(1), 607–628. doi:10.1146/annurev.clinpsy.1.102803.144141 PMID:17716101

Schreier, H., Ladakakos, C., Morabito, D., Chapman, L., & Knudson, M. M. (2005). Posttraumatic stress symptoms in children after mild to moderate pediatric trauma: A longitudinal examination of symptom prevalence, correlates, and parent-child symptom reporting. *The Journal of Trauma and Acute Care Surgery*, *58*(2), 353–363. doi:10.1097/01.TA.0000152537.15672.B7 PMID:15706200

Schroedel, J. (1992). Helping adolescents and young adults who are deaf make career decisions. *The Volta Review*, *94*, 37–46.

Schulten, K. (2015). Skills and strategies: Fake news vs. real news: Determining the reliability of sources. *The New York Times*. Retrieved from https://learning.blogs.nytimes.com/2015/10/02/skills-and-strategies-fake-news-vs-real-news-determining-the-reliability-of-sources/

Scrimin, S., Moscardino, U., Capello, F., & Axia, G. (2009). Attention and memory in school-age children surviving the terrorist attack in Beslan, Russia. *Journal of Clinical Child and Adolescent Psychology*, *38*(3), 402–414. doi:10.1080/15374410902851689 PMID:19437300

Sethi, S. (2013). Treating Youth Depression and Anxiety: A Randomised Controlled Trial Examining the Efficacy of Computerised versus Face-to-face Cognitive Behaviour Therapy. *Australian Psychologist*, *48*(4), 249–257. doi:10.1111/ap.12006

Silver, R. C., Holman, E. A., Andersen, J. P., Poulin, M., McIntosh, D. N., & Gil-Rivas, V. (2013). Mental-and physical-health effects of acute exposure to media images of the September 11, 2001, attacks and the Iraq War. *Psychological Science*, *24*(9), 1623–1634. doi:10.1177/0956797612460406 PMID:23907546

Simons, G., & Strovsky, D. (2006). Censorship in contemporary Russian journalism in the age of the war against terrorism. *European Journal of Communication*, *21*(2), 189–211. doi:10.1177/0267323105064045

Smith, L. B., Quittner, A. I., Osberger, M. J., & Miyamoto, R. (1998). Audition and Visual Attention the developmental trajectory in deaf and hearing populations. *Developmental Psychology*, *34*(5), 840–850. doi:10.1037/0012-1649.34.5.840 PMID:9779732

Snowling, M. J., Adams, J. W., Bishop, D. V. M., & Stohard, S. E. (2001). Educational attainments of school leavers with a preschool history of speech-language impairments. *International Journal of Language & Communication Disorders*, *36*(2), 173–183. doi:10.1080/13682820010019892 PMID:11344593

Sokol, J., & Hyde, M. (2002). Hearing Screening. *Pediatrics*, *23*, 155–161. PMID:11986491

Sowell, E. R., Thompson, P. M., Tessner, K. D., & Toga, A. W. (2001). Mapping continued brain growth and gray matter density reduction in dorsal frontal cortex: Inverse relationships during postadolescent brain maturation. *The Journal of Neuroscience*, *21*(22), 8819–8829. doi:10.1523/JNEUROSCI.21-22-08819.2001 PMID:11698594

Spijkerman, M. P., Pots, W. T., & Bohlmeijer, E. T. (2016). Effectiveness of online mindfulness-based interventions in improving mental health: A review and meta-analysis of randomised controlled trials. *Clinical Psychology Review*, *45*, 102–114. doi:10.1016/j.cpr.2016.03.009 PMID:27111302

Sprung, M., & Harris, P. L. (2010). Intrusive thoughts and young children's knowledge about thinking following a natural disaster. *Journal of Child Psychology and Psychiatry, and Allied Disciplines*, *51*(10), 1115–1124. doi:10.1111/j.1469-7610.2010.02273.x PMID:20840501

Srivistava, K. (2010). A study of Psychological correlates after amputation. *MJAFI*, *66*, 367–373. PMID:27365745

Stahl, S. M. (2013). *Stahl's Essential Psychopharmacology: Neuroscientific Basis and Practical Applications*. New York: Cambridge University Press.

Stallard, P., Velleman, R., & Baldwin, S. (1998). Prospective study of post-traumatic stress disorder in children involved in road traffic accidents. *BMJ (Clinical Research Ed.)*, *317*(7173), 1619–1623. doi:10.1136/bmj.317.7173.1619 PMID:9848900

Stansfeld, S., Roberts, R., & Foot, S. (1997). Assessing the validity of the SF-36 General Health Survey. *Quality of Life Research: An International Journal of Quality of Life Aspects of Treatment, Care and Rehabilitation*, *6*(3), 217–224. doi:10.1023/A:1026406620756 PMID:9226979

Statista. (2018). *News industry - statistics & facts*. Retrieved April 20, 2018 from, https://www.statista.com/topics/1640/news/

Steffen, P. R., Austin, T., & Debarros, A. (2016). Treating chronic stress to address the growing problem of depression and anxiety. *Policy Insights from the Behavioral and Brain Sciences*, *4*(1), 64–70. doi:10.1177/2372732216685333

Stein, M. B., & Ravindran, L. N. (2009). Pharmacotherapy of posttraumatic stress disorder. In Post Traumatic Stress Disorder (pp. 125–135). CRC Press.

Steinberg, A. G., Sullivan, V. J., & Montoya, L. A. (1999). Loneliness and social isolation in the work place for deaf individuals during the transition years: A preliminary investigation. *Journal of Applied Rehabilitation Counseling*, *30*(1), 22–30.

Stein, D., Zungu-Dirwayi, N., & Seedat, S. (2000). Pharmacotherapy for posttraumatic stress disorder. *Cochrane Database of Systematic Reviews*, (4), CD002795. PMID:11034765

Stewart, D. A., & Clarke, B. R. (2003). *Literacy and Your Deaf Child: What Every Parent Should Know*. Washington, DC: Gallaudet University Press.

Stinson, M. S., & Whitmire, K. A. (2000). Adolescents who are deaf or hard of hearing: A Communication Perspective on educational placement. *Topics in Language Disorders*, *20*(2), 58–72. doi:10.1097/00011363-200020020-00006

Stinson, M., & Walter, G. (1997). Improving retention for deaf and hard of hearing students: What the research tells us. *Journal of the American Deafness and Rehabilitation Association*, *30*(4), 14–23.

Stott, R., Wild, J., Grey, N., Liness, S., Warnock-Parkes, E., Commins, S., ... Clark, D. M. (2013). Internet-delivered cognitive therapy for social anxiety disorder: A development pilot series. *Behavioural and Cognitive Psychotherapy*, *41*(4), 383–397. doi:10.1017/S1352465813000404 PMID:23676553

Sullivan, P. M., & Knutson, J. F. (2000). Maltreatment and disabilities: A population-based epidemiological study. *Child Abuse & Neglect*, *24*(10), 1257–1273. doi:10.1016/S0145-2134(00)00190-3 PMID:11075694

Summerfield, D. (2000). Childhood, war, refugeedom and 'trauma': Three core questions for mental health professionals. *Transcultural Psychiatry*, *37*(3), 417–433. doi:10.1177/136346150003700308

Swanson, J. L., & Woitke, M. B. (1997). Theory into practice in career assessment for women: Assessment and interventions regarding perceived career barriers. *Journal of Career Assessment*, *5*(4), 443–462. doi:10.1177/106907279700500405

Szymanski, E. M., & Hershenson, D. B. (2005). An ecological approach to vocational behavior and career development of people with disabilities. In R. Parker, E. M. Szymanski, & J. B. Pattersson (Eds.), *Rehabilitation Counseling: Basics and beyond* (4th ed.; pp. 225–280). Austin, TX: PRO-ED.

Takahashi, B. (2010). Framing and sources: A study of mass media coverage of climate change in Peru during V ALCUE. *Public Understanding of Science (Bristol, England)*, *20*(4), 543–557. doi:10.1177/0963662509356502 PMID:21936267

Tebbutt, J., Swanston, H., Oates, R. K., & O'toole, B. I. (1997). Five years after child sexual abuse: Persisting dysfunction and problems of prediction. *Journal of the American Academy of Child and Adolescent Psychiatry*, *36*(3), 330–339. doi:10.1097/00004583-199703000-00011 PMID:9055513

Teicher, M. H., Samson, J. A., Anderson, C. M., & Ohashi, K. (2016). The effects of childhood maltreatment on brain structure, function and connectivity. *Nature Reviews. Neuroscience*, *17*(10), 652–666. doi:10.1038/nrn.2016.111 PMID:27640984

Terr, L. (1990). *Too scared to cry: How trauma affects children and ultimately us all*. New York: Basic.

Thabet, A. A., Tawahina, A. A., El Sarraj, E., & Vostanis, P. (2008). Exposure to war trauma and PTSD among parents and children in the Gaza strip. *European Child & Adolescent Psychiatry*, *17*(4), 191–199. doi:10.100700787-007-0653-9 PMID:18365135

Thabet, A. A., & Vostanis, P. (2000). Post traumatic stress disorder reactions in children of war: A longitudinal study. *Child Abuse & Neglect*, *24*(2), 291–298. doi:10.1016/S0145-2134(99)00127-1 PMID:10695524

Thilander, B. (1985). *Ronning O.Introduction to Orthodontics*. Tandiakastforlaget.

Titov, N., Dear, B. F., Schwencke, G., Andrews, G., Johnston, L., Craske, M. G., & McEvoy, P. (2011). Transdiagnostic internet treatment for anxiety and depression: A randomised controlled trial. *Behaviour Research and Therapy*, *49*(8), 441–452. doi:10.1016/j.brat.2011.03.007 PMID:21679925

Toppelberg, C. O., & Shapiro, T. (2000). Language disorders: A 10-year research update review. *Journal of the American Academy of Child and Adolescent Psychiatry*, *39*(2), 143–152. doi:10.1097/00004583-200002000-00011 PMID:10673823

Torous, J. B., Chan, S. R., Yellowlees, P. M., & Boland, R. (2016). To Use or Not? Evaluating ASPECTS of Smartphone Apps and Mobile Technology for Clinical Care in Psychiatry. *The Journal of Clinical Psychiatry*, *77*(6), e734–e738. doi:10.4088/JCP.15com10619 PMID:27136691

Torous, J., Kiang, M. V., Lorme, J., & Onnela, J. P. (2016). New Tools for New Research in Psychiatry: A Scalable and Customizable Platform to Empower Data Driven Smartphone Research. *JMIR Ment Health*, *3*(2), e16. doi:10.2196/mental.5165 PMID:27150677

Torous, J., & Roberts, L. W. (2017). Needed Innovation in Digital Health and Smartphone Applications for Mental Health: Transparency and Trust. *JAMA Psychiatry*, *74*(5), 437–438. doi:10.1001/jamapsychiatry.2017.0262 PMID:28384700

Torrance, G. W., & Feeny, D. (1989). Utilities and quality- adjusted life years. *International Journal of Technology Assessment in Health Care*, *5*(04), 559–575. doi:10.1017/S0266462300008461 PMID:2634630

Tottenham, N., & Galván, A. (2016). Stress and the adolescent brain. *Neuroscience and Biobehavioral Reviews*, *70*, 217–227. doi:10.1016/j.neubiorev.2016.07.030 PMID:27473936

Trickey, D., Siddaway, A. P., Meiser-Stedman, R., Serpell, L., & Field, A. P. (2012). A meta-analysis of risk factors for post-traumatic stress disorder in children and adolescents. *Clinical Psychology Review*, *32*(2), 122–138. doi:10.1016/j.cpr.2011.12.001 PMID:22245560

Tucker, B. (1988). Deaf Prison Inmates. Los Angeles, CA: Loyola of Los Angeles School of Law.

Tudo, R. (2017). Psychological Morbidity Associated with Orthopedic Trauma. *American Journal of Psychiatry and Neuroscience*, *5*(6), 22.

Tversky, A., & Shafir, E. (1992). The disjunction effect in choice under uncertainty. *Psychological Science*, *3*(5), 305–309. doi:10.1111/j.1467-9280.1992.tb00678.x

Twenge, J. M., Joiner, T. E., Rogers, M. L., & Martin, G. N. (2017). Increases in depressive symptoms, suicide-related outcomes, and suicide rates among U.S. adolescents after 2010 and links to increased new media screen time. *Clinical Psychological Science*, *6*(1), 3–17. doi:10.1177/2167702617723376

Uhlmann, R. F., Larson, E. B., Rees, T. S., Koepsell, T. D., & Duckert, L. G. (1989). Relation of hearing impairment to dementia and cognitive dysfunction in older adults. *Journal of the American Medical Association*, *261*(13), 1916–1919. doi:10.1001/jama.1989.03420130084028 PMID:2926927

UNHCR. (2015). *UNHCR Global Trends*. Retrieved from http://www.unhcr.org/576408cd7

Vaccan, C., & Marshark, M. (1997). Communication between parents and deaf children: Implications for social-emotional development. *Journal of Child Psychology and Psychiatry, and Allied Disciplines*, *38*(7), 793–801. doi:10.1111/j.1469-7610.1997.tb01597.x PMID:9363578

Valaskivi, K. (2007). *Mapping media and communication research.* Department of Communication: University of Helsinki. Retrieved from www.helsinki.fi/crc /Julkaisut/ReportJapan.pdf

Valmaggia, L. R., Latif, L., Kempton, M. J., & Rus-Calafell, M. (2016). Virtual reality in the psychological treatment for mental health problems: An systematic review of recent evidence. *Psychiatry Research*, *236*, 189–195. doi:10.1016/j.psychres.2016.01.015 PMID:26795129

van Beugen, S., Ferwerda, M., Hoeve, D., Rovers, M. M., Spillekom-van Koulil, S., van Middendorp, H., & Evers, A. W. (2014). Internet-based cognitive behavioral therapy for patients with chronic somatic conditions: A meta-analytic review. *Journal of Medical Internet Research*, *16*(3), e88. doi:10.2196/jmir.2777 PMID:24675372

Van den Noort, M., Lim, S., & Bosch, P. (2016). On the need to unify neuroscience and physics. *Neuroimmunology and Neuroinflammation*, *3*(12), 271–273. doi:10.20517/2347-8659.2016.55

Van der Kolk, B. A., & McFarlane, A. C. (1996). *Traumatic stress: The effects of overwhelming experience on mind, body, and society*. Guilford Press.

Van Eldik, T., Trefferes, P. D. A., Veerman, J. W., & Verhulst, F. C. (2004). Mental health problems of deaf Dutch children as indicated by parents responses to the Child Behavior Checklist. *American Annals of the Deaf*, *148*(5), 390–395. doi:10.1353/aad.2004.0002 PMID:15132019

van Spijker, B. A., van Straten, A., & Kerkhof, A. J. (2014). Effectiveness of online self-help for suicidal thoughts: Results of a randomised controlled trial. *PLoS One*, *9*(2), e90118. doi:10.1371/journal.pone.0090118 PMID:24587233

Vandelanotte, C., Spathonis, K. M., Eakin, E. G., & Owen, N. (2007). Website-delivered physical activity interventions a review of the literature. *American Journal of Preventive Medicine*, *33*(1), 54–64. doi:10.1016/j.amepre.2007.02.041 PMID:17572313

Vasterling, J. J., Brailey K. (2005). *Neuropsychological Findings in Adults With PTSD*. Academic Press.

Venail, I., Vieu, A., Artieres, F., Mondain, M., & Uziel, A. (2010). Educational and Employment Achievements in Prelingually Deaf Children who receive cochlear implants. *Archives of Otolaryngology--Head & Neck Surgery*, *136*(4), 366–372. doi:10.1001/archoto.2010.31 PMID:20403853

von Seth, R. (2011). The language of the press in Soviet and post-Soviet Russia: Creation of the citizen role through newspaper discourse. *Journalism*, *13*(1), 53–70. doi:10.1177/1464884911400844

Walker, C., & Orttung, R. W. (2014). Breaking the news: The role of state-run media. *Journal of Democracy*, *25*(1), 71–85. doi:10.1353/jod.2014.0015

Ward, M. E., Shelley, K., Kaase, K., & Pane, J. F. (2008). Hurricane Katrina: A longitudinal study of the achievement and behavior of displaced students. *Journal of Education for Students Placed at Risk*, *13*(2-3), 297–317. doi:10.1080/10824660802350391

Warshaw, M. G., Fierman, E., Pratt, L., Hunt, M., Yonkers, K. A., Massion, A. O., & .... (1993). Quality of life and dissociation in anxiety disorder patients with histories of trauma or PTSD. *The American Journal of Psychiatry*, *150*(10), 1512–1516. doi:10.1176/ajp.150.10.1512 PMID:8379556

Weems, C. F., Scott, B. G., & Banks, D. M. (2012). Is TV traumatic for all youths? The role of preexisting posttraumatic-stress symptoms in the link between disaster coverage and stress. *Psychological Science, 23*(11), 1293-1297. doi:10.1177 /0956797612446952

Weine, S., Becker, D., McGlashan, T., Laub, D., Lazrove, S., & Vojvoda, D. (1995). Psychiatric consequences of" ethnic cleansing": Clinical assessments and trauma testimonies of newly resettled Bosnian refugees. *The American Journal of Psychiatry*, *152*(4), 536–542. doi:10.1176/ajp.152.4.536 PMID:7694901

Weisel, A., & Cinamon, G. C. (2005). Hearing, deaf and HH Israeli adolescents' evaluation of deaf men and deaf women's occupational competence. *Journal of Deaf Studies and Deaf Education*, *10*(4), 376–389. doi:10.1093/deafed/eni045 PMID:16037482

Weiss, J. M., & Grunert, B. K. (2004). Posttraumatic stress disorder following traumatic injuries in adult. *Wisconsin Medical Journal*, *103*(6).

Weitzer, R. (2015). American policing under fire: Misconduct and reform. *Social Science and Public Policy*, *52*, 475–480.

Welch, M., Price, E., & Yankey, N. (2004). Youth violence and race in the media: The emergence of "wilding" as an invention of the press. *Race, Gender, & Class*, *11*, 36–48.

Wells, K. B. (1989). The functioning and well-being of Depressed Patients: Results from the Medical Outcomes Study. *Journal of the American Medical Association*, *262*(7), 914–919. doi:10.1001/jama.1989.03430070062031 PMID:2754791

What is depression? (n.d.). Retrieved 20 March 2018 from https://www.cdc.gov/tobacco/campaign/tips/diseases/depression-anxiety.html

Whiteman, K. L., Lohman, M. C., Gill, L. E., Bruce, M. L., & Bartels, S. J. (2017). Adapting a Psychosocial Intervention for Smartphone Delivery to Middle-Aged and Older Adults with Serious Mental Illness. *The American Journal of Geriatric Psychiatry*, *25*(8), 819–828. doi:10.1016/j.jagp.2016.12.007 PMID:28169129

WHO. (2015). *Global status report on road safety*. Geneva: World Health Organization.

Wild, J., Warnock-Parkes, E., Grey, N., Stott, R., Wiedemann, M., Canvin, L., ... Ehlers, A. (2016). Internet-delivered cognitive therapy for PTSD: A development pilot series. *European Journal of Psychotraumatology*, *7*(1), 31019. doi:10.3402/ejpt.v7.31019 PMID:27837579

Wu, G., Ren, S., Tang, R., Xu, C., Zhou, J., Lin, S., ... Yang, J. (2017). Antidepressant effect of taurine in chronic unpredictable mild stress-induced depressive rats. *Scientific Reports*, *7*(1). PMID:28694433

Yalın, Ş. S., Uzel, B. T., Öztürk, M., Gözaçanlar, Ö., Yörük, G. Ü., & Özkan, Y. (2017). Immigration-related mental health disorders in refugees 5–18 years old living in Turkey. *Neuropsychiatric Disease and Treatment, 13*, 2813–2821. doi:10.2147/NDT.S150592 PMID:29180867

Yeager, A. (2013). Watching media coverage of disasters linked to stress. *Science News*. Retrieved from https://www.sciencenews.org/blog/science-ticker/watching-media-coverage-disasters-linked-stress

Yeung, N. C. A., Yu, N. X., Xu, Z., Zhang, Q., Lau, J. T. F., Zhang, J., ... Lui, W. W. S. (2016). Media exposure related to the 2008 Sichuan earthquake predicted probable PTSD among Chinese adolescents in Kunming, China: A longitudinal study. *Psychological Trauma: Theory, Research, Practice, and Policy, 10*(2), 253–262. doi:10.1037/tra0000121 PMID:27428553

Young, K. D., Zotev, V., Phillips, R., Misaki, M., Drevets, W. C., & Bodurka, J. (2018). Amygdala Real-Time fMRI Neurofeedback for Major Depressive Disorder: A Review. *Psychiatry and Clinical Neurosciences*. doi:10.1111/pcn.12665

Young, S. (2007). How to increase serotonin in the human brain without drugs. *Journal of Psychiatry & Neuroscience, 32*(6), 394–399. PMID:18043762

Yukalov, V. I., & Sornette, D. (2011). Decision theory with prospect interference and entanglement. *Theory and Decision, 70*(3), 283–328. doi:10.100711238-010-9202-y

Yule, W., Bolton, D., Udwin, O., Boyle, S., O'Ryan, D., & Nurrish, J. (2000). The long-term psychological effects of a disaster experienced in adolescence: I: The incidence and course of PTSD. *Journal of Child Psychology and Psychiatry, and Allied Disciplines, 41*(4), 503–511. doi:10.1111/1469-7610.00635 PMID:10836680

Yule, W., & Smith, P. (2015). Post traumatic stress disorder. In A. Thapar, D. S. Pine, J. F. Leckman, S. Scott, M. J. Snowling, & E. Taylor (Eds.), *Rutter's Child and Adolescent Psychiatry* (6th ed.; pp. 806–821). John Wiley & Sons, Ltd. doi:10.1002/9781118381953.ch59

Yuwen, L., & Goldscmidt, J.E. (2009). *Taking Employment Discrimination Seriously. Chinese and European Perspectives*. Leiden: Martinus Nijhoff Publishers.

Zaidan, S., & Roehrer, E. (2016). Popular mobile phone apps for diet and weight loss: A content analysis. *JMIR mHealth and uHealth*, *4*(3), e80. doi:10.2196/mhealth.5406 PMID:27400806

Zhuo, X., Zhang, P., Kahn, H. S., Bardenheier, B. H., Li, R., & Gregg, E. W. (2015). Change in medical spending attributable to diabetes: National data from 1987 to 2011. *Diabetes Care*, *38*(4), 581–587. doi:10.2337/dc14-1687 PMID:25592194

Related References

To continue our tradition of advancing information science and technology research, we have compiled a list of recommended IGI Global readings. These references will provide additional information and guidance to further enrich your knowledge and assist you with your own research and future publications.

Abu Seman, S. A., & Ramayah, T. (2017). Are We Ready to App?: A Study on mHealth Apps, Its Future, and Trends in Malaysia Context. In J. Pelet (Ed.), *Mobile Platforms, Design, and Apps for Social Commerce* (pp. 69–83). Hershey, PA: IGI Global. doi:10.4018/978-1-5225-2469-4.ch005

Aggarwal, S., & Azad, V. (2017). A Hybrid System Based on FMM and MLP to Diagnose Heart Disease. In S. Bhattacharyya, S. De, I. Pan, & P. Dutta (Eds.), *Intelligent Multidimensional Data Clustering and Analysis* (pp. 293–325). Hershey, PA: IGI Global. doi:10.4018/978-1-5225-1776-4.ch011

Akaichi, J., & Mhadhbi, L. (2016). A Clinical Decision Support System: Ontology-Driven Approach for Effective Emergency Management. In J. Moon & M. Galea (Eds.), *Improving Health Management through Clinical Decision Support Systems* (pp. 270–294). Hershey, PA: IGI Global. doi:10.4018/978-1-4666-9432-3.ch013

Akerkar, R. (2016). Towards an Intelligent Integrated Approach for Clinical Decision Support. In A. Aggarwal (Ed.), *Managing Big Data Integration in the Public Sector* (pp. 187–205). Hershey, PA: IGI Global. doi:10.4018/978-1-4666-9649-5.ch011

Al-Busaidi, S. S. (2018). Interdisciplinary Relationships Between Medicine and Social Sciences. In M. Al-Suqri, A. Al-Kindi, S. AlKindi, & N. Saleem (Eds.), *Promoting Interdisciplinarity in Knowledge Generation and Problem Solving* (pp. 124–137). Hershey, PA: IGI Global. doi:10.4018/978-1-5225-3878-3.ch009

Al Kareh, T., & Thoumy, M. (2018). The Impact of Health Information Digitization on the Physiotherapist-Patient Relationship: A Pilot Study of the Lebanese Community. *International Journal of Healthcare Information Systems and Informatics, 13*(2), 29–53. doi:10.4018/IJHISI.2018040103

Alenzuela, R. (2017). Research, Leadership, and Resource-Sharing Initiatives: The Role of Local Library Consortia in Access to Medical Information. In S. Ram (Ed.), *Library and Information Services for Bioinformatics Education and Research* (pp. 199–211). Hershey, PA: IGI Global. doi:10.4018/978-1-5225-1871-6.ch012

Ameri, H., Alizadeh, S., & Noughabi, E. A. (2017). Application of Data Mining Techniques in Clinical Decision Making: A Literature Review and Classification. In E. Noughabi, B. Raahemi, A. Albadvi, & B. Far (Eds.), *Handbook of Research on Data Science for Effective Healthcare Practice and Administration* (pp. 257–295). Hershey, PA: IGI Global. doi:10.4018/978-1-5225-2515-8.ch012

Anand, S. (2017). Medical Image Enhancement Using Edge Information-Based Methods. In B. Singh (Ed.), *Computational Tools and Techniques for Biomedical Signal Processing* (pp. 123–148). Hershey, PA: IGI Global. doi:10.4018/978-1-5225-0660-7.ch006

Angjellari-Dajci, F., Sapienza, C., Lawless, W. F., & Kavanagh, K. (2016). Human Capital Accumulation in Medical Simulated Learning Environments: A Framework for Economic Evaluation. In M. Russ (Ed.), *Quantitative Multidisciplinary Approaches in Human Capital and Asset Management* (pp. 65–88). Hershey, PA: IGI Global. doi:10.4018/978-1-4666-9652-5.ch004

Anil, M., Ayyildiz-Tamis, D., Tasdemir, S., Sendemir-Urkmez, A., & Gulce-Iz, S. (2016). Bioinspired Materials and Biocompatibility. In M. Bououdina (Ed.), *Emerging Research on Bioinspired Materials Engineering* (pp. 294–322). Hershey, PA: IGI Global. doi:10.4018/978-1-4666-9811-6.ch011

Anton, J. L., Soriano, J. V., Martinez, M. I., & Garcia, F. B. (2018). Comprehensive E-Learning Appraisal System. In M. Khosrow-Pour, D.B.A. (Ed.), Encyclopedia of Information Science and Technology, Fourth Edition (pp. 5787-5799). Hershey, PA: IGI Global. doi:10.4018/978-1-5225-2255-3.ch503

Arabi, M. (2016). Redesigning the Organizational Structure to Reach Efficiency: The Case of Ministry of Health and Medical Education of Iran. In R. Gholipour & K. Rouzbehani (Eds.), *Social, Economic, and Political Perspectives on Public Health Policy-Making* (pp. 257–294). Hershey, PA: IGI Global. doi:10.4018/978-1-4666-9944-1.ch012

Assis-Hassid, S., Heart, T., Reychav, I., & Pliskin, J. S. (2016). Modelling Factors Affecting Patient-Doctor-Computer Communication in Primary Care. *International Journal of Reliable and Quality E-Healthcare*, *5*(1), 1–17. doi:10.4018/IJRQEH.2016010101

Atzori, B., Hoffman, H. G., Vagnoli, L., Messeri, A., & Grotto, R. L. (2018). Virtual Reality as Distraction Technique for Pain Management in Children and Adolescents. In M. Khosrow-Pour, D.B.A. (Ed.), Encyclopedia of Information Science and Technology, Fourth Edition (pp. 5955-5965). Hershey, PA: IGI Global. doi:10.4018/978-1-5225-2255-3.ch518

Audibert, M., Mathonnat, J., Pélissier, A., & Huang, X. X. (2018). The Impact of the New Rural Cooperative Medical Scheme on Township Hospitals' Utilization and Income Structure in Weifang Prefecture, China. In I. Management Association (Ed.), Health Economics and Healthcare Reform: Breakthroughs in Research and Practice (pp. 109-121). Hershey, PA: IGI Global. doi:10.4018/978-1-5225-3168-5.ch007

Ayyachamy, S. (2016). Analysis and Comparison of Developed 2D Medical Image Database Design using Registration Scheme, Retrieval Scheme, and Bag-of-Visual-Words. In N. Dey & A. Ashour (Eds.), *Classification and Clustering in Biomedical Signal Processing* (pp. 149–168). Hershey, PA: IGI Global. doi:10.4018/978-1-5225-0140-4.ch007

Babalola, A. C. (2016). Literacy and Decision Making on Health Issues among Married Women in Southwest Nigeria. In V. Wang (Ed.), *Handbook of Research on Advancing Health Education through Technology* (pp. 191–212). Hershey, PA: IGI Global. doi:10.4018/978-1-4666-9494-1.ch009

Babu, A., & Ayyappan, S. (2017). A Methodological Evaluation of Crypto-Watermarking System for Medical Images. In C. Bhatt & S. Peddoju (Eds.), *Cloud Computing Systems and Applications in Healthcare* (pp. 189–217). Hershey, PA: IGI Global. doi:10.4018/978-1-5225-1002-4.ch010

Bakke, A. (2017). Ethos in E-Health: From Informational to Interactive Websites. In M. Folk & S. Apostel (Eds.), *Establishing and Evaluating Digital Ethos and Online Credibility* (pp. 85–103). Hershey, PA: IGI Global. doi:10.4018/978-1-5225-1072-7.ch005

Bali, S. (2018). Enhancing the Reach of Health Care Through Telemedicine: Status and New Possibilities in Developing Countries. In U. Pandey & V. Indrakanti (Eds.), *Open and Distance Learning Initiatives for Sustainable Development* (pp. 339–354). Hershey, PA: IGI Global. doi:10.4018/978-1-5225-2621-6.ch019

Barrett, T. E. (2018). Essentials for Education and Training for Tomorrow's Physicians. In C. Smith (Ed.), *Exploring the Pressures of Medical Education From a Mental Health and Wellness Perspective* (pp. 230–252). Hershey, PA: IGI Global. doi:10.4018/978-1-5225-2811-1.ch010

Barrett, T. J. (2016). Knowledge in Action: Fostering Health Education through Technology. In V. Wang (Ed.), *Handbook of Research on Advancing Health Education through Technology* (pp. 39–62). Hershey, PA: IGI Global. doi:10.4018/978-1-4666-9494-1.ch003

Berrahal, S., & Boudriga, N. (2017). The Risks of Wearable Technologies to Individuals and Organizations. In A. Marrington, D. Kerr, & J. Gammack (Eds.), *Managing Security Issues and the Hidden Dangers of Wearable Technologies* (pp. 18–46). Hershey, PA: IGI Global. doi:10.4018/978-1-5225-1016-1.ch002

Bhagat, A. P., & Atique, M. (2016). Medical Image Mining Using Fuzzy Connectedness Image Segmentation: Efficient Retrieval of Patients' Stored Images. In W. Karâa & N. Dey (Eds.), *Biomedical Image Analysis and Mining Techniques for Improved Health Outcomes* (pp. 184–209). Hershey, PA: IGI Global. doi:10.4018/978-1-4666-8811-7.ch009

Bhargava, P. (2018). Blended Learning: An Effective Application to Clinical Teaching. In S. Tang & C. Lim (Eds.), *Preparing the Next Generation of Teachers for 21st Century Education* (pp. 302–320). Hershey, PA: IGI Global. doi:10.4018/978-1-5225-4080-9.ch018

Binh, N. T., & Tuyet, V. T. (2016). The Combination of Adaptive Filters to Improve the Quality of Medical Images in New Wavelet Domain. In N. Dey & A. Ashour (Eds.), *Classification and Clustering in Biomedical Signal Processing* (pp. 46–76). Hershey, PA: IGI Global. doi:10.4018/978-1-5225-0140-4.ch003

Bird, J. L. (2017). Writing Healing Narratives. In V. Bryan & J. Bird (Eds.), *Healthcare Community Synergism between Patients, Practitioners, and Researchers* (pp. 1–28). Hershey, PA: IGI Global. doi:10.4018/978-1-5225-0640-9.ch001

Bottrighi, A., Leonardi, G., Piovesan, L., & Terenziani, P. (2016). Knowledge-Based Support to the Treatment of Exceptions in Computer Interpretable Clinical Guidelines. *International Journal of Knowledge-Based Organizations, 6*(3), 1–27. doi:10.4018/IJKBO.2016070101

Bougoulias, K., Kouris, I., Prasinos, M., Giokas, K., & Koutsouris, D. (2017). Ob/Gyn EMR Software: A Solution for Obstetricians and Gynecologists. In A. Moumtzoglou (Ed.), *Design, Development, and Integration of Reliable Electronic Healthcare Platforms* (pp. 101–111). Hershey, PA: IGI Global. doi:10.4018/978-1-5225-1724-5.ch006

Bouslimi, R., Ayadi, M. G., & Akaichi, J. (2018). Medical Image Retrieval in Healthcare Social Networks. *International Journal of Healthcare Information Systems and Informatics, 13*(2), 13–28. doi:10.4018/IJHISI.2018040102

Bouzaabia, O., Bouzaabia, R., & Mejri, K. (2017). Role of Internet in the Development of Medical Tourism Service in Tunisia. In A. Capatina & E. Rancati (Eds.), *Key Challenges and Opportunities in Web Entrepreneurship* (pp. 211–241). Hershey, PA: IGI Global. doi:10.4018/978-1-5225-2466-3.ch009

Briz-Ponce, L., Juanes-Méndez, J. A., & García-Peñalvo, F. J. (2016). The Role of Gender in Technology Acceptance for Medical Education. In M. Cruz-Cunha, I. Miranda, R. Martinho, & R. Rijo (Eds.), *Encyclopedia of E-Health and Telemedicine* (pp. 1013–1027). Hershey, PA: IGI Global. doi:10.4018/978-1-4666-9978-6.ch079

Briz-Ponce, L., Juanes-Méndez, J. A., & García-Peñalvo, F. J. (2016). A Research Contribution to the Analysis of Mobile Devices in Higher Education from Medical Students' Point of View. In L. Briz-Ponce, J. Juanes-Méndez, & F. García-Peñalvo (Eds.), *Handbook of Research on Mobile Devices and Applications in Higher Education Settings* (pp. 196–221). Hershey, PA: IGI Global. doi:10.4018/978-1-5225-0256-2.ch009

Brown-Jackson, K. L. (2018). Telemedicine and Telehealth: Academics Engaging the Community in a Call to Action. In S. Burton (Ed.), *Engaged Scholarship and Civic Responsibility in Higher Education* (pp. 166–193). Hershey, PA: IGI Global. doi:10.4018/978-1-5225-3649-9.ch008

Bwalya, K. J. (2017). Next Wave of Tele-Medicine: Virtual Presence of Medical Personnel. In K. Moahi, K. Bwalya, & P. Sebina (Eds.), *Health Information Systems and the Advancement of Medical Practice in Developing Countries* (pp. 168–180). Hershey, PA: IGI Global. doi:10.4018/978-1-5225-2262-1.ch010

Carlton, E. L., Holsinger, J. W. Jr, & Anunobi, N. (2016). Physician Engagement with Health Information Technology: Implications for Practice and Professionalism. *International Journal of Computers in Clinical Practice*, *1*(2), 51–73. doi:10.4018/IJCCP.2016070103

Castillo-Page, L., Eliason, J., Conrad, S. S., & Nivet, M. A. (2016). Diversity in Undergraduate Medical Education: An Examination of Organizational Culture and Climate in Medical Schools. In C. Scott & J. Sims (Eds.), *Developing Workforce Diversity Programs, Curriculum, and Degrees in Higher Education* (pp. 304–326). Hershey, PA: IGI Global. doi:10.4018/978-1-5225-0209-8.ch016

Cebeci, H. I., & Hiziroglu, A. (2016). Review of Business Intelligence and Intelligent Systems in Healthcare Domain. In N. Celebi (Ed.), *Intelligent Techniques for Data Analysis in Diverse Settings* (pp. 192–206). Hershey, PA: IGI Global. doi:10.4018/978-1-5225-0075-9.ch009

Celik, G. (2018). Determining Headache Diseases With Genetic Algorithm. In U. Kose, G. Guraksin, & O. Deperlioglu (Eds.), *Nature-Inspired Intelligent Techniques for Solving Biomedical Engineering Problems* (pp. 249–262). Hershey, PA: IGI Global. doi:10.4018/978-1-5225-4769-3.ch012

Chakraborty, C., Gupta, B., & Ghosh, S. K. (2016). Mobile Telemedicine Systems for Remote Patient's Chronic Wound Monitoring. In A. Moumtzoglou (Ed.), *M-Health Innovations for Patient-Centered Care* (pp. 213–239). Hershey, PA: IGI Global. doi:10.4018/978-1-4666-9861-1.ch011

Chakraborty, S., Chatterjee, S., Ashour, A. S., Mali, K., & Dey, N. (2018). Intelligent Computing in Medical Imaging: A Study. In N. Dey (Ed.), *Advancements in Applied Metaheuristic Computing* (pp. 143–163). Hershey, PA: IGI Global. doi:10.4018/978-1-5225-4151-6.ch006

Chavez, A., & Kovarik, C. (2017). Open Source Technology for Medical Practice in Developing Countries. In K. Moahi, K. Bwalya, & P. Sebina (Eds.), *Health Information Systems and the Advancement of Medical Practice in Developing Countries* (pp. 33–59). Hershey, PA: IGI Global. doi:10.4018/978-1-5225-2262-1.ch003

Chen, E. T. (2016). Examining the Influence of Information Technology on Modern Health Care. In P. Manolitzas, E. Grigoroudis, N. Matsatsinis, & D. Yannacopoulos (Eds.), *Effective Methods for Modern Healthcare Service Quality and Evaluation* (pp. 110–136). Hershey, PA: IGI Global. doi:10.4018/978-1-4666-9961-8.ch006

Chin, S. (2016). Surviving Sandy: Recovering Collections after a Natural Disaster. In E. Decker & J. Townes (Eds.), *Handbook of Research on Disaster Management and Contingency Planning in Modern Libraries* (pp. 366–388). Hershey, PA: IGI Global. doi:10.4018/978-1-4666-8624-3.ch016

Chojnacki, M., & Wójcik, A. (2016). Security and the Role of New Technologies and Innovation in Medical Ethics. In A. Rosiek & K. Leksowski (Eds.), *Organizational Culture and Ethics in Modern Medicine* (pp. 52–77). Hershey, PA: IGI Global. doi:10.4018/978-1-4666-9658-7.ch003

Cılız, N., Yıldırım, H., & Temizel, Ş. (2016). Structure Development for Effective Medical Waste and Hazardous Waste Management System. In U. Akkucuk (Ed.), *Handbook of Research on Waste Management Techniques for Sustainability* (pp. 303–327). Hershey, PA: IGI Global. doi:10.4018/978-1-4666-9723-2.ch016

Ciufudean, C. (2018). Innovative Formalism for Biological Data Analysis. In M. Khosrow-Pour, D.B.A. (Ed.), Encyclopedia of Information Science and Technology, Fourth Edition (pp. 1814-1824). Hershey, PA: IGI Global. doi:10.4018/978-1-5225-2255-3.ch158

Ciufudean, C., & Ciufudean, O. (2016). Tele-Monitoring for Medical Diagnosis Availability. In M. Cruz-Cunha, I. Miranda, R. Martinho, & R. Rijo (Eds.), *Encyclopedia of E-Health and Telemedicine* (pp. 401–411). Hershey, PA: IGI Global. doi:10.4018/978-1-4666-9978-6.ch032

Colaguori, R., & Danesi, M. (2017). Medical Semiotics: A Revisitation and an Exhortation. *International Journal of Semiotics and Visual Rhetoric*, *1*(1), 11–18. doi:10.4018/IJSVR.2017010102

Cole, A. W., & Salek, T. A. (2017). Adopting a Parasocial Connection to Overcome Professional Kakoethos in Online Health Information. In M. Folk & S. Apostel (Eds.), *Establishing and Evaluating Digital Ethos and Online Credibility* (pp. 104–120). Hershey, PA: IGI Global. doi:10.4018/978-1-5225-1072-7.ch006

Contreras, E. C., & Puente, G. J. (2016). How to Identify Rheumatic Diseases by General Physicians. In T. Gasmelseid (Ed.), *Advancing Pharmaceutical Processes and Tools for Improved Health Outcomes* (pp. 136–166). Hershey, PA: IGI Global. doi:10.4018/978-1-5225-0248-7.ch006

D'Andrea, A., Ferri, F., & Grifoni, P. (2016). RFID Technologies in Healthcare Setting: Applications and Future Perspectives. *International Journal of Computers in Clinical Practice*, *1*(1), 15–27. doi:10.4018/IJCCP.2016010102

Damianakis, A., Kallonis, P., Loudos, G., Tsatsos, D., & Tsoukalis, A. (2016). Exploiting 3D Medical Equipment Simulations to Support Biomedical Engineering Academic Courses: Design Methodology and Implementation in a Small Scale National Project. In B. Khan (Ed.), *Revolutionizing Modern Education through Meaningful E-Learning Implementation* (pp. 277–295). Hershey, PA: IGI Global. doi:10.4018/978-1-5225-0466-5.ch015

Demiroz, E. (2016). Principles of Instructional Design for E-Learning and Online Learning Practices: Implications for Medical Education. In V. Wang (Ed.), *Handbook of Research on Advancing Health Education through Technology* (pp. 419–451). Hershey, PA: IGI Global. doi:10.4018/978-1-4666-9494-1.ch018

Deperlioglu, O. (2018). Intelligent Techniques Inspired by Nature and Used in Biomedical Engineering. In U. Kose, G. Guraksin, & O. Deperlioglu (Eds.), *Nature-Inspired Intelligent Techniques for Solving Biomedical Engineering Problems* (pp. 51–77). Hershey, PA: IGI Global. doi:10.4018/978-1-5225-4769-3.ch003

Dey, N., & Ashour, A. S. (2018). Meta-Heuristic Algorithms in Medical Image Segmentation: A Review. In N. Dey (Ed.), *Advancements in Applied Metaheuristic Computing* (pp. 185–203). Hershey, PA: IGI Global. doi:10.4018/978-1-5225-4151-6.ch008

Dey, N., Ashour, A. S., & Althoupety, A. S. (2017). Thermal Imaging in Medical Science. In V. Santhi (Ed.), *Recent Advances in Applied Thermal Imaging for Industrial Applications* (pp. 87–117). Hershey, PA: IGI Global. doi:10.4018/978-1-5225-2423-6.ch004

Di Virgilio, F., Camillo, A. A., & Camillo, I. C. (2017). The Impact of Social Network on Italian Users' Behavioural Intention for the Choice of a Medical Tourist Destination. *International Journal of Tourism and Hospitality Management in the Digital Age, 1*(1), 36–49. doi:10.4018/IJTHMDA.2017010103

Dias, C. M., Ribeiro, A. G., & Furtado, S. F. (2016). An Overview about the Use of Healthcare Applications on Mobile Devices. In M. Cruz-Cunha, I. Miranda, R. Martinho, & R. Rijo (Eds.), *Encyclopedia of E-Health and Telemedicine* (pp. 285–298). Hershey, PA: IGI Global. doi:10.4018/978-1-4666-9978-6.ch024

Dogra, A. K., & Dogra, P. (2017). The Medical Tourism Industry in the BRIC Nations: An Indian Analysis. In M. Dhiman (Ed.), *Opportunities and Challenges for Tourism and Hospitality in the BRIC Nations* (pp. 320–336). Hershey, PA: IGI Global. doi:10.4018/978-1-5225-0708-6.ch020

Drowos, J. L., & Wood, S. K. (2017). Preparing Future Physicians to Adapt to the Changing Health Care System: Promoting Humanism through Curricular Design. In V. Bryan & J. Bird (Eds.), *Healthcare Community Synergism between Patients, Practitioners, and Researchers* (pp. 106–125). Hershey, PA: IGI Global. doi:10.4018/978-1-5225-0640-9.ch006

Dulam, K. (2017). Medical Patents and Impact on Availability and Affordability of Essential Medicines in India. In R. Aggarwal & R. Kaur (Eds.), *Patent Law and Intellectual Property in the Medical Field* (pp. 41–57). Hershey, PA: IGI Global. doi:10.4018/978-1-5225-2414-4.ch003

Dutta, P. (2017). Decision Making in Medical Diagnosis via Distance Measures on Interval Valued Fuzzy Sets. *International Journal of System Dynamics Applications*, *6*(4), 63–83. doi:10.4018/IJSDA.2017100104

Edoh, T. O., Pawar, P. A., Brügge, B., & Teege, G. (2016). A Multidisciplinary Remote Healthcare Delivery System to Increase Health Care Access, Pathology Screening, and Treatment in Developing Countries: The Case of Benin. *International Journal of Healthcare Information Systems and Informatics*, *11*(4), 1–31. doi:10.4018/IJHISI.2016100101

El Guemhioui, K., & Demurjian, S. A. (2017). Semantic Reconciliation of Electronic Health Records Using Semantic Web Technologies. *International Journal of Information Technology and Web Engineering*, *12*(2), 26–48. doi:10.4018/IJITWE.2017040102

Ellouze, N., Rekhis, S., & Boudriga, N. (2016). Forensic Investigation of Digital Crimes in Healthcare Applications. In O. Isafiade & A. Bagula (Eds.), *Data Mining Trends and Applications in Criminal Science and Investigations* (pp. 169–210). Hershey, PA: IGI Global. doi:10.4018/978-1-5225-0463-4.ch007

Eneanya, A. N. (2016). Health Policy Implementation and Its Barriers: The Case Study of US Health System. In R. Gholipour & K. Rouzbehani (Eds.), *Social, Economic, and Political Perspectives on Public Health Policy-Making* (pp. 42–63). Hershey, PA: IGI Global. doi:10.4018/978-1-4666-9944-1.ch003

Entico, G. J. (2016). Knowledge Management and the Medical Health Librarians: A Perception Study. In J. Yap, M. Perez, M. Ayson, & G. Entico (Eds.), *Special Library Administration, Standardization and Technological Integration* (pp. 52–77). Hershey, PA: IGI Global. doi:10.4018/978-1-4666-9542-9.ch003

Ferradji, M. A., & Zidani, A. (2016). Collaborative Environment for Remote Clinical Reasoning Learning. *International Journal of E-Health and Medical Communications, 7*(4), 62–81. doi:10.4018/IJEHMC.2016100104

Fisher, J. (2018). Sociological Perspectives on Improving Medical Diagnosis Emphasizing CAD. In M. Khosrow-Pour, D.B.A. (Ed.), Encyclopedia of Information Science and Technology, Fourth Edition (pp. 1017-1024). Hershey, PA: IGI Global. doi:10.4018/978-1-5225-2255-3.ch088

Flores, C. D., Respício, A., Coelho, H., Bez, M. R., & Fonseca, J. M. (2016). Simulation for Medical Training. In M. Cruz-Cunha, I. Miranda, R. Martinho, & R. Rijo (Eds.), *Encyclopedia of E-Health and Telemedicine* (pp. 827–842). Hershey, PA: IGI Global. doi:10.4018/978-1-4666-9978-6.ch064

Frank, E. M. (2018). Healthcare Education: Integrating Simulation Technologies. In V. Bryan, A. Musgrove, & J. Powers (Eds.), *Handbook of Research on Human Development in the Digital Age* (pp. 163–182). Hershey, PA: IGI Global. doi:10.4018/978-1-5225-2838-8.ch008

Garner, G. (2018). Foundations for Yoga Practice in Rehabilitation. In S. Telles & N. Singh (Eds.), *Research-Based Perspectives on the Psychophysiology of Yoga* (pp. 263–307). Hershey, PA: IGI Global. doi:10.4018/978-1-5225-2788-6.ch015

Gasmelseid, T. M. (2016). Improving Pharmaceutical Care through the Use of Intelligent Pharmacoinformatics. In T. Gasmelseid (Ed.), *Advancing Pharmaceutical Processes and Tools for Improved Health Outcomes* (pp. 167–188). Hershey, PA: IGI Global. doi:10.4018/978-1-5225-0248-7.ch007

Gavurová, B., Kováč, V., & Šoltés, M. (2018). Medical Equipment and Economic Determinants of Its Structure and Regulation in the Slovak Republic. In M. Khosrow-Pour, D.B.A. (Ed.), Encyclopedia of Information Science and Technology, Fourth Edition (pp. 5841-5852). Hershey, PA: IGI Global. doi:10.4018/978-1-5225-2255-3.ch508

Ge, X., Wang, Q., Huang, K., Law, V., & Thomas, D. C. (2017). Designing Simulated Learning Environments and Facilitating Authentic Learning Experiences in Medical Education. In J. Stefaniak (Ed.), *Advancing Medical Education Through Strategic Instructional Design* (pp. 77–100). Hershey, PA: IGI Global. doi:10.4018/978-1-5225-2098-6.ch004

Gewald, H., & Gewald, C. (2018). Inhibitors of Physicians' Use of Mandatory Hospital Information Systems (HIS). *International Journal of Healthcare Information Systems and Informatics, 13*(1), 29–44. doi:10.4018/IJHISI.2018010103

Ghosh, D., & Dinda, S. (2017). Health Infrastructure and Economic Development in India. In R. Das (Ed.), *Social, Health, and Environmental Infrastructures for Economic Growth* (pp. 99–119). Hershey, PA: IGI Global. doi:10.4018/978-1-5225-2364-2.ch006

Ghosh, K., & Sen, K. C. (2017). The Potential of Crowdsourcing in the Health Care Industry. In N. Wickramasinghe (Ed.), *Handbook of Research on Healthcare Administration and Management* (pp. 418–427). Hershey, PA: IGI Global. doi:10.4018/978-1-5225-0920-2.ch024

Ghrab, S., & Saad, I. (2016). Identifying Crucial Know-How and Knowing-That for Medical Decision Support. *International Journal of Decision Support System Technology, 8*(4), 14–33. doi:10.4018/IJDSST.2016100102

Giokas, K., Tsirmpas, C., Anastasiou, A., Iliopoulou, D., Costarides, V., & Koutsouris, D. (2016). Contemporary Heart Failure Treatment Based on Improved Knowledge and Personalized Care of Comorbidities. In D. Fotiadis (Ed.), *Handbook of Research on Trends in the Diagnosis and Treatment of Chronic Conditions* (pp. 301–314). Hershey, PA: IGI Global. doi:10.4018/978-1-4666-8828-5.ch014

Gopalan, V., Chan, E., & Ho, D. T. (2018). Deliberate Self-Harm and Suicide Ideology in Medical Students. In C. Smith (Ed.), *Exploring the Pressures of Medical Education From a Mental Health and Wellness Perspective* (pp. 122–143). Hershey, PA: IGI Global. doi:10.4018/978-1-5225-2811-1.ch005

Goswami, S., Dey, U., Roy, P., Ashour, A., & Dey, N. (2017). Medical Video Processing: Concept and Applications. In N. Dey, A. Ashour, & P. Patra (Eds.), *Feature Detectors and Motion Detection in Video Processing* (pp. 1–17). Hershey, PA: IGI Global. doi:10.4018/978-1-5225-1025-3.ch001

Goswami, S., Mahanta, K., Goswami, S., Jigdung, T., & Devi, T. P. (2018). Ageing and Cancer: The Epigenetic Basis, Alternative Treatment, and Care. In B. Prasad & S. Akbar (Eds.), *Handbook of Research on Geriatric Health, Treatment, and Care* (pp. 206–235). Hershey, PA: IGI Global. doi:10.4018/978-1-5225-3480-8.ch012

Gouva, M. I. (2017). The Psychological Impact of Medical Error on Patients, Family Members, and Health Professionals. In M. Riga (Ed.), *Impact of Medical Errors and Malpractice on Health Economics, Quality, and Patient Safety* (pp. 171–196). Hershey, PA: IGI Global. doi:10.4018/978-1-5225-2337-6.ch007

Gürcü, M., & Tengilimoğlu, D. (2017). Health Tourism-Based Destination Marketing. In A. Bayraktar & C. Uslay (Eds.), *Strategic Place Branding Methodologies and Theory for Tourist Attraction* (pp. 308–331). Hershey, PA: IGI Global. doi:10.4018/978-1-5225-0579-2.ch015

Gürsel, G. (2016). Mobility in Healthcare: M-Health. In A. Panagopoulos (Ed.), *Handbook of Research on Next Generation Mobile Communication Systems* (pp. 485–511). Hershey, PA: IGI Global. doi:10.4018/978-1-4666-8732-5.ch019

Gürsel, G. (2017). For Better Healthcare Mining Health Data. In S. Bhattacharyya, S. De, I. Pan, & P. Dutta (Eds.), *Intelligent Multidimensional Data Clustering and Analysis* (pp. 135–158). Hershey, PA: IGI Global. doi:10.4018/978-1-5225-1776-4.ch006

Guzman-Lugo, G., Lopez-Martinez, M., Lopez-Ramirez, B., & Avila-Vazquez, D. (2016). City-Driven Approach to Determine Health Services Based on Current User Location and Collaborative Information. *International Journal of Knowledge Society Research*, *7*(1), 53–62. doi:10.4018/IJKSR.2016010104

Gyaase, P. O., Darko-Lartey, R., William, H., & Borkloe, F. (2017). Towards an Integrated Electronic Medical Records System for Quality Healthcare in Ghana: An Exploratory Factor Analysis. *International Journal of Computers in Clinical Practice*, *2*(2), 38–55. doi:10.4018/IJCCP.2017070103

Handayani, P. W., Sandhyaduhita, P. I., Hidayanto, A. N., Pinem, A. A., Fajrina, H. R., Junus, K. M., ... Ayuningtyas, D. (2016). Integrated Hospital Information System Architecture Design in Indonesia. In T. Iyamu & A. Tatnall (Eds.), *Maximizing Healthcare Delivery and Management through Technology Integration* (pp. 207–236). Hershey, PA: IGI Global. doi:10.4018/978-1-4666-9446-0.ch013

Hanel, P. (2017). Is China Catching Up?: Health-Related Applications of Biotechnology. In T. Bas & J. Zhao (Eds.), *Comparative Approaches to Biotechnology Development and Use in Developed and Emerging Nations* (pp. 465–520). Hershey, PA: IGI Global. doi:10.4018/978-1-5225-1040-6.ch016

Harmsen, C. A., & Royle, R. N. (2016). St. Stephen's Hospital Hervey Bay: Study of Developing a Digital Hospital. In J. Moon & M. Galea (Eds.), *Improving Health Management through Clinical Decision Support Systems* (pp. 127–153). Hershey, PA: IGI Global. doi:10.4018/978-1-4666-9432-3.ch006

Harp, D., Shim, R. S., Johnson, J., Harp, J. A., Wilcox, W. C., & Wilcox, J. K. (2016). Race and Gender Inequalities in Medicine and Biomedical Research. In U. Thomas & J. Drake (Eds.), *Critical Research on Sexism and Racism in STEM Fields* (pp. 115–134). Hershey, PA: IGI Global. doi:10.4018/978-1-5225-0174-9.ch006

Hartman, A., & Brown, S. (2017). Synergism through Therapeutic Visual Arts. In V. Bryan & J. Bird (Eds.), *Healthcare Community Synergism between Patients, Practitioners, and Researchers* (pp. 29–48). Hershey, PA: IGI Global. doi:10.4018/978-1-5225-0640-9.ch002

Hazra, J., Chowdhury, A. R., & Dutta, P. (2016). Cluster Based Medical Image Registration Using Optimized Neural Network. In S. Bhattacharyya, P. Banerjee, D. Majumdar, & P. Dutta (Eds.), *Handbook of Research on Advanced Hybrid Intelligent Techniques and Applications* (pp. 551–581). Hershey, PA: IGI Global. doi:10.4018/978-1-4666-9474-3.ch018

Hung, S., Huang, W., Yen, D. C., Chang, S., & Lu, C. (2016). Effect of Information Service Competence and Contextual Factors on the Effectiveness of Strategic Information Systems Planning in Hospitals. *Journal of Global Information Management*, *24*(1), 14–36. doi:10.4018/JGIM.2016010102

Iltchev, P., Śliwczyński, A., Szynkiewicz, P., & Marczak, M. (2016). Mobile Health Applications Assisting Patients with Chronic Diseases: Examples from Asthma Care. In A. Moumtzoglou (Ed.), *M-Health Innovations for Patient-Centered Care* (pp. 170–196). Hershey, PA: IGI Global. doi:10.4018/978-1-4666-9861-1.ch009

Iqbal, S., Ahmad, S., & Willis, I. (2017). Influencing Factors for Adopting Technology Enhanced Learning in the Medical Schools of Punjab, Pakistan. *International Journal of Information and Communication Technology Education, 13*(3), 27–39. doi:10.4018/IJICTE.2017070103

Jagan, J., Dalkiliç, Y., & Samui, P. (2016). Utilization of SVM, LSSVM and GP for Predicting the Medical Waste Generation. In G. Hua (Ed.), *Smart Cities as a Solution for Reducing Urban Waste and Pollution* (pp. 224–251). Hershey, PA: IGI Global. doi:10.4018/978-1-5225-0302-6.ch008

Jagiello, K., Sosnowska, A., Mikolajczyk, A., & Puzyn, T. (2017). Nanomaterials in Medical Devices: Regulations' Review and Future Perspectives. *Journal of Nanotoxicology and Nanomedicine, 2*(2), 1–11. doi:10.4018/JNN.2017070101

Jena, T. K. (2018). Skill Training Process in Medicine Through Distance Mode. In U. Pandey & V. Indrakanti (Eds.), *Optimizing Open and Distance Learning in Higher Education Institutions* (pp. 228–243). Hershey, PA: IGI Global. doi:10.4018/978-1-5225-2624-7.ch010

Jesus, Â., & Gomes, M. J. (2016). Web 2.0 Tools in Biomedical and Pharmaceutical Education: Updated Review and Commentary. In T. Gasmelseid (Ed.), *Advancing Pharmaceutical Processes and Tools for Improved Health Outcomes* (pp. 52–78). Hershey, PA: IGI Global. doi:10.4018/978-1-5225-0248-7.ch003

Joseph, V., & Miller, J. M. (2018). Medical Students' Perceived Stigma in Seeking Care: A Cultural Perspective. In C. Smith (Ed.), *Exploring the Pressures of Medical Education From a Mental Health and Wellness Perspective* (pp. 44–67). Hershey, PA: IGI Global. doi:10.4018/978-1-5225-2811-1.ch002

Joyce, B. L., & Swanberg, S. M. (2017). Using Backward Design for Competency-Based Undergraduate Medical Education. In J. Stefaniak (Ed.), *Advancing Medical Education Through Strategic Instructional Design* (pp. 53–76). Hershey, PA: IGI Global. doi:10.4018/978-1-5225-2098-6.ch003

Kaljo, K., & Jacques, L. (2018). Flipping the Medical School Classroom. In M. Khosrow-Pour, D.B.A. (Ed.), Encyclopedia of Information Science and Technology, Fourth Edition (pp. 5800-5809). Hershey, PA: IGI Global. doi:10.4018/978-1-5225-2255-3.ch504

Karon, R. (2016). Utilisation of Health Information Systems for Service Delivery in the Namibian Environment. In T. Iyamu & A. Tatnall (Eds.), *Maximizing Healthcare Delivery and Management through Technology Integration* (pp. 169–183). Hershey, PA: IGI Global. doi:10.4018/978-1-4666-9446-0.ch011

Kasina, H., Bahubalendruni, M. V., & Botcha, R. (2017). Robots in Medicine: Past, Present and Future. *International Journal of Manufacturing, Materials, and Mechanical Engineering*, *7*(4), 44–64. doi:10.4018/IJMMME.2017100104

Katehakis, D. G. (2018). Electronic Medical Record Implementation Challenges for the National Health System in Greece. *International Journal of Reliable and Quality E-Healthcare*, *7*(1), 16–30. doi:10.4018/IJRQEH.2018010102

Katz, A., & Shtub, A. (2016). Design and Build a Wizard of Oz (WOZ) Telemedicine Simulator Platform. In M. Cruz-Cunha, I. Miranda, R. Martinho, & R. Rijo (Eds.), *Encyclopedia of E-Health and Telemedicine* (pp. 128–141). Hershey, PA: IGI Global. doi:10.4018/978-1-4666-9978-6.ch011

Kaur, P. D., & Sharma, P. (2017). Success Dimensions of ICTs in Healthcare. In B. Singh (Ed.), *Computational Tools and Techniques for Biomedical Signal Processing* (pp. 149–173). Hershey, PA: IGI Global. doi:10.4018/978-1-5225-0660-7.ch007

Kaushik, P. (2018). Comorbidity of Medical and Psychiatric Disorders in Geriatric Population: Treatment and Care. In B. Prasad & S. Akbar (Eds.), *Handbook of Research on Geriatric Health, Treatment, and Care* (pp. 448–474). Hershey, PA: IGI Global. doi:10.4018/978-1-5225-3480-8.ch025

Khachane, M. Y. (2017). Organ-Based Medical Image Classification Using Support Vector Machine. *International Journal of Synthetic Emotions*, *8*(1), 18–30. doi:10.4018/IJSE.2017010102

Kirci, P. (2018). Intelligent Techniques for Analysis of Big Data About Healthcare and Medical Records. In N. Shah & M. Mittal (Eds.), *Handbook of Research on Promoting Business Process Improvement Through Inventory Control Techniques* (pp. 559–582). Hershey, PA: IGI Global. doi:10.4018/978-1-5225-3232-3.ch029

Kldiashvili, E. (2016). Cloud Computing as the Useful Resource for Application of the Medical Information System for Quality Assurance Purposes. *International Journal of Computers in Clinical Practice*, *1*(2), 1–23. doi:10.4018/IJCCP.2016070101

Kldiashvili, E. (2018). Cloud Approach for the Medical Information System: MIS on Cloud. In M. Khosrow-Pour (Ed.), *Incorporating Nature-Inspired Paradigms in Computational Applications* (pp. 238–261). Hershey, PA: IGI Global. doi:10.4018/978-1-5225-5020-4.ch008

Kldiashvili, E., Burduli, A., Ghortlishvili, G., & Sheklashvili, I. (2016). Georgian Experience in Telecytology. In M. Cruz-Cunha, I. Miranda, R. Martinho, & R. Rijo (Eds.), *Encyclopedia of E-Health and Telemedicine* (pp. 62–71). Hershey, PA: IGI Global. doi:10.4018/978-1-4666-9978-6.ch006

Ko, H., Mesicek, L., Choi, J., Choi, J., & Hwang, S. (2018). A Study on Secure Contents Strategies for Applications With DRM on Cloud Computing. *International Journal of Cloud Applications and Computing*, *8*(1), 143–153. doi:10.4018/IJCAC.2018010107

Komendziński, T., Dreszer-Drogorób, J., Mikołajewska, E., Mikołajewski, D., & Bałaj, B. (2016). Interdisciplinary Education for Research and Everyday Clinical Practice: Lessons Learned from InteRDoCTor Project. In A. Rosiek & K. Leksowski (Eds.), *Organizational Culture and Ethics in Modern Medicine* (pp. 78–110). Hershey, PA: IGI Global. doi:10.4018/978-1-4666-9658-7.ch004

Komendziński, T., Mikołajewska, E., & Mikołajewski, D. (2018). Cross-Cultural Decision-Making in Healthcare: Theory and Practical Application in Real Clinical Conditions. In A. Rosiek-Kryszewska & K. Leksowski (Eds.), *Healthcare Administration for Patient Safety and Engagement* (pp. 276–298). Hershey, PA: IGI Global. doi:10.4018/978-1-5225-3946-9.ch015

Konecny, L. T. (2018). Medical School Wellness Initiatives. In C. Smith (Ed.), *Exploring the Pressures of Medical Education From a Mental Health and Wellness Perspective* (pp. 209–228). Hershey, PA: IGI Global. doi:10.4018/978-1-5225-2811-1.ch009

Konieczna, A., & Słomkowski, P. (2016). Confrontation of Human Rights in Daily Clinical Situations. In A. Rosiek & K. Leksowski (Eds.), *Organizational Culture and Ethics in Modern Medicine* (pp. 255–281). Hershey, PA: IGI Global. doi:10.4018/978-1-4666-9658-7.ch011

Kromrei, H., Solomonson, W. L., & Juzych, M. S. (2017). Teaching Residents How to Teach. In J. Stefaniak (Ed.), *Advancing Medical Education Through Strategic Instructional Design* (pp. 164–185). Hershey, PA: IGI Global. doi:10.4018/978-1-5225-2098-6.ch008

Kulkarni, S., Savyanavar, A., Kulkarni, P., Stranieri, A., & Ghorpade, V. (2018). Framework for Integration of Medical Image and Text-Based Report Retrieval to Support Radiological Diagnosis. In M. Kolekar & V. Kumar (Eds.), *Biomedical Signal and Image Processing in Patient Care* (pp. 86–122). Hershey, PA: IGI Global. doi:10.4018/978-1-5225-2829-6.ch006

Kumar, A., & Sarkar, B. K. (2018). Performance Analysis of Nature-Inspired Algorithms-Based Bayesian Prediction Models for Medical Data Sets. In U. Singh, A. Tiwari, & R. Singh (Eds.), *Soft-Computing-Based Nonlinear Control Systems Design* (pp. 134–155). Hershey, PA: IGI Global. doi:10.4018/978-1-5225-3531-7.ch007

Kurtz, R. S. (2016). Fortitude: A Study of African Americans in Surgery in New York City. In U. Thomas & J. Drake (Eds.), *Critical Research on Sexism and Racism in STEM Fields* (pp. 153–169). Hershey, PA: IGI Global. doi:10.4018/978-1-5225-0174-9.ch009

Labbadi, W., & Akaichi, J. (2017). Efficient Algorithm for Answering Fuzzy Medical Requests in Pervasive Healthcare Information Systems. *International Journal of Healthcare Information Systems and Informatics*, *12*(2), 46–64. doi:10.4018/IJHISI.2017040103

Lagumdzija, A., & Swing, V. K. (2017). Health, Digitalization, and Individual Empowerment. In F. Topor (Ed.), *Handbook of Research on Individualism and Identity in the Globalized Digital Age* (pp. 380–402). Hershey, PA: IGI Global. doi:10.4018/978-1-5225-0522-8.ch017

Lamey, T. W., & Davidson-Shivers, G. V. (2017). Instructional Strategies and Sequencing. In J. Stefaniak (Ed.), *Advancing Medical Education Through Strategic Instructional Design* (pp. 30–52). Hershey, PA: IGI Global. doi:10.4018/978-1-5225-2098-6.ch002

Leon, G. (2017). The Role of Forensic Medicine in Medical Errors. In M. Riga (Ed.), *Impact of Medical Errors and Malpractice on Health Economics, Quality, and Patient Safety* (pp. 144–170). Hershey, PA: IGI Global. doi:10.4018/978-1-5225-2337-6.ch006

Lidia, B., Federica, G., & Maria, V. E. (2016). The Patient-Centered Medicine as the Theoretical Framework for Patient Engagement. In G. Graffigna (Ed.), *Promoting Patient Engagement and Participation for Effective Healthcare Reform* (pp. 25–39). Hershey, PA: IGI Global. doi:10.4018/978-1-4666-9992-2.ch002

Love, L., & McDowelle, D. (2018). Developing a Comprehensive Wellness Program for Medical Students. In C. Smith (Ed.), *Exploring the Pressures of Medical Education From a Mental Health and Wellness Perspective* (pp. 190–208). Hershey, PA: IGI Global. doi:10.4018/978-1-5225-2811-1.ch008

Lovell, K. L. (2017). Development and Evaluation of Neuroscience Computer-Based Modules for Medical Students: Instructional Design Principles and Effectiveness. In J. Stefaniak (Ed.), *Advancing Medical Education Through Strategic Instructional Design* (pp. 262–276). Hershey, PA: IGI Global. doi:10.4018/978-1-5225-2098-6.ch013

Lubin, R., & Hamlin, M. D. (2018). Medical Student Burnout: A Social Cognitive Learning Perspective on Medical Student Mental Health and Wellness. In C. Smith (Ed.), *Exploring the Pressures of Medical Education From a Mental Health and Wellness Perspective* (pp. 92–121). Hershey, PA: IGI Global. doi:10.4018/978-1-5225-2811-1.ch004

Luk, C. Y. (2018). Moving Towards Universal Health Coverage: Challenges for the Present and Future in China. In B. Fong, A. Ng, & P. Yuen (Eds.), *Sustainable Health and Long-Term Care Solutions for an Aging Population* (pp. 19–45). Hershey, PA: IGI Global. doi:10.4018/978-1-5225-2633-9.ch002

Mahat, M., & Pettigrew, A. (2017). The Regulatory Environment of Non-Profit Higher Education and Research Institutions and Its Implications for Managerial Strategy: The Case of Medical Education and Research. In L. West & A. Worthington (Eds.), *Handbook of Research on Emerging Business Models and Managerial Strategies in the Nonprofit Sector* (pp. 336–351). Hershey, PA: IGI Global. doi:10.4018/978-1-5225-2537-0.ch017

Maitra, I. K., & Bandhyopadhyaay, S. K. (2017). Adaptive Edge Detection Method towards Features Extraction from Diverse Medical Imaging Technologies. In S. Bhattacharyya, S. De, I. Pan, & P. Dutta (Eds.), *Intelligent Multidimensional Data Clustering and Analysis* (pp. 159–192). Hershey, PA: IGI Global. doi:10.4018/978-1-5225-1776-4.ch007

Mangu, V. P. (2017). Mobile Health Care: A Technology View. In C. Bhatt & S. Peddoju (Eds.), *Cloud Computing Systems and Applications in Healthcare* (pp. 1–18). Hershey, PA: IGI Global. doi:10.4018/978-1-5225-1002-4.ch001

Manirabona, A., Fourati, L. C., & Boudjit, S. (2017). Investigation on Healthcare Monitoring Systems: Innovative Services and Applications. *International Journal of E-Health and Medical Communications*, *8*(1), 1–18. doi:10.4018/IJEHMC.2017010101

Mannai, M. M., & Karâa, W. B. (2016). Biomedical Image Processing Overview. In W. Karâa & N. Dey (Eds.), *Biomedical Image Analysis and Mining Techniques for Improved Health Outcomes* (pp. 1–12). Hershey, PA: IGI Global. doi:10.4018/978-1-4666-8811-7.ch001

Manzoor, A. (2016). RFID in Health Care-Building Smart Hospitals for Quality Healthcare. *International Journal of User-Driven Healthcare*, *6*(2), 21–45. doi:10.4018/IJUDH.2016070102

Marwan, M., Kartit, A., & Ouahmane, H. (2018). A Framework to Secure Medical Image Storage in Cloud Computing Environment. *Journal of Electronic Commerce in Organizations*, *16*(1), 1–16. doi:10.4018/JECO.2018010101

Masoud, M. P., Nejad, M. K., Darebaghi, H., Chavoshi, M., & Farahani, M. (2018). The Decision Support System and Conventional Method of Telephone Triage by Nurses in Emergency Medical Services: A Comparative Investigation. *International Journal of E-Business Research*, *14*(1), 77–88. doi:10.4018/IJEBR.2018010105

McDonald, W. G., Martin, M., & Salzberg, L. D. (2018). From Medical Student to Medical Resident: Graduate Medical Education and Mental Health in the United States. In C. Smith (Ed.), *Exploring the Pressures of Medical Education From a Mental Health and Wellness Perspective* (pp. 145–169). Hershey, PA: IGI Global. doi:10.4018/978-1-5225-2811-1.ch006

Medhekar, A. (2017). The Role of Social Media for Knowledge Dissemination in Medical Tourism: A Case of India. In R. Chugh (Ed.), *Harnessing Social Media as a Knowledge Management Tool* (pp. 25–54). Hershey, PA: IGI Global. doi:10.4018/978-1-5225-0495-5.ch002

Medhekar, A., & Haq, F. (2018). Urbanization and New Jobs Creation in Healthcare Services in India: Challenges and Opportunities. In U. Benna & I. Benna (Eds.), *Urbanization and Its Impact on Socio-Economic Growth in Developing Regions* (pp. 198–218). Hershey, PA: IGI Global. doi:10.4018/978-1-5225-2659-9.ch010

Mehta, G., Dutta, M. K., & Kim, P. S. (2016). An Efficient and Lossless Cryptosystem for Security in Tele-Ophthalmology Applications Using Chaotic Theory. *International Journal of E-Health and Medical Communications*, 7(4), 28–47. doi:10.4018/IJEHMC.2016100102

Mehta, P. (2017). Framework of Indian Healthcare System and its Challenges: An Insight. In V. Bryan & J. Bird (Eds.), *Healthcare Community Synergism between Patients, Practitioners, and Researchers* (pp. 247–271). Hershey, PA: IGI Global. doi:10.4018/978-1-5225-0640-9.ch011

Metelmann, B., & Metelmann, C. (2016). M-Health in Prehospital Emergency Medicine: Experiences from the EU funded Project LiveCity. In A. Moumtzoglou (Ed.), *M-Health Innovations for Patient-Centered Care* (pp. 197–212). Hershey, PA: IGI Global. doi:10.4018/978-1-4666-9861-1.ch010

Mi, M. (2017). Informal Learning in Medical Education. In J. Stefaniak (Ed.), *Advancing Medical Education Through Strategic Instructional Design* (pp. 225–244). Hershey, PA: IGI Global. doi:10.4018/978-1-5225-2098-6.ch011

Miglioretti, M., Mariani, F., & Vecchio, L. (2016). Could Patient Engagement Promote a Health System Free From Malpractice Litigation Risk? In G. Graffigna (Ed.), *Promoting Patient Engagement and Participation for Effective Healthcare Reform* (pp. 240–264). Hershey, PA: IGI Global. doi:10.4018/978-1-4666-9992-2.ch012

Misra, S. C., & Bisui, S. (2016). Feasibility of Large Scale Implementation of Personalized Medicine in the Current Scenario. *International Journal of E-Health and Medical Communications*, *7*(2), 30–49. doi:10.4018/IJEHMC.2016040103

Misra, S. C., Bisui, S., & Fantazy, K. (2016). Identifying Critical Changes in Adoption of Personalized Medicine (PM) in Healthcare Management. *International Journal of E-Health and Medical Communications*, *7*(3), 1–15. doi:10.4018/IJEHMC.2016070101

Mohammadian, M., Hatzinakos, D., Spachos, P., & Jentzsh, R. (2016). An Intelligent and Secure Framework for Wireless Information Technology in Healthcare for User and Data Classification in Hospitals. In V. Wang (Ed.), *Handbook of Research on Advancing Health Education through Technology* (pp. 452–479). Hershey, PA: IGI Global. doi:10.4018/978-1-4666-9494-1.ch019

Mokeddem, S., & Atmani, B. (2016). Assessment of Clinical Decision Support Systems for Predicting Coronary Heart Disease. *International Journal of Operations Research and Information Systems*, *7*(3), 57–73. doi:10.4018/IJORIS.2016070104

Mokrzycka, A., & Kowalska-Bobko, I. (2016). Public Health Legislation and Patient's Rights: Health2020 Strategy, European Perspective. In A. Rosiek & K. Leksowski (Eds.), *Organizational Culture and Ethics in Modern Medicine* (pp. 298–322). Hershey, PA: IGI Global. doi:10.4018/978-1-4666-9658-7.ch013

Moon, J. D., & Galea, M. P. (2016). Overview of Clinical Decision Support Systems in Healthcare. In J. Moon & M. Galea (Eds.), *Improving Health Management through Clinical Decision Support Systems* (pp. 1–27). Hershey, PA: IGI Global. doi:10.4018/978-1-4666-9432-3.ch001

Mosadeghrad, A. M., & Woldemichael, A. (2017). Application of Quality Management in Promoting Patient Safety and Preventing Medical Errors. In M. Riga (Ed.), *Impact of Medical Errors and Malpractice on Health Economics, Quality, and Patient Safety* (pp. 91–112). Hershey, PA: IGI Global. doi:10.4018/978-1-5225-2337-6.ch004

Moumtzoglou, A. (2017). Digital Medicine: The Quality Standpoint. In A. Moumtzoglou (Ed.), *Design, Development, and Integration of Reliable Electronic Healthcare Platforms* (pp. 179–195). Hershey, PA: IGI Global. doi:10.4018/978-1-5225-1724-5.ch011

Moumtzoglou, A., & Pouliakis, A. (2018). Population Health Management and the Science of Individuality. *International Journal of Reliable and Quality E-Healthcare*, *7*(2), 1–26. doi:10.4018/IJRQEH.2018040101

Mpofu, C. (2016). International Medical Experiences Outbound New Zealand: An Economic and Medical Workforce Strategy. In D. Velliaris & D. Coleman-George (Eds.), *Handbook of Research on Study Abroad Programs and Outbound Mobility* (pp. 446–469). Hershey, PA: IGI Global. doi:10.4018/978-1-5225-0169-5.ch018

Mukhtar, W. F., & Abuelyaman, E. S. (2017). Opportunities and Challenges of Big Data in Healthcare. In N. Wickramasinghe (Ed.), *Handbook of Research on Healthcare Administration and Management* (pp. 47–58). Hershey, PA: IGI Global. doi:10.4018/978-1-5225-0920-2.ch004

Munugala, S., Brar, G. K., Syed, A., Mohammad, A., & Halgamuge, M. N. (2018). The Much Needed Security and Data Reforms of Cloud Computing in Medical Data Storage. In M. Lytras & P. Papadopoulou (Eds.), *Applying Big Data Analytics in Bioinformatics and Medicine* (pp. 99–113). Hershey, PA: IGI Global. doi:10.4018/978-1-5225-2607-0.ch005

Narasimhamurthy, A. (2016). An Overview of Machine Learning in Medical Image Analysis: Trends in Health Informatics. In N. Dey & A. Ashour (Eds.), *Classification and Clustering in Biomedical Signal Processing* (pp. 23–45). Hershey, PA: IGI Global. doi:10.4018/978-1-5225-0140-4.ch002

Ngara, R. (2017). Multiple Voices, Multiple Paths: Towards Dialogue between Western and Indigenous Medical Knowledge Systems. In P. Ngulube (Ed.), *Handbook of Research on Theoretical Perspectives on Indigenous Knowledge Systems in Developing Countries* (pp. 332–358). Hershey, PA: IGI Global. doi:10.4018/978-1-5225-0833-5.ch015

O'Connor, Y., & Heavin, C. (2018). Defining and Characterising the Landscape of eHealth. In M. Khosrow-Pour, D.B.A. (Ed.), Encyclopedia of Information Science and Technology, Fourth Edition (pp. 5864-5875). Hershey, PA: IGI Global. doi:10.4018/978-1-5225-2255-3.ch510

Ochonogor, W. C., & Okite-Amughoro, F. A. (2018). Building an Effective Digital Library in a University Teaching Hospital (UTH) in Nigeria. In A. Tella & T. Kwanya (Eds.), *Handbook of Research on Managing Intellectual Property in Digital Libraries* (pp. 184–204). Hershey, PA: IGI Global. doi:10.4018/978-1-5225-3093-0.ch010

Olaniran, B. A. (2016). ICTs, E-health, and Multidisciplinary Healthcare Teams: Promises and Challenges. *International Journal of Privacy and Health Information Management*, *4*(2), 62–75. doi:10.4018/IJPHIM.2016070105

Olaniran, B. A. (2016). ICT Use and Multidisciplinary Healthcare Teams in the Age of e-Health. *International Journal of Reliable and Quality E-Healthcare*, *5*(1), 18–31. doi:10.4018/IJRQEH.2016010102

Olivares, S. L., Cruz, A. G., Cabrera, M. V., Regalado, A. I., & García, J. E. (2017). An Assessment Study of Quality Model for Medical Schools in Mexico. In S. Mukerji & P. Tripathi (Eds.), *Handbook of Research on Administration, Policy, and Leadership in Higher Education* (pp. 404–439). Hershey, PA: IGI Global. doi:10.4018/978-1-5225-0672-0.ch016

Omidoyin, E. O., Opeke, R. O., & Osagbemi, G. K. (2016). Utilization Pattern and Privacy Issues in the use of Health Records for Research Practice by Doctors: Selected Nigerian Teaching Hospitals as Case Study. *International Journal of Privacy and Health Information Management*, *4*(1), 1–11. doi:10.4018/IJPHIM.2016010101

Omoruyi, E. A., & Omidele, F. (2018). Resident Physician and Medical Academic Faculty Burnout: A Review of Current Literature. In C. Smith (Ed.), *Exploring the Pressures of Medical Education From a Mental Health and Wellness Perspective* (pp. 171–189). Hershey, PA: IGI Global. doi:10.4018/978-1-5225-2811-1.ch007

Osop, H., & Sahama, T. (2016). Data-Driven and Practice-Based Evidence: Design and Development of Efficient and Effective Clinical Decision Support System. In J. Moon & M. Galea (Eds.), *Improving Health Management through Clinical Decision Support Systems* (pp. 295–328). Hershey, PA: IGI Global. doi:10.4018/978-1-4666-9432-3.ch014

Ossowski, R., & Izdebski, P. (2016). Ethical Aspects of Talking to a Patient. In A. Rosiek & K. Leksowski (Eds.), *Organizational Culture and Ethics in Modern Medicine* (pp. 203–235). Hershey, PA: IGI Global. doi:10.4018/978-1-4666-9658-7.ch009

Pandian, P. S. (2016). An Overview of Telemedicine Technologies for Healthcare Applications. *International Journal of Biomedical and Clinical Engineering*, *5*(2), 29–52. doi:10.4018/IJBCE.2016070103

Papadopoulou, P., Lytras, M., & Marouli, C. (2018). Bioinformatics as Applied to Medicine: Challenges Faced Moving from Big Data to Smart Data to Wise Data. In M. Lytras & P. Papadopoulou (Eds.), *Applying Big Data Analytics in Bioinformatics and Medicine* (pp. 1–25). Hershey, PA: IGI Global. doi:10.4018/978-1-5225-2607-0.ch001

Paraskou, A., & George, B. P. (2018). An Overview of Reproductive Tourism. In *Legal and Economic Considerations Surrounding Reproductive Tourism: Emerging Research and Opportunities* (pp. 1–17). Hershey, PA: IGI Global. doi:10.4018/978-1-5225-2694-0.ch001

Park, S., & Moon, J. (2016). Strategic Approach towards Clinical Information Security. In J. Moon & M. Galea (Eds.), *Improving Health Management through Clinical Decision Support Systems* (pp. 329–359). Hershey, PA: IGI Global. doi:10.4018/978-1-4666-9432-3.ch015

Pereira, D., Castro, A., Gomes, P., Areias, J. C., Reis, Z. S., Coimbra, M. T., & Cruz-Correia, R. (2016). Digital Auscultation: Challenges and Perspectives. In M. Cruz-Cunha, I. Miranda, R. Martinho, & R. Rijo (Eds.), *Encyclopedia of E-Health and Telemedicine* (pp. 910–927). Hershey, PA: IGI Global. doi:10.4018/978-1-4666-9978-6.ch070

Peters, R. A., & Cruz, M. (2016). The States as Generators of Incremental Change in American Health Care Policy: 1935 to 1965. In R. Gholipour & K. Rouzbehani (Eds.), *Social, Economic, and Political Perspectives on Public Health Policy-Making* (pp. 86–114). Hershey, PA: IGI Global. doi:10.4018/978-1-4666-9944-1.ch005

Phuritsabam, B., & Devi, A. B. (2017). Information Seeking Behavior of Medical Scientists at Jawaharlal Nehru Institute of Medical Science: A Study. In S. Ram (Ed.), *Library and Information Services for Bioinformatics Education and Research* (pp. 177–187). Hershey, PA: IGI Global. doi:10.4018/978-1-5225-1871-6.ch010

Pieczka, B. (2018). Management of Risk and Adverse Events in Medical Entities. In A. Rosiek-Kryszewska & K. Leksowski (Eds.), *Healthcare Administration for Patient Safety and Engagement* (pp. 31–46). Hershey, PA: IGI Global. doi:10.4018/978-1-5225-3946-9.ch003

Poduval, J. (2016). Curriculum Development. In *Optimizing Medicine Residency Training Programs* (pp. 45–102). Hershey, PA: IGI Global. doi:10.4018/978-1-4666-9527-6.ch003

Poduval, J. (2016). Ethics and Professionalism. In *Optimizing Medicine Residency Training Programs* (pp. 103–133). Hershey, PA: IGI Global. doi:10.4018/978-1-4666-9527-6.ch004

Poduval, J. (2016). Management Skills and Leadership. In *Optimizing Medicine Residency Training Programs* (pp. 182–205). Hershey, PA: IGI Global. doi:10.4018/978-1-4666-9527-6.ch008

Poduval, J. (2016). Medicine Residency Training. In *Optimizing Medicine Residency Training Programs* (pp. 1–27). Hershey, PA: IGI Global. doi:10.4018/978-1-4666-9527-6.ch001

Poduval, J. (2016). Personal Issues. In *Optimizing Medicine Residency Training Programs* (pp. 206–221). Hershey, PA: IGI Global. doi:10.4018/978-1-4666-9527-6.ch009

Poduval, J. (2017). Medical Errors: Impact on Health Care Quality. In M. Riga (Ed.), *Impact of Medical Errors and Malpractice on Health Economics, Quality, and Patient Safety* (pp. 33–60). Hershey, PA: IGI Global. doi:10.4018/978-1-5225-2337-6.ch002

Politis, D., Stagiopoulos, P., Aidona, S., Kyriafinis, G., & Constantinidis, I. (2018). Autonomous Learning and Skill Accreditation: A Paradigm for Medical Studies. In A. Kumar (Ed.), *Optimizing Student Engagement in Online Learning Environments* (pp. 266–296). Hershey, PA: IGI Global. doi:10.4018/978-1-5225-3634-5.ch012

Pomares-Quimbaya, A., Gonzalez, R. A., Quintero, S., Muñoz, O. M., Bohórquez, W. R., García, O. M., & Londoño, D. (2016). A Review of Existing Applications and Techniques for Narrative Text Analysis in Electronic Medical Records. In M. Cruz-Cunha, I. Miranda, R. Martinho, & R. Rijo (Eds.), *Encyclopedia of E-Health and Telemedicine* (pp. 796–811). Hershey, PA: IGI Global. doi:10.4018/978-1-4666-9978-6.ch062

Pomares-Quimbaya, A., González, R. A., Sierra, A., Daza, J. C., Muñoz, O., García, A., ... Bohórquez, W. R. (2017). ICT for Enabling the Quality Evaluation of Health Care Services: A Case Study in a General Hospital. In A. Moumtzoglou (Ed.), *Design, Development, and Integration of Reliable Electronic Healthcare Platforms* (pp. 196–210). Hershey, PA: IGI Global. doi:10.4018/978-1-5225-1724-5.ch012

Pouliakis, A., Margari, N., Karakitsou, E., Archondakis, S., & Karakitsos, P. (2018). Emerging Technologies Serving Cytopathology: Big Data, the Cloud, and Mobile Computing. In I. El Naqa (Ed.), *Emerging Developments and Practices in Oncology* (pp. 114–152). Hershey, PA: IGI Global. doi:10.4018/978-1-5225-3085-5.ch005

Queirós, A., Silva, A. G., Ferreira, A., Caravau, H., Cerqueira, M., & Rocha, N. P. (2016). Assessing Mobile Applications Considered Medical Devices. In M. Cruz-Cunha, I. Miranda, R. Martinho, & R. Rijo (Eds.), *Encyclopedia of E-Health and Telemedicine* (pp. 111–127). Hershey, PA: IGI Global. doi:10.4018/978-1-4666-9978-6.ch010

Raffaeli, L., Spinsante, S., & Gambi, E. (2016). Integrated Smart TV-Based Personal e-Health System. *International Journal of E-Health and Medical Communications*, *7*(1), 48–64. doi:10.4018/IJEHMC.2016010103

Rai, A., Kothari, R., & Singh, D. P. (2017). Assessment of Available Technologies for Hospital Waste Management: A Need for Society. In R. Singh, A. Singh, & V. Srivastava (Eds.), *Environmental Issues Surrounding Human Overpopulation* (pp. 172–188). Hershey, PA: IGI Global. doi:10.4018/978-1-5225-1683-5.ch010

Ramamoorthy, S., & Sivasubramaniam, R. (2018). Image Processing Including Medical Liver Imaging: Medical Image Processing from Big Data Perspective, Ultrasound Liver Images, Challenges. In M. Lytras & P. Papadopoulou (Eds.), *Applying Big Data Analytics in Bioinformatics and Medicine* (pp. 380–392). Hershey, PA: IGI Global. doi:10.4018/978-1-5225-2607-0.ch016

Rathor, G. P., & Gupta, S. K. (2017). Improving Multimodality Image Fusion through Integrate AFL and Wavelet Transform. In V. Tiwari, B. Tiwari, R. Thakur, & S. Gupta (Eds.), *Pattern and Data Analysis in Healthcare Settings* (pp. 143–157). Hershey, PA: IGI Global. doi:10.4018/978-1-5225-0536-5.ch008

Rawat, D. B., & Bhattacharya, S. (2016). Wireless Body Area Network for Healthcare Applications. In N. Meghanathan (Ed.), *Advanced Methods for Complex Network Analysis* (pp. 343–358). Hershey, PA: IGI Global. doi:10.4018/978-1-4666-9964-9.ch014

Rea, P. M. (2016). Advances in Anatomical and Medical Visualisation. In M. Pinheiro & D. Simões (Eds.), *Handbook of Research on Engaging Digital Natives in Higher Education Settings* (pp. 244–264). Hershey, PA: IGI Global. doi:10.4018/978-1-5225-0039-1.ch011

Rexhepi, H., & Persson, A. (2017). Challenges to Implementing IT Support for Evidence Based Practice Among Nurses and Assistant Nurses: A Qualitative Study. *Journal of Electronic Commerce in Organizations, 15*(2), 61–76. doi:10.4018/JECO.2017040105

Reychav, I., & Azuri, J. (2016). Including Elderly Patients in Decision Making via Electronic Health Literacy. In M. Cruz-Cunha, I. Miranda, R. Martinho, & R. Rijo (Eds.), *Encyclopedia of E-Health and Telemedicine* (pp. 241–249). Hershey, PA: IGI Global. doi:10.4018/978-1-4666-9978-6.ch020

Richards, D., & Caldwell, P. H. (2016). Gamification to Improve Adherence to Clinical Treatment Advice: Improving Adherence to Clinical Treatment. In D. Novák, B. Tulu, & H. Brendryen (Eds.), *Handbook of Research on Holistic Perspectives in Gamification for Clinical Practice* (pp. 47–77). Hershey, PA: IGI Global. doi:10.4018/978-1-4666-9522-1.ch004

Rissman, B. (2016). Medical Conditions Associated with NLD. In B. Rissman (Ed.), *Medical and Educational Perspectives on Nonverbal Learning Disability in Children and Young Adults* (pp. 27–66). Hershey, PA: IGI Global. doi:10.4018/978-1-4666-9539-9.ch002

Rosiek, A. (2018). The Assessment of Actions of the Environment and the Impact of Preventive Medicine for Public Health in Poland. In A. Rosiek-Kryszewska & K. Leksowski (Eds.), *Healthcare Administration for Patient Safety and Engagement* (pp. 106–119). Hershey, PA: IGI Global. doi:10.4018/978-1-5225-3946-9.ch006

Rosiek, A., Leksowski, K., Goch, A., Rosiek-Kryszewska, A., & Leksowski, Ł. (2016). Medical Treatment and Difficult Ethical Decisions in Interdisciplinary Hospital Teams. In A. Rosiek & K. Leksowski (Eds.), *Organizational Culture and Ethics in Modern Medicine* (pp. 121–153). Hershey, PA: IGI Global. doi:10.4018/978-1-4666-9658-7.ch006

Rosiek, A., & Rosiek-Kryszewska, A. (2018). Managed Healthcare: Doctor Life Satisfaction and Its Impact on the Process of Communicating With the Patient. In A. Rosiek-Kryszewska & K. Leksowski (Eds.), *Healthcare Administration for Patient Safety and Engagement* (pp. 244–261). Hershey, PA: IGI Global. doi:10.4018/978-1-5225-3946-9.ch013

Rosiek-Kryszewska, A., Leksowski, Ł., Rosiek, A., Leksowski, K., & Goch, A. (2016). Clinical Communication in the Aspect of Development of New Technologies and E-Health in the Doctor-Patient Relationship. In A. Rosiek & K. Leksowski (Eds.), *Organizational Culture and Ethics in Modern Medicine* (pp. 18–51). Hershey, PA: IGI Global. doi:10.4018/978-1-4666-9658-7.ch002

Rosiek-Kryszewska, A., & Rosiek, A. (2018). The Involvement of the Patient and his Perspective Evaluation of the Quality of Healthcare. In A. Rosiek-Kryszewska & K. Leksowski (Eds.), *Healthcare Administration for Patient Safety and Engagement* (pp. 121–144). Hershey, PA: IGI Global. doi:10.4018/978-1-5225-3946-9.ch007

Rosiek-Kryszewska, A., & Rosiek, A. (2018). The Impact of Management and Leadership Roles in Building Competitive Healthcare Units. In A. Rosiek-Kryszewska & K. Leksowski (Eds.), *Healthcare Administration for Patient Safety and Engagement* (pp. 13–30). Hershey, PA: IGI Global. doi:10.4018/978-1-5225-3946-9.ch002

Roşu, S. M., Păvăloiu, I. B., Dragoi, G., Apostol, C. G., & Munteanu, D. (2016). Telemedicine Based on LMDS in the Urban/Metropolitan Area: A Romanian Case Study. In M. Cruz-Cunha, I. Miranda, R. Martinho, & R. Rijo (Eds.), *Encyclopedia of E-Health and Telemedicine* (pp. 96–109). Hershey, PA: IGI Global. doi:10.4018/978-1-4666-9978-6.ch009

Rouzbehani, K. (2017). Health Policy Implementation: Moving Beyond Its Barriers in United States. In N. Wickramasinghe (Ed.), *Handbook of Research on Healthcare Administration and Management* (pp. 541–552). Hershey, PA: IGI Global. doi:10.4018/978-1-5225-0920-2.ch032

Ruiz, I. M., Cohen, D. S., & Marco, Á. M. (2016). ISO/IEEE11073 Family of Standards: Trends and Applications on E-Health Monitoring. In M. Cruz-Cunha, I. Miranda, R. Martinho, & R. Rijo (Eds.), *Encyclopedia of E-Health and Telemedicine* (pp. 646–660). Hershey, PA: IGI Global. doi:10.4018/978-1-4666-9978-6.ch050

Sam, S. (2017). Mobile Phones and Expanding Human Capabilities in Plural Health Systems. In K. Moahi, K. Bwalya, & P. Sebina (Eds.), *Health Information Systems and the Advancement of Medical Practice in Developing Countries* (pp. 93–114). Hershey, PA: IGI Global. doi:10.4018/978-1-5225-2262-1.ch006

Sankaranarayanan, S., & Ganesan, S. (2016). Applications of Intelligent Agents in Health Sector-A Review. *International Journal of E-Health and Medical Communications*, *7*(1), 1–30. doi:10.4018/IJEHMC.2016010101

Santos-Trigo, M., Suaste, E., & Figuerola, P. (2018). Technology Design and Routes for Tool Appropriation in Medical Practices. In M. Khosrow-Pour, D.B.A. (Ed.), Encyclopedia of Information Science and Technology, Fourth Edition (pp. 3794-3804). Hershey, PA: IGI Global. doi:10.4018/978-1-5225-2255-3.ch329

Sarivougioukas, J., Vagelatos, A., Parsopoulos, K. E., & Lagaris, I. E. (2018). Home UbiHealth. In M. Khosrow-Pour, D.B.A. (Ed.), Encyclopedia of Information Science and Technology, Fourth Edition (pp. 7765-7774). Hershey, PA: IGI Global. doi:10.4018/978-1-5225-2255-3.ch675

Sarkar, B. K. (2017). Big Data and Healthcare Data: A Survey. *International Journal of Knowledge-Based Organizations*, *7*(4), 50–77. doi:10.4018/IJKBO.2017100104

Saxena, K., & Banodha, U. (2017). An Essence of the SOA on Healthcare. In R. Bhadoria, N. Chaudhari, G. Tomar, & S. Singh (Eds.), *Exploring Enterprise Service Bus in the Service-Oriented Architecture Paradigm* (pp. 283–304). Hershey, PA: IGI Global. doi:10.4018/978-1-5225-2157-0.ch018

Schmeida, M., & McNeal, R. (2016). Consulting Online Healthcare Information: E-Caregivers as Knowledgeable Decision Makers. *International Journal of Computers in Clinical Practice*, *1*(1), 42–52. doi:10.4018/IJCCP.2016010104

Sen, K., & Ghosh, K. (2018). Incorporating Global Medical Knowledge to Solve Healthcare Problems: A Framework for a Crowdsourcing System. *International Journal of Healthcare Information Systems and Informatics*, *13*(1), 1–14. doi:10.4018/IJHISI.2018010101

Shakdher, A., & Pandey, K. (2017). REDAlert+: Medical/Fire Emergency and Warning System using Android Devices. *International Journal of E-Health and Medical Communications*, *8*(1), 37–51. doi:10.4018/IJEHMC.2017010103

Shekarian, E., Abdul-Rashid, S. H., & Olugu, E. U. (2017). An Integrated Fuzzy VIKOR Method for Performance Management in Healthcare. In M. Tavana, K. Szabat, & K. Puranam (Eds.), *Organizational Productivity and Performance Measurements Using Predictive Modeling and Analytics* (pp. 40–61). Hershey, PA: IGI Global. doi:10.4018/978-1-5225-0654-6.ch003

Shi, J., Erdem, E., & Liu, H. (2016). Expanding Role of Telephone Systems in Healthcare: Developments and Opportunities. In A. Dwivedi (Ed.), *Reshaping Medical Practice and Care with Health Information Systems* (pp. 87–131). Hershey, PA: IGI Global. doi:10.4018/978-1-4666-9870-3.ch004

Shijina, V., & John, S. J. (2017). Multiple Relations and its Application in Medical Diagnosis. *International Journal of Fuzzy System Applications, 6*(4), 47–62. doi:10.4018/IJFSA.2017100104

Shipley, N., & Chakraborty, J. (2018). Big Data and mHealth: Increasing the Usability of Healthcare Through the Customization of Pinterest – Literary Perspective. In J. Machado, A. Abelha, M. Santos, & F. Portela (Eds.), *Next-Generation Mobile and Pervasive Healthcare Solutions* (pp. 46–66). Hershey, PA: IGI Global. doi:10.4018/978-1-5225-2851-7.ch004

Singh, A., & Dutta, M. K. (2017). A Reversible Data Hiding Scheme for Efficient Management of Tele-Ophthalmological Data. *International Journal of E-Health and Medical Communications, 8*(3), 38–54. doi:10.4018/IJEHMC.2017070103

Sivaji, A., Radjo, H. K., Amin, M., & Abu Hashim, M. A. (2016). Design of a Hospital Interactive Wayfinding System: Designing for Malaysian Users. In N. Mohamed, T. Mantoro, M. Ayu, & M. Mahmud (Eds.), *Critical Socio-Technical Issues Surrounding Mobile Computing* (pp. 88–123). Hershey, PA: IGI Global. doi:10.4018/978-1-4666-9438-5.ch005

Skourti, P. K., & Pavlakis, A. (2017). The Second Victim Phenomenon: The Way Out. In M. Riga (Ed.), *Impact of Medical Errors and Malpractice on Health Economics, Quality, and Patient Safety* (pp. 197–222). Hershey, PA: IGI Global. doi:10.4018/978-1-5225-2337-6.ch008

Smith, C. R. (2018). Medical Students' Quest Towards the Long White Coat: Impact on Mental Health and Well-Being. In C. Smith (Ed.), *Exploring the Pressures of Medical Education From a Mental Health and Wellness Perspective* (pp. 1–42). Hershey, PA: IGI Global. doi:10.4018/978-1-5225-2811-1.ch001

Smith, S. I., & Dandignac, M. (2018). Perfectionism: Addressing Lofty Expectations in Medical School. In C. Smith (Ed.), *Exploring the Pressures of Medical Education From a Mental Health and Wellness Perspective* (pp. 68–91). Hershey, PA: IGI Global. doi:10.4018/978-1-5225-2811-1.ch003

Sobrinho, Á. A., Dias da Silva, L., Perkusich, A., Cunha, P., Pinheiro, M. E., & Melo de Medeiros, L. (2016). Towards Medical Systems to Aid the Detection and Treatment of Chronic Diseases. In D. Fotiadis (Ed.), *Handbook of Research on Trends in the Diagnosis and Treatment of Chronic Conditions* (pp. 50–69). Hershey, PA: IGI Global. doi:10.4018/978-1-4666-8828-5.ch003

Soczywko, J., & Rutkowska, D. (2018). The Patient/Provider Relationship in Emergency Medicine: Organization, Communication, and Understanding. In A. Rosiek-Kryszewska & K. Leksowski (Eds.), *Healthcare Administration for Patient Safety and Engagement* (pp. 74–105). Hershey, PA: IGI Global. doi:10.4018/978-1-5225-3946-9.ch005

Sołtysik-Piorunkiewicz, A., Furmankiewicz, M., & Ziuziański, P. (2016). Web Healthcare Applications in Poland: Trends, Standards, Barriers and Possibilities of Implementation and Usage of E-Health Systems. In I. Deliyannis, P. Kostagiolas, & C. Banou (Eds.), *Experimental Multimedia Systems for Interactivity and Strategic Innovation* (pp. 258–283). Hershey, PA: IGI Global. doi:10.4018/978-1-4666-8659-5.ch013

Soni, P. (2018). Implications of HIPAA and Subsequent Regulations on Information Technology. In M. Gupta, R. Sharman, J. Walp, & P. Mulgund (Eds.), *Information Technology Risk Management and Compliance in Modern Organizations* (pp. 71–98). Hershey, PA: IGI Global. doi:10.4018/978-1-5225-2604-9.ch004

Spinelli, R., & Benevolo, C. (2016). From Healthcare Services to E-Health Applications: A Delivery System-Based Taxonomy. In A. Dwivedi (Ed.), *Reshaping Medical Practice and Care with Health Information Systems* (pp. 205–245). Hershey, PA: IGI Global. doi:10.4018/978-1-4666-9870-3.ch007

Srivastava, A., & Aggarwal, A. K. (2018). Medical Image Fusion in Spatial and Transform Domain: A Comparative Analysis. In M. Anwar, A. Khosla, & R. Kapoor (Eds.), *Handbook of Research on Advanced Concepts in Real-Time Image and Video Processing* (pp. 281–300). Hershey, PA: IGI Global. doi:10.4018/978-1-5225-2848-7.ch011

Srivastava, S. K., & Roy, S. N. (2018). Recommendation System: A Potential Tool for Achieving Pervasive Health Care. In J. Machado, A. Abelha, M. Santos, & F. Portela (Eds.), *Next-Generation Mobile and Pervasive Healthcare Solutions* (pp. 111–127). Hershey, PA: IGI Global. doi:10.4018/978-1-5225-2851-7.ch008

Stancu, A. (2016). Correlations and Patterns of Food and Health Consumer Expenditure. In A. Jean-Vasile (Ed.), *Food Science, Production, and Engineering in Contemporary Economies* (pp. 44–101). Hershey, PA: IGI Global. doi:10.4018/978-1-5225-0341-5.ch003

Stanimirovic, D. (2017). Digitalization of Death Certification Model: Transformation Issues and Implementation Concerns. In S. Saeed, Y. Bamarouf, T. Ramayah, & S. Iqbal (Eds.), *Design Solutions for User-Centric Information Systems* (pp. 22–43). Hershey, PA: IGI Global. doi:10.4018/978-1-5225-1944-7.ch002

Stavros, A., Vavoulidis, E., & Nasioutziki, M. (2016). The Use of Mobile Health Applications for Quality Control and Accreditational Purposes in a Cytopathology Laboratory. In A. Moumtzoglou (Ed.), *M-Health Innovations for Patient-Centered Care* (pp. 262–283). Hershey, PA: IGI Global. doi:10.4018/978-1-4666-9861-1.ch013

Sukkird, V., & Shirahada, K. (2018). E-Health Service Model for Asian Developing Countries: A Case of Emergency Medical Service for Elderly People in Thailand. In M. Khosrow-Pour (Ed.), *Optimizing Current Practices in E-Services and Mobile Applications* (pp. 214–232). Hershey, PA: IGI Global. doi:10.4018/978-1-5225-5026-6.ch011

Sygit, B., & Wąsik, D. (2016). Patients' Rights and Medical Personnel Duties in the Field of Hospital Care. In A. Rosiek & K. Leksowski (Eds.), *Organizational Culture and Ethics in Modern Medicine* (pp. 282–297). Hershey, PA: IGI Global. doi:10.4018/978-1-4666-9658-7.ch012

Sygit, B., & Wąsik, D. (2016). The Idea of Human Rights in Conditions of Hospital Treatment. In A. Rosiek & K. Leksowski (Eds.), *Organizational Culture and Ethics in Modern Medicine* (pp. 236–254). Hershey, PA: IGI Global. doi:10.4018/978-1-4666-9658-7.ch010

Talbot, T. B. (2017). Making Lifelike Medical Games in the Age of Virtual Reality: An Update on "Playing Games with Biology" from 2013. In B. Dubbels (Ed.), *Transforming Gaming and Computer Simulation Technologies across Industries* (pp. 103–119). Hershey, PA: IGI Global. doi:10.4018/978-1-5225-1817-4.ch006

Tamposis, I., Pouliakis, A., Fezoulidis, I., & Karakitsos, P. (2016). Mobile Platforms Supporting Health Professionals: Need, Technical Requirements, and Applications. In A. Moumtzoglou (Ed.), *M-Health Innovations for Patient-Centered Care* (pp. 91–114). Hershey, PA: IGI Global. doi:10.4018/978-1-4666-9861-1.ch005

Tiago, M. T., Tiago, F., Amaral, F. E., & Silva, S. (2016). Healthy 3.0: Healthcare Digital Dimensions. In A. Dwivedi (Ed.), *Reshaping Medical Practice and Care with Health Information Systems* (pp. 287–322). Hershey, PA: IGI Global. doi:10.4018/978-1-4666-9870-3.ch010

Tripathy, B. (2016). Application of Rough Set Based Models in Medical Diagnosis. In S. Dash & B. Subudhi (Eds.), *Handbook of Research on Computational Intelligence Applications in Bioinformatics* (pp. 144–168). Hershey, PA: IGI Global. doi:10.4018/978-1-5225-0427-6.ch008

Turcu, C. E., & Turcu, C. O. (2017). Social Internet of Things in Healthcare: From Things to Social Things in Internet of Things. In C. Reis & M. Maximiano (Eds.), *Internet of Things and Advanced Application in Healthcare* (pp. 266–295). Hershey, PA: IGI Global. doi:10.4018/978-1-5225-1820-4.ch010

Unwin, D. W., Sanzogni, L., & Sandhu, K. (2017). Developing and Measuring the Business Case for Health Information Technology. In K. Moahi, K. Bwalya, & P. Sebina (Eds.), *Health Information Systems and the Advancement of Medical Practice in Developing Countries* (pp. 262–290). Hershey, PA: IGI Global. doi:10.4018/978-1-5225-2262-1.ch015

Urooj, S., & Singh, S. P. (2016). Wavelet Transform-Based Soft Computational Techniques and Applications in Medical Imaging. In P. Saxena, D. Singh, & M. Pant (Eds.), *Problem Solving and Uncertainty Modeling through Optimization and Soft Computing Applications* (pp. 339–363). Hershey, PA: IGI Global. doi:10.4018/978-1-4666-9885-7.ch016

Vasant, P. (2018). A General Medical Diagnosis System Formed by Artificial Neural Networks and Swarm Intelligence Techniques. In U. Kose, G. Guraksin, & O. Deperlioglu (Eds.), *Nature-Inspired Intelligent Techniques for Solving Biomedical Engineering Problems* (pp. 130–145). Hershey, PA: IGI Global. doi:10.4018/978-1-5225-4769-3.ch006

Waegemann, C. P. (2016). mHealth: History, Analysis, and Implementation. In A. Moumtzoglou (Ed.), M-Health Innovations for Patient-Centered Care (pp. 1-19). Hershey, PA: IGI Global. doi:10.4018/978-1-4666-9861-1.ch001

Watfa, M. K., Majeed, H., & Salahuddin, T. (2016). Computer Based E-Healthcare Clinical Systems: A Comprehensive Survey. *International Journal of Privacy and Health Information Management*, *4*(1), 50–69. doi:10.4018/IJPHIM.2016010104

Wietholter, J. P., Coetzee, R., Nardella, B., Kincaid, S. E., & Slain, D. (2016). International Healthcare Experiences: Caring While Learning and Learning While Caring. In D. Velliaris & D. Coleman-George (Eds.), *Handbook of Research on Study Abroad Programs and Outbound Mobility* (pp. 470–496). Hershey, PA: IGI Global. doi:10.4018/978-1-5225-0169-5.ch019

Witzke, K., & Specht, O. (2017). M-Health Telemedicine and Telepresence in Oral and Maxillofacial Surgery: An Innovative Prehospital Healthcare Concept in Structurally Weak Areas. *International Journal of Reliable and Quality E-Healthcare*, *6*(4), 37–48. doi:10.4018/IJRQEH.2017100105

Wójcik, A., & Chojnacki, M. (2016). Behavior and Ethical Problems in the Functioning of the Operating Theater (Case Study). In A. Rosiek & K. Leksowski (Eds.), *Organizational Culture and Ethics in Modern Medicine* (pp. 154–179). Hershey, PA: IGI Global. doi:10.4018/978-1-4666-9658-7.ch007

Wolk, K., & Marasek, K. P. (2016). Translation of Medical Texts using Neural Networks. *International Journal of Reliable and Quality E-Healthcare*, *5*(4), 51–66. doi:10.4018/IJRQEH.2016100104

Wong, A. K., & Lo, M. F. (2018). Using Pervasive Computing for Sustainable Healthcare in an Aging Population. In B. Fong, A. Ng, & P. Yuen (Eds.), *Sustainable Health and Long-Term Care Solutions for an Aging Population* (pp. 187–202). Hershey, PA: IGI Global. doi:10.4018/978-1-5225-2633-9.ch010

Wu, W., Martin, B. C., & Ni, C. (2017). A Systematic Review of Competency-Based Education Effort in the Health Professions: Seeking Order Out of Chaos. In K. Rasmussen, P. Northrup, & R. Colson (Eds.), *Handbook of Research on Competency-Based Education in University Settings* (pp. 352–378). Hershey, PA: IGI Global. doi:10.4018/978-1-5225-0932-5.ch018

Yadav, N., Aliasgari, M., & Poellabauer, C. (2016). Mobile Healthcare in an Increasingly Connected Developing World. *International Journal of Privacy and Health Information Management*, *4*(2), 76–97. doi:10.4018/IJPHIM.2016070106

Yadav, S., Ekbal, A., Saha, S., Pathak, P. S., & Bhattacharyya, P. (2017). Patient Data De-Identification: A Conditional Random-Field-Based Supervised Approach. In S. Saha, A. Mandal, A. Narasimhamurthy, S. V, & S. Sangam (Eds.), Handbook of Research on Applied Cybernetics and Systems Science (pp. 234-253). Hershey, PA: IGI Global. doi:10.4018/978-1-5225-2498-4.ch011

Yu, B., Wijesekera, D., & Costa, P. C. (2017). Informed Consent in Healthcare: A Study Case of Genetic Services. In A. Moumtzoglou (Ed.), *Design, Development, and Integration of Reliable Electronic Healthcare Platforms* (pp. 211–242). Hershey, PA: IGI Global. doi:10.4018/978-1-5225-1724-5.ch013

Yu, B., Wijesekera, D., & Costa, P. C. (2017). Informed Consent in Electronic Medical Record Systems. In I. Management Association (Ed.), Healthcare Ethics and Training: Concepts, Methodologies, Tools, and Applications (pp. 1029-1049). Hershey, PA: IGI Global. doi:10.4018/978-1-5225-2237-9.ch049

Yu, M., Li, J., & Wang, W. (2017). Creative Life Experience among Students in Medical Education. In C. Zhou (Ed.), *Handbook of Research on Creative Problem-Solving Skill Development in Higher Education* (pp. 158–184). Hershey, PA: IGI Global. doi:10.4018/978-1-5225-0643-0.ch008

Zarour, K. (2017). Towards a Telehomecare in Algeria: Case of Diabetes Measurement and Remote Monitoring. *International Journal of E-Health and Medical Communications*, *8*(4), 61–80. doi:10.4018/IJEHMC.2017100104

Zavyalova, Y. V., Korzun, D. G., Meigal, A. Y., & Borodin, A. V. (2017). Towards the Development of Smart Spaces-Based Socio-Cyber-Medicine Systems. *International Journal of Embedded and Real-Time Communication Systems*, *8*(1), 45–63. doi:10.4018/IJERTCS.2017010104

Zeinali, A. A. (2018). Word Formation Study in Developing Naming Guidelines in the Translation of English Medical Terms Into Persian. In M. Khosrow-Pour, D.B.A. (Ed.), Encyclopedia of Information Science and Technology, Fourth Edition (pp. 5136-5147). Hershey, PA: IGI Global. doi:10.4018/978-1-5225-2255-3.ch446

Ziminski, T. B., Demurjian, S. A., Sanzi, E., & Agresta, T. (2016). Toward Integrating Healthcare Data and Systems: A Study of Architectural Alternatives. In T. Iyamu & A. Tatnall (Eds.), *Maximizing Healthcare Delivery and Management through Technology Integration* (pp. 270–304). Hershey, PA: IGI Global. doi:10.4018/978-1-4666-9446-0.ch016

Ziminski, T. B., Demurjian, S. A., Sanzi, E., Baihan, M., & Agresta, T. (2016). An Architectural Solution for Health Information Exchange. *International Journal of User-Driven Healthcare*, *6*(1), 65–103. doi:10.4018/IJUDH.2016010104

Zineldin, M., & Vasicheva, V. (2018). Reducing Medical Errors and Increasing Patient Safety: TRM and 5 Q's Approaches for Better Quality of Life. In *Technological Tools for Value-Based Sustainable Relationships in Health: Emerging Research and Opportunities* (pp. 87–115). Hershey, PA: IGI Global. doi:10.4018/978-1-5225-4091-5.ch005

About the Contributors

Sophia Aidona is a Speech Pathologist and a Dyslexia Specialist, Research Associate of the Center of Cochlear Implantation, 1st Academic ENT Department, AHEPA Hospital, Aristotle University of Thessaloniki, Greece. Webpage: http://www.ahepaci.gr.

Veysi Çeri currently works at the Department of Child and Adolescent Psychiatry at Marmara University school of medicine. Dr. Ceri conducts research in the fields of Child Development, Adverse Childhood Experiences, Autism, Accident Proneness in ADHD, PTSD, Speech and Language Pathology and mental wellbeing of refugee children. He is the executive head of 'Refugee Children Outpatient Treatment Unit' at Marmara University. Their current project is 'Trauma and stressor related disorders' and he is working on the idea of psychological vaccinations which might be used to prevent development of PTSD in children after traumatic exposure.

Richard Louis currently is the Manager of Student Support Services for the Bachelor of Applied Science Programs at Broward College in Fort Lauderdale, Florida. Dr. Louis is also an adjunct professor at Broward College teaching courses such as Training & Development, Entrepreneurship, and Applied Organizational Behavior & Leadership. Dr. Louis is originally from Cambria Heights, New York where he attended and graduated with his Bachelor of Science in Athletic Administration from St. John's University. Dr. Louis is the recipient of two Master's degrees, a Master of Arts in Sports Administration from Wayne State University (Detroit, Michigan) and a Master of Business Administration in Human Resources Management from Nova Southeastern University (Fort Lauderdale, Florida). In May 2018, Dr. Louis earned his Doctor of Education in Organizational Leadership from Nova Southeastern University as his dissertation topic was The Relationship Between Recidivism Rates and Post-Release Employment. Over a 25-year plus career,

Dr. Louis has held numerous leadership positions in education, non-profits, and criminal justice reform advocacy. Dr. Louis also serves as a Governing Board Member of the Regional Board of Directors for Charter Schools USA and is a member of the Human Resources Association of Broward County. In addition to his work in higher education, Dr. Louis is also the Founder and President of Springfield Heights Associates, LLC which is a consulting firm designed to assist formerly incarcerated individuals re-integrate into the workplace and assist companies, colleges, and universities to effectively service formerly incarcerated individuals that become their employees and students respectively.

Danielle McKain is a High School Mathematics Teacher at Beaver Area High School. She has taught a variety of courses including Algebra I, Algebra II, Integrated Math, Probability and Statistics, Trigonometry, and Computer Assisted Algebra. Additionally, she has years of experience preparing students for the SAT. Dr. McKain earned her Ph.D in Instructional Management and Leadership from Robert Morris University. She holds a Master of Science degree in Instructional Leadership with a concentration in Mathematics Education and a Bachelor of Science degree in Applied Mathematics. Her research interests include real world math, test preparation, math anxiety, remedial math, and preparing future teachers.

Igor Pantic, Docent/As. Professor at the Department of Medical Physiology at the Faculty of Medicine, University of Belgrade. Affiliated Professor at the University of Haifa, Israel. Psychiatrist with experience in the field of depression, anxiety disorders and addiction. The author of a number of scientific papers in psychophysiology and psychiatry in prestigious international journals such as Psychiatry Research, European Psychiatry, and Computers in Human Behavior. Visiting Scholar at the Israeli Interdisciplinary Center of Herzliya, Laboratory for Social Cognition and Psychophysiology in August 2017. In December 2017, also a Visiting Professor at the Ben-Gurion University - Zlotowski Center for Neuroscience ". Since July 2015, a member of the Special Work Group of the Serbian Ministry of Health for the education of doctors and health care workers in primary health care, specialized professions and related disciplines in the field of diagnostics, treatment, rehabilitation and prevention of addiction diseases. Since December 2017, a member of the Supervisory Board of the Clinic for psychiatric illness "Dr Laza Lazarevic" in Belgrade. From April 2018 serves as a member of the Board of Directors of the Gynecology and Obstetric Clinic "Narodni Front" in Belgrade.

Dionysios Politis is an Assistant Professor at the Software and Interactive Technologies Lab, Dept. of Informatics, Aristotle University of Thessaloniki, Greece. His research interests focus on Computer Music, Multimedia Learning, Byzantine Music, Cognitive Neurosciences and Special Education (in conjunction with the Cochlear Implantation Center, AHEPA University Hospital, Thessaloniki, Greece). Webpage: http://dipolitis.github.io.

David B. Ross has many years of experience in adult education, leadership, operations management, ethics, policy, government, critical thinking and decision making, curriculum development, classroom instruction, and research. In his present role as an Associate Professor at the Abraham S. Fischler College of Education, Nova Southeastern University, he teaches doctoral level courses in educational, instructional, and organizational leadership as well as higher education to prepare today's practitioners who will assume leadership positions in any profession for current and future challenges. His courses focus on current trends and issues that influence society on both the national and global level. Learning from many perspectives and philosophies from mentors while attending Northern Illinois University, the University of Alabama, and Florida Atlantic University, has assisted him in guiding students in the learning process. Dr. Ross earned his Doctorate in Educational Leadership, with an emphasis in Leadership, Research, Curriculum, and Adult Education; and a Master of Justice Policy Management with a Professional Certificate in Public Administration at Florida Atlantic University. He earned his Bachelor of Science Degree in Computer Science at Northern Illinois University. Dr. Ross regularly speaks at conferences and provides consultation and training in the areas of leadership and management, policy issues, critical thinking, team building, professional development, academic writing, education, and behavior management. He has written articles and book chapters on leadership, power, narcissism, organizational stress, academic integrity, plagiarism and fraud, Gerontechnology, policy development, professional development, and areas of homeland security. Dr. Ross is a dissertation chair and committee member of various methodologies: quantitative, qualitative, and mixed methods. In addition, he is a reviewer for the university's Institutional Review Board. Dr. Ross was named Professor of the Year 2015-2016 for the Abraham S. Fischler College of Education.

Melissa T. Sasso is an Italian Canadian native who grew up in Montreal, Quebec and went to preparatory school throughout her elementary and high school years. She then moved to Florida, at the age of 16. Dr. Sasso attained her Bachelor of Arts in Psychology at Florida International University where she graduated with Cum Laude and joined PSI CHI, the International Honour Society in Psychology as well as Golden Key International Honour Society and Delta Epsilon Iota Academic Honor Society. She received both her Master's of Science in Exceptional Student Education and Doctorate in Education with a concentration in Organizational Leadership at Nova Southeastern University, where she graduated with a 4.0 GPA in both degrees and joined Kappa Delta Pi, an International Honor Society in Education. Dr. Sasso has several years of experience working with exceptional students who suffer from disabilities from Pre-K to Grade 5 and is still interested in remaining within the education field, with her final goal of opening a school for students who suffer from disabilities. She has written articles with her dissertation chair, Dr. David B. Ross, which can be found in NSUWorks and has her published dissertation entitled How Narcissists Cannot Hold an Organization Together: A Mixed Method Approach to a Fictitious Puzzle Factory located in ProQuest. Her dissertation received a Dr. Charles L. Faires distinction award. This award is created to honor Dr. Charles L. Faires and is presented to graduating doctoral students whose dissertations have been nominated by their dissertation chair as outstanding, and meet the rigorous criteria set forth by the review committee. She will be presenting her dissertation at the TQR's 10th annual conference with her dissertation chair, where she will share the strategic methodology of her study. In addition, she is an article reviewer and has also commenced editing various works. Her research interests include stress, and she is a passionate researcher in the fields of toxic workplace environments, and narcissistic leadership.

Petros Stagiopoulos is a Counselor for Elementary Education, working for the Ministry of Education in Greece. He is a Research Associate of the Center of Cochlear Implantation, 1st Academic ENT Department, AHEPA Hospital, Aristotle University of Thessaloniki, Greece. Webpage: http://www.ahepaci.gr.

Aleksandra Stanimirovic, PhD, is a postdoctoral fellow, supervised by Dr. Valeria E. Rac. She is currently involved in several mixed method studies focused on evaluation of interventions for prevention and management of chronic diseases. Aleksandra attended Medical School, University of

Belgrade, Serbia. She completed her undergraduate degree at the University of Western Ontario and received her Masters degree from School of Health Policy and Management, York University. Aleksandra completed her PhD at the Institute of Health Policy, Management and Evaluation, University of Toronto. Aleksandra's research focuses on health services utilization, economic models, quality of care and patient outcomes as related to chronic disease management. In addition, Aleksandra's interests focus on policy interventions designed to improve the overall quality of care for Canadians, to improve patients' experiences of care, to achieve better value for money and to design innovative ways to integrate health care between hospital and community providers. Aleksandra is a recipient of several awards including Faculty of Medicine, Queen Elizabeth Science and Technology Award, and Diabetes Action Canada and Mentoring Group & Patient-Oriented Research Network Training Grant.

Branislav Starcevic is an orthopaedic surgeon who works with polytraumatized patients as well as elective procedures such as hip and knee arthroplasty. Dr Starcevic is also very dedicated in investigating new approaches and procedures in orthopaedic surgery. He is an author of many scientific papers.

Aleksandar Stojanovic worked in Teleinformatics engineering, Federal University of Ceara, Brazil His PhD Thesis title was: ''Complete Security Model for Authentication of DV-QKD Protocols''. He is also M.Sc. in Electrical engineering and Computer science (Telecommunication and Information Technology), faculty of Electrical engineering, University of Belgrade, Serbia with thesis title: "The Estimation of Impact of Quantum Effects on the Complexity of Communication Systems." His research interests: Zero error theory, QKD protocol.

Mirka Stojanovic is an orthodontist, before private practice she was working for more than 30 years in primary care, Primary Health center Paracin. She is also a dedicated scientific as well as practitioner specialist in Orthodontics with more scientific papers from national and international orthodontic congresses. Dr Stojanovic also emphasizes the importance of psychological basis of the individual in every condition and irregularity in orthodontics and the importance of stress impact which can cause a great damage in individual life such as orthodontic irregularity.

Index

M

N

O

P

Q

R

S

T